Neurology: A Case-Based Approach

Neurology: A Case-Based Approach

Editor: Isabella Holmes

AMERICAN
MEDICAL PUBLISHERS
www.americanmedicalpublishers.com

AMERICAN
MEDICAL PUBLISHERS
www.americanmedicalpublishers.com

Cataloging-in-Publication Data

Neurology: a case-based approach / edited by Isabella Holmes.
p. cm.
Includes bibliographical references and index.
ISBN 979-8-88740-647-3
1. Neurology. 2. Nervous system--Diseases. 3. Nervous system--Diseases--Case studies.
I. Holmes, Isabella.
RC346 .N48 2023
616.8--dc23

American Medical Publishers,
41 Flatbush Avenue,
1st Floor, New York,
NY 11217, USA

ISBN 979-8-88740-647-3 (Hardback)

Contents

Preface

Neurology is a medical specialty that focuses on the diagnosis and treatment of diseases and disorders of the nervous system. Some of the diagnostic approaches which are used within this field are neuroimaging, electrophysiological tests and genetic testing. Neuroimaging techniques such as magnetic resonance imaging (MRI), computed tomography (CT), and positron emission tomography (PET) scans help in visualizing the structure and function of the brain and spinal cord. Electrophysiological tests include tests such as electroencephalography (EEG), electromyography (EMG), and nerve conduction studies (NCS), and they measure the electrical activity of the brain, nerves, and muscles. Some of the common treatment approaches which are used within this field are rehabilitation therapies, interventional procedures and surgical interventions. This book includes some of the vital pieces of work being conducted across the world, on various topics related to neurology. It will serve as a valuable source of reference for graduate and postgraduate students.

The information contained in this book is the result of intensive hard work done by researchers in this field. All due efforts have been made to make this book serve as a complete guiding source for students and researchers. The topics in this book have been comprehensively explained to help readers understand the growing trends in the field.

I would like to thank the entire group of writers who made sincere efforts in this book and my family who supported me in my efforts of working on this book. I take this opportunity to thank all those who have been a guiding force throughout my life.

Editor

1

Peculiar Presentation of COVID-19: A Case Report of Concurrent Stroke and Guillain–Barré Syndrome

Behnaz Ansari and **Helia Hemasian**

Isfahan Neuroscience Research Center, Department of Neurology, Al Zahra Research Institute, Isfahan University of Medical Sciences, Isfahan, Iran

Correspondence should be addressed to Helia Hemasian; helia_h22@yahoo.com

Academic Editor: Mathias Toft

Background. Coronavirus disease 2019 (COVID-19) is a newly recognized infectious disease that has turned into a pandemic. There are few studies reporting Guillain–Barré syndrome (GBS) and stroke separately associated with COVID-19. In this study, we report an unusual case of COVID-19 with stroke and GBS concurrently. *Case Report.* A 59-year-old woman presented with left-sided weakness of two weeks' duration followed by right-sided weakness and foot paresthesia. She also complained of cough, myalgia, and respiratory distress of three weeks' duration. On examination, the patient had respiratory distress. The limb examination revealed asymmetric weakness. All limb reflexes were absent. Pinprick sensation was impaired. The chest CT scan and PCR of nasopharyngeal swab confirmed the diagnosis of COVID-19. Further evaluation revealed acute cerebral infarction and GBS. Consequently, the patient was treated by plasmapheresis, and her symptoms partially improved. *Conclusion.* According to reports, 36.4% of COVID-19 cases display neurological complications. The neurological manifestations of the disease can involve both the central and peripheral nervous systems. Previously, a few cases of GBS and cerebrovascular disease have been reported in association with COVID-19 separately, while in the present case, CNS and PNS involvement occurred concurrently. It is hypothesized that this concurrence is related to the imbalance of the systemic inflammatory responses and blood vessel autonomous dysfunction.

1. Introduction

Coronavirus disease 2019 (COVID-19), originated in China, is rapidly spreading throughout the world. This is an infectious disease caused by the severe acute respiratory syndrome coronavirus 2 (SARS-CoV-2). Evidence increasingly shows that SARS-CoV-2 is not always confined to the respiratory system and can induce neurological disorders as well. Both central and peripheral nervous system disorders have been reported following COVID-19 [1]. Acute clinical neurological syndromes of COVID-19 fall into three main categories: stroke, Guillain–Barré syndrome (GBS), and meningoencephalitis, encephalopathy, or encephalitis [2]. About one-third of COVID-19 patients develop neurological symptoms. Damage to the CNS or PNS could be caused by the virus directly or by the body's adaptive immune responses to the infection [1].

There are several case reports of stroke and GBS separately in association with COVID-19. In this study, we report an unusual case of COVID-19 with CNS and PNS involvement concurrently.

2. Case Report

A 59-year-old woman with a past medical history of hypertension and stroke presented to the emergency department with left-sided weakness of two weeks' duration followed by right-sided weakness and foot paresthesia. She

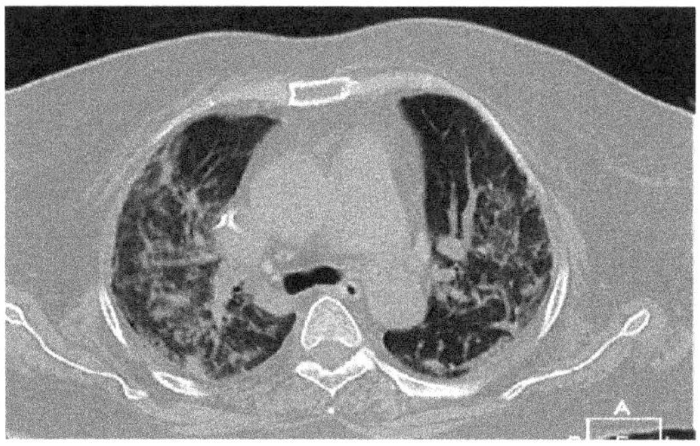

Figure 1: Chest computed tomography on admission showed multilobar ground-glass opacity with reticulation and consolidation in the center and periphery of both lungs.

also complained of cough, myalgia, and respiratory distress of three weeks' duration and reported dizziness and falling down 2 days before admission. She had no bladder symptoms of note.

On examination, the patient was afebrile. Oxygen saturation was 90% on air and respiratory rate was 26 breaths/min. The limb examination revealed an asymmetric weakness of −3/5 in the right upper and lower limbs and 2/5 on the left side. All limb reflexes were absent. No Babinski sign was found. Pinprick sensation was impaired to the ankle on both sides, with impaired vibration and position senses in the left lower limb. Cranial nerves were intact.

On admission, white blood cell count was 12300 cells per microliter (neutrophils: 80.9%; lymphocytes: 12.7%). The renal profile, electrolytes, FBS, HbA1C, serum angiotensin converting enzyme (ACE), B12, and thyroid and clotting functions were all within the normal range. Vasculitis, HIV, and hepatitis B and C tests were negative.

CRP was mildly positive, and D-dimer and IL-6 levels had not increased.

The patient's chest CT scan on admission (Figure 1) showed multilobar ground-glass opacity with reticulation and consolidation in the center and periphery of both lungs. The nasopharyngeal swab PCR test was positive for SARS-CoV-2. Because of the asymmetric and unusual presentation, brain and spinal cord imaging were performed. In the brain MRI, acute infarct in the left centrum semiovale, as well as an old infarct on the right side, was detected (Figure 2). Cardiac and carotid investigation results were within the normal limits. No obvious intracranial stenosis was detected in the transcranial duplex study.

The patient was admitted with suspected GBS secondary to COVID-19. Lumbar puncture was tried but failed. Nerve conduction studies were performed and revealed reduced amplitude and velocity in all tested sensory nerves in the upper limbs, increased latency in both median nerves, and absence of response in the lower limbs. Reduced amplitude and conduction velocity with an asymmetric pattern (left->right) and prolonged distal latency in both median and left ulnar motor nerves, as well as the absence of response in the lower limbs, were noticed. No *F* waves could be elicited from either of the median nerves and the left ulnar nerve (Table 1). In electromyography, no spontaneous activity was detected; moreover, reduced recruitment in both tibialis anterior and left gastrocnemius muscles and a normal pattern in the upper limbs were observed. These results meet the electrodiagnostic criteria for acute inflammatory demyelinating polyneuropathy, and consequently, treatment was started with plasma exchange (PLEX), ASA (80 mg/day), and enoxaparin (1 mg/kg). In follow-up, the patient's weakness obviously improved with PLEX. Written consent was obtained from the patient for publishing the contents of this study.

3. Discussion

COVID-19 presents with a variety of symptoms, ranging from asymptomatic to severe, rapid multiorgan dysfunction and death. Although the predominant clinical presentation is respiratory disease, neurological manifestations are being increasingly recognized.

In an analysis of 214 cases of COVID-19 in Wuhan, China, 36.4% had neurological complications [3]. These manifestations may be direct effects of the virus on the nervous system, parainfectious or postinfectious immune-mediated disease, or neurological complications of the systemic effects of COVID-19 [1]. The neurological manifestations of this disease involve either the central or peripheral nervous system. Surprisingly, in the case presented here, CNS and PNS involvement occurred concurrently.

One of the peripheral nervous system complications of COVID-19 is the Guillain–Barré syndrome; also, one of its central nervous complications is cerebrovascular accident. A number of cases of GBS have been reported in patients with COVID-19 [4–10]. GBS is an infrequent complication of COVID-19. Short interval between viral infection and the onset of weakness, as in the present case, suggests a parainfectious rather than a postinfectious nature for it [5]. One possible immunological explanation for this phenomenon is the cytokine release syndrome (CRS) in response to COVID-19 [11, 12], which can produce extensive tissue damage, including in the peripheral nervous system [13].

Acute cerebrovascular disease is emerging as a significant complication of COVID-19, with cohort studies reporting stroke in 2–6% of hospitalized patients with the disease [1]. Cerebrovascular disease in COVID-19 might be due to abnormalities in the coagulation cascade; SARS-CoV-2 can cause damage to endothelial cells and activate inflammatory and thrombotic pathways. Hence, cytokines have been implicated in the pathogenesis of cerebrovascular disease in COVID-19 through a systemic inflammatory response syndrome and induction of a proinflammatory condition [14]. There are reports of various types of stroke in COVID-19 [1], including intracerebral hemorrhage [15, 16] and cerebral sinus venous thrombosis [17, 18], but not of watershed infarct.

Both GBS and cerebral stroke are critical neurological diseases, and their clinical symptoms may be obscured by each other. However, the exact mechanism of their relationship is not known. Wu et al. discussed patients with both hemorrhagic infarct and GBS and attributed this concurrence to the imbalance of systemic inflammatory responses,

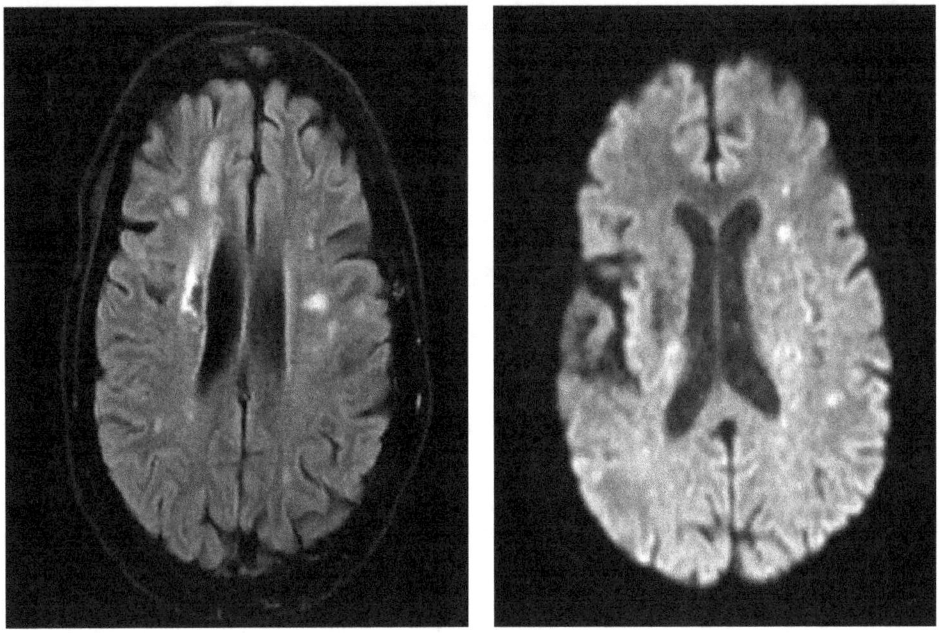

(a) (b)

Figure 2: Magnetic resonance imaging. (a) Fluid-attenuated inversion recovery (FLAIR) and (b) diffusion-weighted sequence (DWI) revealed acute infarct in the left centrum semiovale and old infarct on the right side.

Table 1: Results of the neurophysiologic study.

Motor nerve conduction	Distal latency (ms)	Amplitude (mV)	Conduction velocity (m/s)	*F* waves
Median nerve				
Wrist-abductor pollicis brevis	*R* = 5.42; *L* = 4.69 (n.v. < 4.2)	*R* = 2.1; *L* = 1.2 (n.v. > 4)	*R* = 35; *L* = 38 (n.v. > 50)	*R* = *A*; *L* = *A*
Antecubital fossa-wrist	*R* = 10.10; *L* = 9.27	*R* = 2.1; *L* = 1.2		
Ulnar nerve				
Wrist-abductor digiti minimi	*R* = 3.7; *L* = 6.77 (n.v. < 3.2)	*R* = 4.3; *L* = 0.5 (n.v. > 6)	*R* = 35; *L* = *A* (n.v. > 50)	*R* = 24; *L* = *A*
Below elbow-wrist	*R* = 6.61; *L* = *a*	*R* = 3.3; *L* = *a*		
Tibial nerve				
Medial malleolus-abductor hallucis brevis	*R* = *a*; *L* = *a* (n.v. < 5)	*R* = *a*; *L* = *a* (n.v. > 4)	*R* = A; *L* = A (n.v. > 40)	*R* = A; *L* = A
Popliteal fossa-medial malleolus	*R* = *a*; *L* = *a*	*R* = *a*; *L* = *a*		
Peroneal nerve				
Ankle-extensor digitorum brevis	*R* = *a*; *L* = *a* (n.v. < 6.5)	*R* = *a*; *L* = *a* (n.v. > 2)	*R* = *A*; *L* = *A* (n.v. > 40)	*R* = *A*; *L* = *A*
Below fibula-ankle	*R* = *a*; *L* = *a*	*R* = *a*; *L* = *a*		
Antidromic sensory nerve conduction studies				
Median nerve digit 2-wrist	*R* = 3.80; *L* = 3.7 (n.v. < 3.5)	*R* = 8.9; *L* = 10.7 (n.v. > 20)	*R* = 34; *L* = 44 (n.v. > 45)	
Ulnar nerve digit 5-wrist	*R* = 2.60; *L* = 2.50 (n.v. < 3.2)	*R* = 15.1; *L* = 9.2 (n.v. > 17)	*R* = 42, *L* = 44 (n.v. > 45)	
Sural nerve posterior ankle-calf	*R* = *A*; *L* = *A* (n.v. < 4.4)	*R* = *A*; *L* = *A* (n.v. > 6)	*R* = *A*; *L* = *A* (n.v. > 40)	

R, right; *L*, left; n.v., normal values adjusted for age; *A*, absent.

blood vessel autonomous dysfunction, and the use of intravenous immunoglobulin (IVIg) [19].

Rarely, cases of cerebral infarction have been reported after the management of GBS with IVIg [20]. These cases are believed to be due to hyperviscosity, thromboembolism, vasculitis, or cerebral vasospasm; however, our patient had not received IVIg. As mentioned, she experienced hypotension and falling prior to admission. Furthermore, dysautonomia due to GBS results in fluctuations of hemodynamic parameters, which could be the cause of cerebral infarct of watershed areas in our patient. Another possible cause is the imbalance of inflammatory responses due to COVID-19.

4. Conclusion

Neurologic complications of COVID-19 vary from a mild headache to severe disorders, and as discussed, it is not inconceivable that they could involve the CNS and PNS concurrently, in which case, clinical symptoms of the two involvements may cover each other, leading to confusion in diagnosis. Generally, limited case reports only suggest a possible association, and more cases with epidemiological data are necessary to support a causal relationship.

References

[1] M. Ellul and L. Benjamin, "Neurological associations of COVID-19," *The Lancet Neurology*, vol. 19, 2020.

[2] A. Pryce-Roberts, M. Talaei, and N. P. Robertson, "Neurological complications of COVID-19: a preliminary review," *Journal of Neurology*, vol. 267, no. 6, pp. 1870–1873, 2020.

[3] L. Mao, H. Jin, M. Wang et al., "Neurologic manifestations of hospitalized patients with coronavirus disease 2019 in Wuhan, China," *JAMA Neurology*, vol. 77, Article ID e201127, 2020.

[4] R. W. Paterson, R. L. Brown, L. Benjamin et al., "The emerging spectrum of COVID-19 neurology: clinical, radiological and laboratory findings," *Brain*, vol. 143, 2020.

[5] G. Toscano, F. Palmerini, S. Ravaglia et al., "Guillain-Barré syndrome associated with SARS-CoV-2," *New England Journal of Medicine*, vol. 382, no. 26, p. 2574, 2020.

[6] H. Zhao, D. Shen, H. Zhou, J. Liu, and S. Chen, "Guillain-Barré syndrome associated with SARS-CoV-2 infection: causality or coincidence?" *The Lancet Neurology*, vol. 19, no. 5, p. 383, 2020.

[7] A. Virani, E. Rabold, T. Hanson et al., "Guillain-Barré syndrome associated with SARS-CoV-2 infection," *ID Cases*, Article ID e00771, 2020.

[8] P. Alberti, S. Beretta, M. Piatti et al., "Guillain-Barré syndrome related to COVID-19 infection," *Neurol Neuroimmunol Neuroinflamm*, vol. 7, 2020.

[9] H. El Otmani, B. El Moutawakil, M.-A. Rafai et al., "Covid-19 and Guillain-Barré syndrome: more than a coincidence!" *Revue Neurologique*, vol. 176, no. 6, p. 518, 2020.

[10] J. P. Camdessanche, J. Morel, B. Pozzetto et al., "COVID-19 may induce Guillain-Barré syndrome COVID-19 and guillain-barré syndrome: response," *Revue Neurologique*, vol. 176, 2020.

[11] J. B. Moore and C. H. June, "Cytokine release syndrome in severe COVID-19," *Science*, vol. 368, no. 6490, pp. 473-474, 2020.

[12] Y. Jamilloux, T. Henry, A. Belot et al., "Should we stimulate or suppress immune responses in COVID-19? Cytokine and anti-cytokine interventions," *Autoimmunity Reviews*, vol. 19, no. 7, Article ID 102567, 2020.

[13] J. Lyons-Weiler, "Pathogenic priming likely contributes to serious and critical illness and mortality in COVID-19 via autoimmunity," *Journal of Translational Autoimmunity*, vol. 3, no. 3, Article ID 100051, 2020.

[14] S. T. Reddy, T. Garg, C. Shah et al., "Cerebrovascular disease in patients with COVID-19: a review of the literature and case series," *Case Reports in Neurology*, vol. 12, no. 2, pp. 199–209, 2020.

[15] M. Morassi, D. Bagatto, M. Cobelli et al., "Stroke in patients with SARS-CoV-2 infection: case series," *Journal of Neurology*, vol. 267, no. 8, p. 2185, 2020.

[16] F. A. Saiegh, R. Ghosh, A. Leibold et al., "Status of SARS-CoV-2 in cerebrospinal fluid of patients with COVID-19 and stroke," *Journal of Neurology, Neurosurgery, and Psychiatry*, vol. 91, 2020.

[17] H. Hemasian and B. Ansari, "First case of Covid-19 presented with cerebral venous thrombosis: a rare and dreaded case," *Revue Neurologique*, vol. 176, 2020.

[18] Y. Li, M. Wang, Y. Zhou et al., "Acute cerebrovascular disease following COVID-19: a single center, retrospective, observational study," *Stroke and Vascular Neurology*, vol. 5, 2020.

[19] Q. Wu, N. Liu, C. Pan, B. Bu, and Z. Tang, "Guillain-Barré syndrome and cerebral hemorrhage: two cases and literature review," *European Neurology*, vol. 76, no. 3, pp. 182–186, 2016.

[20] U. Katz and Y. Shoenfeld, "Review: intravenous immunoglobulin therapy and thromboembolic complications," *Lupus*, vol. 14, no. 10, pp. 802–808, 2005.

2

Clinical and Radiological Characterization of an Infant with Caudal Regression Syndrome Type III

Kavinda Dayasiri,[1] V. Thadchanamoorthy,[2] Kaushika Thudugala,[1] Aruni Ranaweera,[1] and N. Parthipan[3]

[1]*Department of Paediatrics, Base Hospital Mahaoya, Maha Oya, Sri Lanka*
[2]*Faculty of Health Care Science, Eastern University, Chenkalady, Sri Lanka*
[3]*Department of Radiology, Base Hospital Mahaoya, Maha Oya, Sri Lanka*

Correspondence should be addressed to Kavinda Dayasiri; kavindadayasiri@gmail.com

Academic Editor: Mehmet Turgut

Caudal regression syndrome is a rare disorder of developmental failure of lumbosacral vertebra and corresponding spinal cord during notochord formation. The severity varies from absent coccyx to complete absence of lumbosacral vertebra and caudal spinal cord. Both genetic and environmental factors are believed to play roles in aetiopathogenesis of caudal regression. The authors report a two-month-old child born to a diabetic mother, in whom the diagnosis of caudal regression syndrome type III was confirmed based on clinical and radiological characteristics. The child was managed by the multidisciplinary team to continue supportive care and screen and monitor for long-term complications. The long-term prognosis for mobility was less favourable given the presence of bilateral hip dysplasia and involvement of lumbar vertebra in addition to sacral agenesis.

1. Introduction

Caudal regression syndrome is a rare congenital anomaly, which has an incidence of approximately 1 per 100,000 newborns [1]. The clinical features of this condition were first reported by Geoffroy Saint-Hilaire and Hohl in 1852 [2]. However, it was first proposed as a distinct clinical entity by Duhamel in 1960 [3]. Although the precise aetiology is unknown, poorly controlled maternal diabetes, vascular hypoperfusion, and genetic factors are thought to be contributory factors [4].

Caudal regression syndrome characteristically involves lumbosacral vertebra and corresponding segments of the spinal cord, which innervate structures in the pelvis and lower limbs due to a developmental failure [5]. Caudal agenesis is associated with malformations such as renal and ureter agenesis, duplex ureters, neuropathic bladder, vesicoureteric reflux, hydronephrosis, anorectal atresia, and imperforated anus [6]. Severe variants are often associated with cardiovascular, pulmonary, gastrointestinal, and musculoskeletal abnormalities. The authors report a two-month-old child, in whom the diagnosis of caudal regression syndrome type III was confirmed based on clinical and radiological characteristics.

2. Case Presentation

A two-month-old child was referred for evaluation of multiple congenital abnormalities. He was third born to nonconsanguineous parents with two healthy elder siblings. Antenatal period was uncomplicated apart from gestational diabetes, which was not controlled during the second trimester and before the diagnosis was made. Mother was on folic acid supplementation as recommended, and there was no history of radiation exposure or ingestion of long-term medications apart from being on antidiabetic medications.

He had been having constant leakage of urine and stools since birth. Growth was age appropriate. Physical examination revealed a narrow pelvis, bilateral knee flexion contractures, bilateral leg muscle atrophy, and bilateral

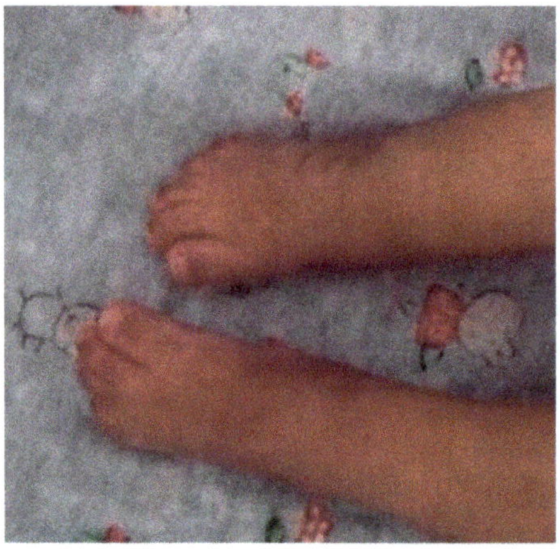

FIGURE 1: Bilateral congenital talipes equinovarus deformity.

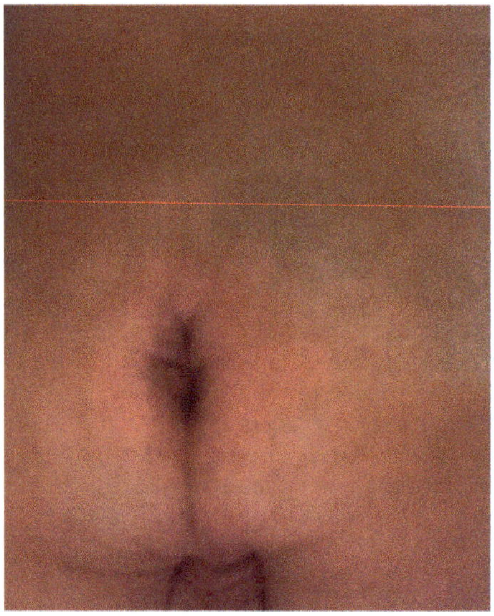

FIGURE 2: Displaced, patulous anus with flat, dimpled buttocks and no evidence of meningocele/meningomyelocele.

congenital talipes equinovarus deformity with diminished ankle joint creases. He had clinical evidence of bilateral hip dysplasia with positive Ortolani's and Barlow's test. Other abnormalities included micropenis (stretched penile length: 1 cm) and displaced patulous anus with tiny pressure sores and flat, dimpled buttocks. Figures 1–3 show bilateral congenital talipes equinovarus deformity, appearance of the buttocks, and micropenis noticed in the reported child.

He was investigated with X-ray of whole/spine and ultrasound of lumbosacral spine. Ultrasound revealed complete agenesis of the sacrum and L5 vertebra. The iliac bones were articulated with L4 vertebral body. The cord had terminated abruptly at the L1 level. Thickened conus medullaris was seen. There was no evidence of either meningomyelocele or meningocele. Ultrasound of hips revealed bilateral hip dysplasia with shallow acetabula. Overall, the findings were in keeping with type III caudal regression syndrome. Figures 4 and 5 show anteroposterior and lateral views of lumbosacral spine, and Figure 6 shows ultrasound appearance of abrupt termination of spinal cord at the L1 level. Figure 7 demonstrates abrupt termination of spinal cord at the L1 vertebra level and a syrinx involving lower thoracic spine.

Abdominopelvic ultrasound showed no evidence of renal agenesis, neurogenic bladder, vesicoureteric reflux, and bowel malrotation. Serum creatinine was within the normal range. 2D echocardiogram was normal. MRI brain was also normal.

Parents were counseled regarding long-term prognosis and available supportive treatment options. Long-term follow-up was arranged with the general paediatrician to monitor for growth, development, and screen for long-term health issues including the neurogenic bladder. Early interventions were commenced to ensure sitting stability; however, the probability of ambulation was low as he had bilateral hip dysplasia, leg muscle wasting, and fixed knee contractures resulting from an advanced lumbosacral vertebral defect. The child was referred to orthopedic surgeon to discuss treatment options to improve pelvic stability. Follow-up was also arranged with the paediatric neurologist.

3. Discussion

Caudal regression syndrome is characterised by failure of development of lumbosacral vertebra and caudal spinal cord, and the severity could range from absent coccyx to total absence of lumbar and sacral vertebra. The aetiology is complex with implication of both environmental and genetic factors in aetiopathogenesis [7]. The underlying defect is failure of notochord formation during the gastrulation phase of embryogenesis [8]. The mother of this child had undetected and hence uncontrolled diabetes during the second trimester of pregnancy. Hyperglycemia is considered to be a strong risk factor for caudal regression syndrome. This is due to its negative impact on oxidative stress and DNA structure of which both can increase the risk of malformations in the fetus [9].

Clinical features of sirenomelia and VACTERL (vertebral defects, anal atresia, cardiac defects, tracheoesophageal fistula, renal anomalies, and limb anomalies) association overlap with clinical features of caudal regression syndrome [10]. Cardiac evaluation of this child was normal, and there were no tracheaesophageal malformations. Similarly, there was no fusion of soft tissues of lower limbs as seen in reported children with sirenomelia [11].

The current classification of caudal regression syndrome to four distinct types was proposed by Renshaw in 1978 based on the type of vertebral defect and nature of attachment of iliac bones to lowest vertebra [12]. Type I is characterized by either partial or complete unilateral sacral agenesis. Type II is the most common form, and in addition to partial sacral agenesis, there is a bilaterally symmetrical defect between ilia and either normal or hypoplastic first sacral vertebra. Type III is characterised by total sacral agenesis and variable lumbar vertebral agenesis. The two iliac bones are attached to the sides of the lowest vertebra. Type IV is the worst type, and either fusion of iliac bones or iliac amphiarthrosis is seen in addition to features described in type III. High abrupt termination of spinal cord as seen in this child is considered to be a hall mark of caudal regression syndrome [13].

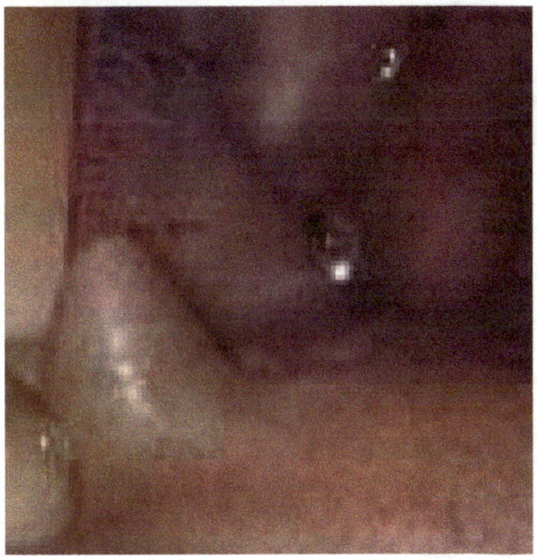

FIGURE 3: Micropenis (stretched penile length at 2 months of age: 1 cm).

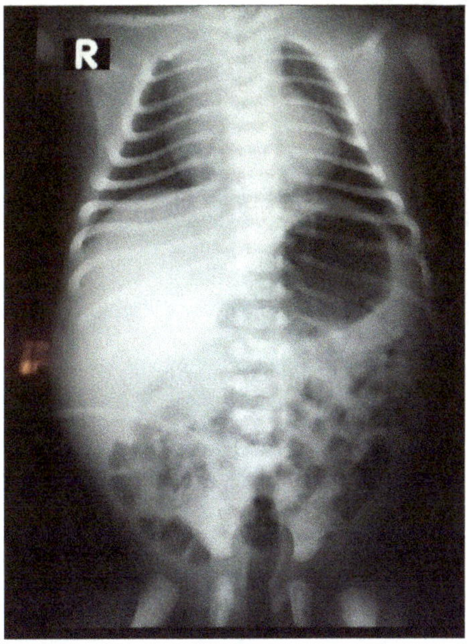

FIGURE 4: X-ray spine anteroposterior view: absent L5 vertebra and sacrum and bilateral iliac bones attaching to L4 vertebra.

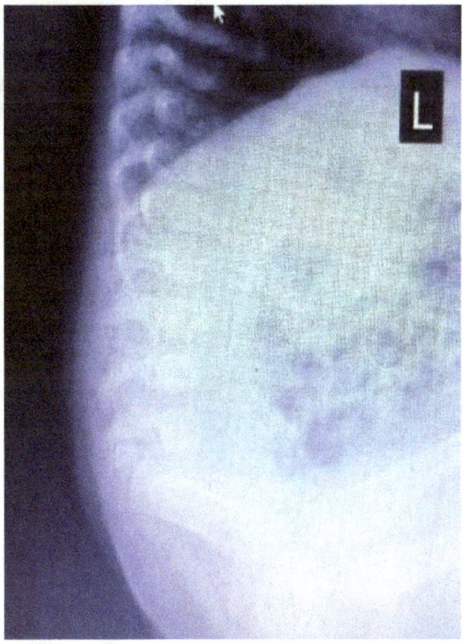

FIGURE 5: X-ray spine lateral view: absent L5 vertebra and sacrum.

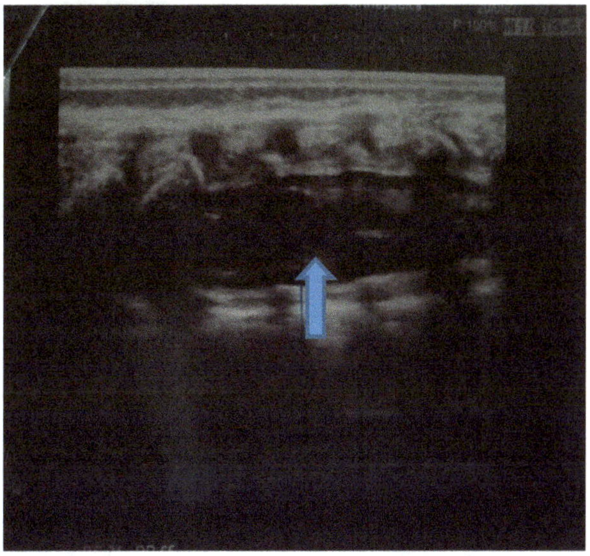

FIGURE 6: Ultrasound view: abrupt termination of spinal cord at the L1 vertebra level (arrow) and thickened conus medullaris.

Type III caudal regression syndrome as proposed by Renshaw is rarely described in literature. Its clinical features are largely similar to type I caudal regression described in Pang's classification [5]. Table 1 illustrates previously reported children/fetuses that had radiological features of type III caudal regression syndrome.

Management of types III and IV caudal regression is supportive, and aim of rehabilitation is to improve functionality rather than correcting deformities. There are limited data on optimal correction of deformities by orthopedic interventions for children with types III and IV caudal regression. Multilevel pedicular screw fixation combined with spinopelvic fusion to improve stability and sagittal spine balance was associated with enhanced quality of life [18].

The severity of defect in vertebra and spinal cord and associated malformations determines long-term prognosis [20]. Caudal regression is associated with long-term neurological, orthopedic, and urologic complications. Although there were no associated malformations in this child, the long-term outcome for functionality is less favourable given he had both lumbar and complete sacral agenesis and bilaterally dysplastic hips.

4. Conclusion

Type III caudal regression syndrome is characterised by complete sacral agenesis, lumbar vertebral agenesis, and articulation of two separate iliac bones on either side of

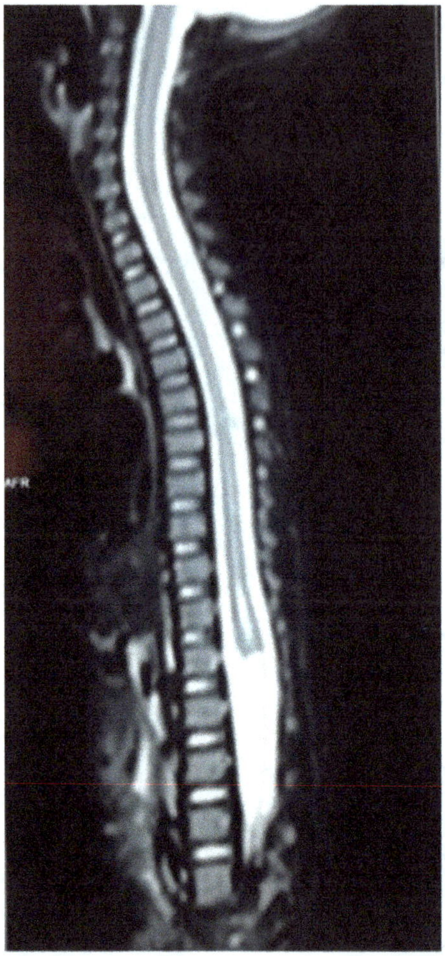

FIGURE 7: MRI spine: abrupt termination of spinal cord at the L1 vertebra level, syrinx involving D11-L1 measuring 17 mm in length and 1 mm in diameter.

TABLE 1: Previously reported children/fetuses with radiological features of type III caudal regression syndrome.

	Associated clinical findings	Reported risk factors
Boruah et al. [14]	Triangular pelvis	Diabetes
Kumar et al. [15]	Bilateral grade V vesicoureteric reflux and situs inversus totalis	Diabetes
Zaw et al. [16]	—	Diabetes
Hashami et al. [17]	Partial agenesis of the corpus callosum and partial lobar holoprosencephaly	Diabetes
Vissarionov et al. [18]	Kyphosis, bilateral hip dysplasia	—
Balioglu et al. [19]	—	—

the lowest vertebra. High abrupt termination of spinal cord is a hall mark of caudal regression syndrome. It is important to rule out VACTERL association as a differential diagnosis given the involvement of multiple organ malformations in both conditions. Long-term rehabilitation in caudal regression types III and IV is aimed at improving functionality rather than correcting deformities.

Consent

Written consent was obtained from the legal guardian of the child to publish the image and clinical information.

Disclosure

No funding was received.

Authors' Contributions

KD led clinical management of the patient, performed literature survey, and wrote the manuscript. KT and AR participated in clinical management of the patient. NP performed and interpreted radiological investigations. All authors approved the final version of the manuscript.

References

[1] A. D. Thottungal, A. K. Charles, J. E. Dickinson, and C. Bower, "Caudal dysgenesis and sirenomelia: single centre experience suggests common pathogenic basis," *American Journal of Medical Genetics Part A*, vol. 152A, no. 10, pp. 2578–2587, 2010.

[2] S. Bhatt, A. Tandon, A. Kumar Singh, S. Manchanda, S. Jain, and N. Meena, "Caudal regression syndrome: a case study with associated review of common differential diagnoses made with antenatal sonography," *Journal of Diagnostic Medical Sonography*, vol. 33, no. 2, pp. 130–133, 2017.

[3] P. Sharma, S. Kumar, and A. Jaiswal, "Clinico-radiologic findings in group II caudal regression syndrome," *Journal of Clinical Imaging Science*, vol. 3, p. 26, 2013.

[4] M. M. Boulas, "Recognition of caudal regression syndrome," *Advances in Neonatal Care*, vol. 9, no. 2, pp. 61–69, 2009.

[5] D. Pang, "Sacral agenesis and caudal spinal cord malformations," *Neurosurgery*, vol. 32, no. 5, pp. 755–778, 1993.

[6] Ö Özdemir, T. Çalisaneller, A. Gülsen, A. Gerilmez, E. Karadeli, and H. Caner, "Sakral ageneziye bagli gergin omurilik sendromu ve dekstrokardi birlikteligi: olgu sunumu," *Türk Nörosirürji Dergisi*.vol. 19, pp. 61–65, 2009.

[7] T. Warner, T. A. Scullen, J. Iwanaga et al., "Caudal regression syndrome-a review focusing on genetic associations," *World Neurosurgery*, vol. 138, pp. 461–467, 2020.

[8] C. L. Harlow, M. D. Partington, and G. A. Thieme, "Lumbosacral agenesis: clinical characteristics, imaging, and embryogenesis," *Pediatric Neurosurgery*, vol. 23, pp. 140–147, 1995.

[9] A. C. Polanco Ponce, M. C. Revilla Monsalve, M. A. Palomino Garibay, and S. Islas Andrade, "[Effect of maternal diabetes on human and rat fetal development]," *Ginecol Obstet Mex*, vol. 73, no. 10, pp. 544–552, 2005.

[10] M. Castori, E. Silvestri, S. Cappellacci, F. Binni, G. S. Sforzolini, and P. Grammatico, "Sirenomelia and VACTERL association in the offspring of a woman with diabetes," *American Journal of Medical Genetics Part A*, vol. 152, no. 7, pp. 1803–1807, 2010.

[11] E. K. Kavunga, G. K. Bunduki, M. Mumbere et al., "Sirenomelia associated with an anterior abdominal wall defect: a case report," *ournal of Medical Case Reports*, vol. 13, p. 213, 2019.

[12] T. S. Renshaw, "Sacral agenesis," *The Journal of Bone & Joint Surgery*, vol. 60, no. 3, pp. 373–383, 1978.

[13] K. T. Puneeth, A. Goyal, and M. Jana, "High abrupt cord termination: a hallmark of caudal regression syndrome," *BMJ Case Reports*, vol. 2014, Article ID bcr2013201770, 2014.

[14] D. K. Boruah, D. D. Dhingani, S. Achar et al., "Magnetic resonance imaging analysis of caudal regression syndrome and concomitant anomalies in pediatric patients," *Journal of Clinical Imaging Science*, vol. 6, p. 36, 2016.

[15] Y. Kumar, N. Gupta, K. Hooda et al., "Caudal regression syndrome: a case series of a rare congenital anomaly," *Polish Journal of Radiology*, vol. 82, pp. 188–192, 2017.

[16] W. Zaw and D. Stone, "Caudal regression syndrome in twin pregnancy with type II diabetes," *Journal of Perinatology*, vol. 22, no. 2, pp. 171–174, 2002.

[17] H. A. Hashami, M. F. Bataclan, M. Mathew, and L. Krishnan, "Caudal regression syndrome with partial agenesis of the corpus callosum and partial lobar holoprosencephaly: case report," *Sultan Qaboos University Medical Journal*, vol. 10, no. 1, pp. 89–93, 2010.

[18] S. Vissarionov, J. E. Schroder, D. Kokushin, V. Murashko, S. Belianchikov, and L. Kaplan, "Surgical correction of spinopelvic instability in children with caudal regression syndrome," *Global Spine Journal*, vol. 9, no. 3, pp. 260–265, 2019.

[19] M. B. Balioglu, A. Albayrak, Y. Atici et al., "Caudal regression syndorme (sacra agenesis) with associated anomalies," *The Journal of Turkish Spinal Surgery*, vol. 24, no. 3, pp. 191–198, 2013.

[20] K. Semba, "Etiology of caudal regression syndrome," *Human Genetics and Embryology*, vol. 3, no. 2, p. 107, 2013.

3

Referred Trigeminal Facial Pain from Occipital Neuralgia Occurring Much Earlier than Occipital Neuralgia

Byung-chul Son[1,2]

[1]*Department of Neurosurgery, Seoul St. Mary's Hospital, Seoul, The Catholic University of Korea, Republic of Korea*
[2]*Catholic Neuroscience Institute, College of Medicine, The Catholic University of Korea, Seoul, Republic of Korea*

Correspondence should be addressed to Byung-chul Son; sbc@catholic.ac.kr

Academic Editor: Tapas Kumar Banerjee

We report a very rare case in which a patient believed to have auriculotemporal neuralgia due to the repeated recurrence of paroxysmal stabbing pain in the preauricular temporal region for four years developed occipital neuralgia, which finally improved with decompression of the greater occipital nerve (GON). The pain of occipital neuralgia has been suggested to be referred to the frontoorbital (V1) region through trigeminocervical interneuronal connections in the trigeminal spinal nucleus. However, the reports of such cases are very rare. In occipital neuralgia, the pain referred to the ipsilateral facial trigeminal region reportedly also occurs in the V2 and V3 distributions in addition to that in the V1 region. In the existing cases of referred trigeminal pain from occipital neuralgia, continuous aching pain is usually induced, but in the present case, typical neuralgic pain was induced and diagnosed as idiopathic auriculotemporal neuralgia. In addition, recurrent trigeminal pain occurred for four years before the onset of occipital neuralgia. If the typical occipital neuralgia did not develop in four years, it would be impossible to infer an association with the GON. This case shows that the clinical manifestations of referred trigeminal pain caused by the sensitization of the trigeminocervical complex by chronic entrapment of the GON can be very diverse.

1. Introduction

Occipital neuralgia is characterized by paroxysmal shooting or stabbing pain in the posterior part of the scalp with distributions of the greater and lesser occipital nerves (GON and LON) [1]. Although it has been suggested that the pain of occipital neuralgia can reach the frontoorbital (V1) area through trigeminocervical interneuronal connections in the trigeminal spinal nucleus [1], reports of referred trigeminal pain from occipital neuralgia are rare [2]. However, recently, pain referred to the facial trigeminal nerve distribution by occipital neuralgia due to GON entrapment has been reported [2–5]. Referral to the facial trigeminal distribution occurred not only in the V1 region but also in the V2 and V3 regions and even caused hemifacial sensory changes [2–5]. The referred trigeminal facial pain was immediately improved by decompression of the GON. In the previous reports, the nature of the referred facial trigeminal pain caused by GON entrapment showed continuous aching pain and occurred months after the symptoms of occipital neuralgia [2–5]. However, the authors experienced a very rare case where referred facial trigeminal pain appeared in the form of severe paroxysmal stabbing pain in the preauricular temporal area rather than aching pain. In addition, this facial pain occurred years before the symptoms of occipital neuralgia and continued to recur. These aspects made the diagnosis very difficult.

The natural course of untreated occipital neuralgia due to chronic entrapment of the GON remains unknown [5]. The GON originates from the medial branch of the dorsal rami of the second cervical nerve root [6–9]. Therefore, the GON constitutes the main sensory afferent nerve through the C2 root, and this afferent input is directly relayed to the C2 dorsal horn [10–12]. The etiology of primary occipital neuralgia is mostly unknown [2]. However, entrapment of the GON at its piercing point of the tendinous aponeurotic attachment of the trapezius at the superior nuchal line is known as the most common cause [2, 8, 13]. The chronic continuous and noxious afferent input of occipital neuralgia caused by GON entrapment seems to be associated with sensitization and hypersensitivity of the second-order neurons in the trigeminocervical complex, a population of neurons in the C2 dorsal horn characterized by receiving convergent input from dural and cervical structures [10–12].

2. Case Report

In December 2014, a 78-year-old female presented with severe paroxysmal stabbing pain in the front of the left ear and anterior temporal region. The pain initially began with persistent aching pain in the left molars and gums, and severe paroxysmal stabbing pain occurred at 5 to 10 second intervals over a day or two. Paroxysmal pain continued to occur even when she was resting and was more severe when she moved her jaw or spoke or lightly touched the front part of her left ear and temporal region (Figure 1(a)). The left facial pain was severe (7 to 8 out of 10 on the numerical rating scale (NRS-11)). Physical examination showed no changes in facial sensation and no abnormal findings in the cranial nerve, but pulsatile pain and tenderness of the superficial temporal artery in the anterior temporal region were observed.

Under the preliminary diagnosis of trigeminal neuralgia or temporal vasculitis, she was prescribed carbamazepine and gabapentin and consulted with the Rheumatology department. The laboratory examinations showed normal findings, including an elevated sedimentation rate (ESR) of 6 mm/hr. Magnetic resonance imaging (MRI) scans suspected for trigeminal neuralgia but did not show vascular compression or abnormal enhancement of the trigeminal nerve. After about 10 days, her severe pain gradually disappeared with medication and no special sequelae were observed.

Nine months later, in September 2015, her severe pain suddenly recurred without any special event. As in the past, the paroxysmal stabbing pains in the preauricular and temporal areas continued. Especially when she moved her chin, the pain in her lower gum was so severe that she could hardly eat. Nonsteroidal anti-inflammatory drugs (NSAIDs) were ineffective, and the pain did not decrease with gabapentin 1600 mg/day, pregabalin 450 mg/day, tramadol 450 mg/day, and amitriptyline 30 mg/day. Her pain was so severe (NRS-11, 7-8/10) that she had to be hospitalized for pain control three weeks after she became sick. The neurological examination showed no abnormalities, and severe tenderness of the temporal area was present, but no swelling was observed. IR-codon® (40 mg/day) added to the anticonvulsants had little effect on pain control, and only an intramuscular injection of diclofenac sodium could reduce the pain by half for three hours. There were no abnormal findings on laboratory tests including ESR and C-reactive protein (CRP). No abnormal findings of the temporal artery and trigeminal nerve were observed in color-duplex ultrasonography and contrast-enhanced MRI. No sinus, ear, tooth, and temporomandibular joint (TMJ) problems were found upon in otolaryngology and dental consultations.

Unusually, the patient reported the paroxysmal pain was as if the temporal artery's pulse was beating. The rheumatologist did not conduct a biopsy of the temporal artery because there were no signs of inflammation and no imaging problems. Excluding the possibility of temporal arteritis, we tentatively determined that it is rare but an auriculotemporal neuralgia for pain distribution. Blocks with 1% lidocaine (3 ml) were used near the temporal artery. Pain relief was observed for about one hour after the injection, but the pain in the temporal region and gums continued. Even when the patient was hospitalized for 10 days and visited the hospital two weeks after her discharge, she said she was sick enough to have trouble sleeping at night. Her severe pain gradually diminished after a month and a half. No more medication was needed.

In September 2016, the same pain suddenly recurred. This time, the patient had been tired for several days before the pain occurred. The pain also occurred spontaneously in the preauricular temporal area, and she said that the aching pain occurred surprisingly suddenly. This time, paroxysmal pain occurred in the left vertex and deep in the left ear at the same time as the left temporal region (Figure 1(b)). No ear abnormalities were identified in the otolaryngology consultation. A temporal local block and mandibular nerve block were ineffective. Again gabapentin, carbamazepine, tramadol, and amitriptyline were administered, and the pain improved after two weeks. A month later, it reappeared for about two weeks and improved.

In November 2017, she visited our outpatient clinic after receiving treatment at another hospital for the same pain in the preauricular temporal area and vertex. She received similar medications and nerve blocks in other clinic, and resection of the superficial temporal artery was recommanded but she did not have surgery. After about three weeks of medication, the pain disappeared spontaneously. Two months later, in January 2019, pain of the same nature recurred to the left temporal and gum region, inside the ear canal, and parieto-occipital vertex (Figure 1(b)). Her pain was so severe (NRS-11, 6-8/10) and unremitting that she was hospitalized for a week with regular diclofenac sodium injections. Neurological and laboratory testing and MRI were performed again, but no abnormal findings were found. The pain subsided spontaneously after three weeks after discharge.

The patient experienced no pain for the next seven months, but in August 2018, her severe paroxysmal pain recurred again in the left temporal, parieto-occipital vertex, and inside the left ear. The same stabbing pain occurred in the same manner as before, and pain occurred when she moved her head. Specifically, this time, the pain also occurred in the occipital area behind the ear, in the distribution area of the greater occipital nerve (Figure 1(c)). With the possibility of referred trigeminal facial pain from occipital neuralgia in mind, an occipital nerve block (ONB) was performed using 2 ml of 1% lidocaine for the left GON. The effect of the ONB was dramatic for two hours. In addition to the pain in the occipital and vertex area, the paroxysmal pain in the anterior temporal region and deep ear area was significantly improved. She estimated that the pain was reduced by 90% (9/10 for the NRS-11 scale improved to 2-3/10 after one hour). However, the effect of the ONB

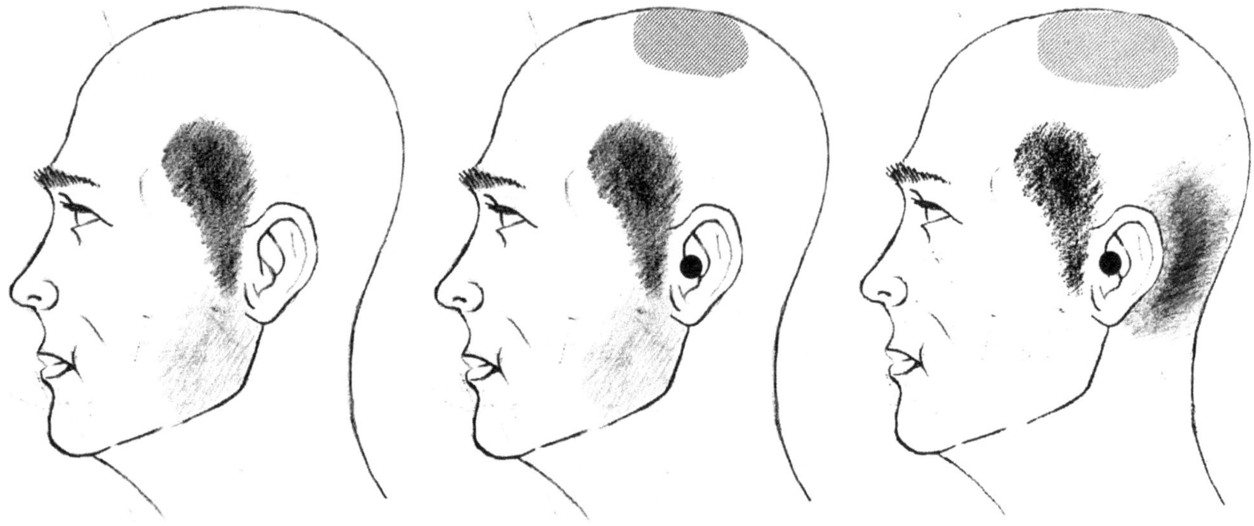

(a) (b) (c)

Figure 1: Schematic diagram demonstrating the distribution and characteristics of pain over the years. (a) The gray areas over the left preauricular temporal area indicate the distribution of paroxysmal lancinating pain that started in 2014. Pain initially began as a persistent aching pain in the left molars and gums (light gray area). (b) In 2016, paroxysmal pain occurred in the left preauricular temporal region, and at the same time in the left vertex (obliquely hatched area) and the left deep ear (black circle). (c) It was not until 2018, four years after the occurrence of paroxysmal pain, that the stabbing pain in the retroauricular occipital area (transversely hatched area) occurred as pain in the left temporal region (gray area), left vertex (obliquely hatched area), and left deep ear (black circle).

disappeared completely after two hours and she became ill again. Transient hypesthesia due to ONB was observed in the occipital and parietal vertex area and the GON distribution area but not in the temporal region.

No abnormalities were detected in the computed tomographic (CT) scan of the cervical spine performed to check for structural lesions in the path from the C2 nerve root to the GON. Two ONBs were performed after admission, and pain reduction in the same occipital and preauricular areas was repeatedly confirmed. Considering the intractability and the possibility of referred trigeminal pain of occipital neuralgia, GON decompression was explained to the patient and her caregivers, and informed consent was obtained.

A 4 cm-sized linear incision was made obliquely along the course of the left GON. The incision was then developed over the trapezius fascia. The GON was found to be severely entrapped by the aponeurotic arch of the trapezius, showing an indentation of chronic entrapment (Figures 2(a) and 2(b)). After the circumferential release of the GON from the tendinous aponeurotic arch, the proximal and distal courses of the GON were dissected. A small tributary of the occipital artery was found to constrict the distal course of the GON, which was cut off, resulting in complete decompression of the left GON (Figure 2(c)). The patient's pain attacks persisted for two days after surgery, and then the instances and intensity of pain decreased from day three. From seven days after surgery, the number of paroxysmal pain attacks decreased by more than 80%, and numbness was observed in the left occipital area. A month later, the paresthesia of the left occipital disappeared, and there was no more painful paroxysm of the left temporal lateral temporal region, inside the ear canal or the occipital area. The patient's pain attack no longer occurred until a year and a half after surgery.

3. Discussion

3.1. Atypical Manifestation of Occipital Neuralgia: Referred Ipsilateral Trigeminal Pain. Occipital neuralgia is defined as paroxysmal, shooting, or stabbing pain in the posterior part of the scalp, in the distribution(s) area of the greater, lesser, and/or third occipital nerves [1]. Occipital neuralgia pain has been suggested to be referred to the frontoorbital (V1) area through trigeminocervical interneuronal connections in the trigeminal spinal nucleus [1], but reports of such cases are very rare [2]. However, in occipital neuralgia, referred pain in the ipsilateral facial trigeminal region has been reported to occur in the V2 region as well as in the V2 and V3 regions and the frontal-orbital (V1) region [2–5]. Occipital neuralgia caused by chronic GON entrapment has been reported to cause not only facial pain but also hemisensory changes throughout the ipsilateral face [2, 3]. These findings provide clinical affirmation of the existence of trigeminal/cervical convergence and hypersensitivity [2, 10, 11].

The trigeminocervical complex (TCC) is a population of neurons in the C2 dorsal horn that receive convergent input from facial skin corresponding to the trigeminal nerve and cervical structures innervated by the high cervical C1-3 roots [10–12]. Convergence of nociceptive afferents and sensitization of TCC neurons have clinical correlates, including hypersensitivity and the spread and referral of pain frequently seen in patients with primary headaches such as migraines [10, 11]. Patients with primary headaches often report pain not only involving the frontal head innervated by

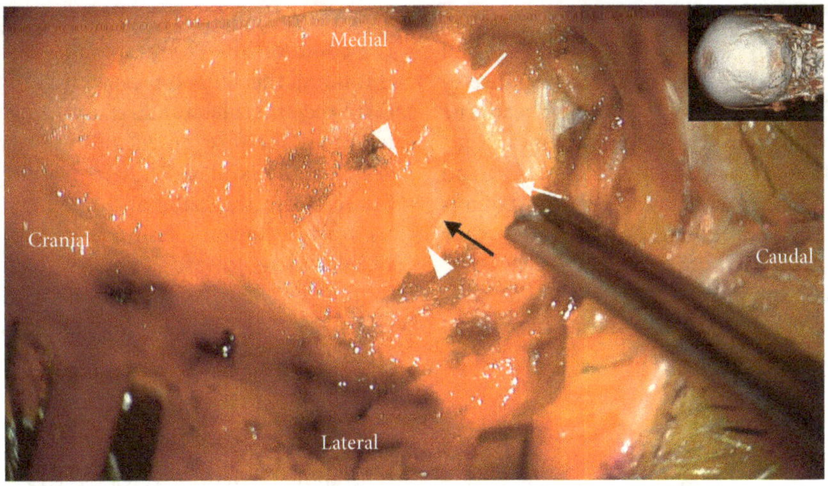

(a)

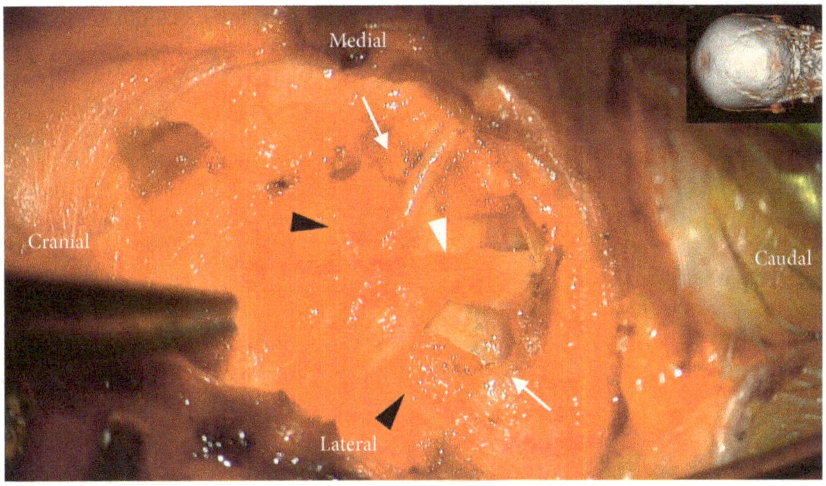

(b)

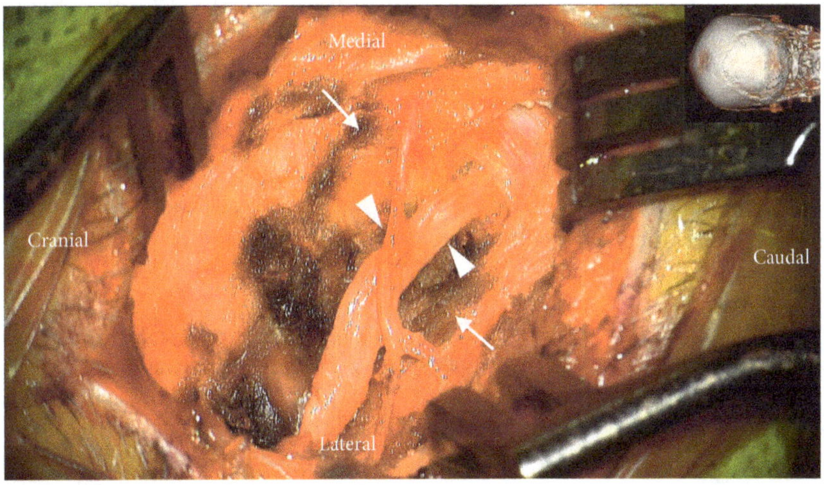

(c)

Figure 2: Intraoperative photographs during the decompression of the greater occipital nerve (GON). (a) Intraoperative photograph showing severe entrapment of the GON (white arrowheads) by the aponeurotic fibrous attachment of the trapezius (white arrows) at the superior nuchal line. The maximal compression point (black arrow) is seen by lifting the trapezial aponeurotic edge. The inset shows the direction of the photo and the location of the incision. (b) Intraoperative photograph after decompression of the left GON (white arrow heads) with the division of the trapezial aponeurosis (white arrows). Even after decompressing the upper side, the GON was still depressed by the lower fascial aponeurosis (black arrowheads). (c) Intraoperative photograph after complete decompression of the left GON (white arrowheads). Its proximal and distal courses are addressed.

the trigeminal nerve but also involving the occipital region innervated by the GON [10]. The sensitization of central nociceptive neurons in the TCC takes place in response to strong dural noxious input seen in secondary headache syndromes such as meningitis, subarachnoid hemorrhage, and experimental headaches [12]. Chronic compression and adhesion of the GON by the occipital artery and its constriction by the aponeurotic fibrous aperture of the trapezius muscle can cause chronic occipital neuralgia [2–5, 13]. The chronic noxious afferent input of occipital neuralgia may lead to central sensitization of the TCC, resulting in referred hemifacial trigeminal pain [2, 4, 10, 11].

3.2. Preauricular Temporal Pain and Deep Ear Canal Pain as Referred Pain. Although initially accompanied by pain in the lower and upper gums, specifically, the main pain in this patient occurred in the temporal region in front of the ear. Due to this unusual distribution of pain, it was considered rare but auriculotemporal neuralgia (ATN). The auriculotemporal nerve is a terminal branch of the mandibular nerve (third division of the trigeminal nerve). ATN neuralgia is characterized by paroxysmal attacks that are strictly unilateral and lancinating, moderate to severe pain on the preauricular area often spreading to the ipsilateral temple [14, 15]. The pain in this patient showed typical neuralgic pain, and the location of pain was the same as that of the ATN distribution. However, blocks around the ATN were not effective for pain in the preauricular temporal area, and ONB performed after the occurrence of occipital neuralgia was effective for pain in the preauricular temporal area. It is difficult for us to explain this phenomenon. We speculated that the referred pain in the trigeminal distribution could to be reduced by blocking the area that caused the referred pain.

Another peculiarity was the pain inside the ear canal that accompanied the occurrence of the typical occipital neuralgia in the temporooccipital area. The pain inside the ear canal was also typical neuralgic pain and was present in the auditory canal not the eardrum. It was not related to any activities, such as drinking, sneezing, or coughing. The anterior wall of the ear canal is innervated by the ATN, and the posterior wall is made by the auricular branch of the vagal nerve (ABVN) [16]. It is difficult to identify which of the two nerves was involved. However, it was reasonable to think of the pain in the deep ear as pain referred to the ATN, a branch of the trigeminal nerve, because typical pain occurred in the ATN of the preauricular temporal area. This was confirmed by temporary improvement of the deep ear pain with the ONB.

3.3. Entrapment Neuropathy of the Greater Occipital Nerve. The GON originates from the medial branch of the dorsal rami of the second cervical nerve root [7–9]. It also receives a branch from the dorsal rami of the C3 nerve. It ascends through the semispinalis muscle and then runs rostrolaterally before emerging into the scalp by piercing the aponeurotic fibrous sling between the trapezius and the sternocleidomastoid near their occipital attachment to the superior nuchal line [17, 18]. This aperture (trapezial tunnel) is a common site of entrapment of the GON [8, 17, 18]. At this point, the GON travels with the occipital artery, running form the anterolateral direction beneath the splenius capitis to supply the integument of the scalp as far anterior as the vertex of the skull [6–9]. After piercing the aponeurotic sling between the trapezius and the sternocleidomastoideus, in contrast to common findings in other peripheral nerves, the GON widens toward its course to the periphery [6]. This finding is regarded as relevant to the entrapment of the GON, as widening of the nerve makes it susceptible to entrapment especially in the firm trapezius muscle aponeurosis [6].

We think that the term "entrapment" is more appropriate than simple compression of the GON. The term "entrapment neuropathies" refers to isolated peripheral nerve injuries that occur at specific locations where a nerve is mechanically constricted in a fibrous or fibro-osseous tunnel or deformed by a fibrous band [19].

3.4. Difficulty in Diagnosing Referred Trigeminal Pain due to Chronic Entrapment of the GON. The natural course of occipital neuralgia due to chronic entrapment of the GON remains unknown. As shown in the present case, chronic entrapment of the GON can cause pain in the V2 and V3 dermatomes. In past cases [2–5, 13], continuous aching pain was induced, but in the present case, typical neuralgic pain was induced and diagnosed as idiopathic ATN neuralgia. Moreover, facial pain preceded occipital pain four years earlier. If the neuralgic pain, which recurred every year for several years, was not accompanied by occipital pain later, it would not be possible to infer GON involvement. Also, unlike trigeminal neuralgia, in which neurovascular contact can be confirmed by MRI, it is difficult to determine the degree of entrapment of the GON within the small trapezial canal. Thus, when unexplained facial pain is accompanied by typical paroxysmal stabbing pain in the occipital area, we recommended confirming that there is no structural lesion through a detailed MRI examination and checking whether facial pain decreases through repeated ONBs.

4. Conclusions

We report a case of occipital neuralgia due to chronic GON entrapment, which was preceded by neuralgic pain in the face. The pain in the distribution of the ATN, the third branch of the trigeminal nerve, was very severe and recurred, and occipital nerve involvement was not suspected until the occurrence of occipital neuralgia. This case shows that the clinical manifestations of referred trigeminal pain caused by the sensitization of the trigeminocervical complex by the chronic entrapment of the GON can be very diverse.

References

[1] Headache Classification Committee of the International Headache Society (IHS), "The International classification of headache disorders," *Cephalalgia*, vol. 38, pp. 1–211, 2018.

[2] B. C. Son and J. G. Choi, "Hemifacial pain and hemisensory disturbance referred from occipital neuralgia caused by pathological vascular contact of the greater occipital nerve," *Case Reports in Neurological Medicine*, vol. 2017, Article ID 3827369, 5 pages, 2017.

[3] H. C. Ko, J. G. Choi, and B. C. Son, "Hemifacial trigeminal pain referred from occipital neuralgia due to compression of the greater occipital nerve by the occipital artery," *Journal of Neurological Surgery Part A: Central European Neurosurgery*, vol. 79, no. 5, pp. 442–446, 2018.

[4] C. I. Lee and B. C. Son, "V2 trigeminal referred pain from chronic occipital neuralgia caused by entrapment of the greater occipital nerve," *Indian Journal of Neurosurgery*, vol. 8, no. 1, pp. 76–80, 2019.

[5] C. I. Lee and B. C. Son, "Chronic craniofacial pain from entrapment of the greater occipital nerve misdiagnosed as chronic migraine, idiopathic odontalgia, and atypical facial pain," *The Nerve*, vol. 5, no. 2, pp. 78–82, 2019.

[6] K. Natsis, X. Baraliakos, H. J. Appell, P. Tsikaras, I. Gigis, and J. Koebke, "The course of the greater occipital nerve in the suboccipital region: a proposal for setting landmarks for local anesthesia in patients with occipital neuralgia," *Clinical Anatomy*, vol. 19, no. 4, pp. 332–336, 2006.

[7] R. S. Tubbs, E. G. Salter, J. C. Wellons III, J. P. Blount, and W. J. Oakes, "Landmarks for the identification of the cutaneous nerves of the occiput and nuchal regions," *Clinical Anatomy*, vol. 20, no. 3, pp. 235–238, 2007.

[8] A. Cesmebasi, M. A. Muhleman, P. Hulsberg et al., "Occipital neuralgia: anatomic considerations," *Clinical Anatomy*, vol. 28, no. 1, pp. 101–108, 2015.

[9] S. Gielecki, "Spinal cord and spinal nerves: gross anatomy," in *Gray's Anatomy: The Anatomical Basis of Clinical Practice*, S. Standring, Ed., Elsevier, Amsterdam, Netherlands, 41th edition, 2008.

[10] E. Piovesan, P. Kowacs, C. Tatsui, M. Lange, L. Ribas, and L. Werneck, "Referred pain after painful stimulation of the greater occipital nerve in humans: evidence of convergence of cervical afferences on trigeminal nuclei," *Cephalalgia*, vol. 21, no. 2, pp. 107–109, 2001.

[11] T. Bartsch and P. J. Goadsby, "Stimulation of the greater occipital nerve induces increased central excitability of dural afferent input," *Brain*, vol. 125, no. 7, pp. 1496–1509, 2002.

[12] T. Bartsch and P. J. Goadsby, "The trigeminocervical complex and migraine: current concepts and synthesis," *Current Pain and Headache Reports*, vol. 7, no. 5, pp. 371–376, 2003.

[13] C. Cornely, M. Fischer, G. Ingianni, and S. Isenmann, "Greater occipital nerve neuralgia caused by pathological arterial contact: treatment by surgical decompression," *Headache: The Journal of Head and Face Pain*, vol. 51, no. 4, pp. 609–616, 2010.

[14] J. G. Speciali and D. A. G. Gonçalves, "Auriculotemporal neuralgia," *Current Pain and Headache Reports*, vol. 9, no. 4, pp. 277–280, 2005.

[15] M. Ruiz, J. Porta-Etessam, S. Garcia-Ptacek, C. de la Cruz, M. L. Cuadrado, and A. L. Guerrero, "Auriculotemporal neuralgia: eight new cases report: table 1," *Pain Medicine*, vol. 17, no. 9, pp. 1744–1748, 2016.

[16] K. Watanabe, R. S. Tubbs, S. Satoh et al., "Isolated deep ear canal pain: possible role of auricular branch of vagus nerve-case Illustrations with cadaveric correlation," *World Neurosurgery*, vol. 96, pp. 293–301, 2016.

[17] S. W. Mosser, B. Guyuron, J. E. Janis, and R. J. Rohrich, "The anatomy of the greater occipital nerve: implications for the etiology of migraine headaches," *Plastic and Reconstructive Surgery*, vol. 113, no. 2, pp. 693–697, 2004.

[18] I. Ducic, M. Moriarty, and A. Al-Attar, "Anatomical variations of the occipital nerves: implications for the treatment of chronic headaches," *Plastic and Reconstructive Surgery*, vol. 123, no. 3, pp. 859–863, 2009.

[19] J. D. England, "Entrapment neuropathies," *Current Opinion in Neurology*, vol. 12, no. 5, pp. 597–602, 1999.

4

Unilateral Upper Cervical Cord Infarction: A Report of Two Cases with Mild Neurological Symptoms Accompanying a Small Ischemic Lesion Detected by Brain MRI

Manabu Wada, Hikaru Nagasawa, and Yoshitaka Yamaguchi

Department of Neurology, Yamagata Prefectural Central Hospital, 1800 Aoyagi, Yamagata, Japan

Correspondence should be addressed to Manabu Wada; mwada@ypch.gr.jp

Academic Editor: Peter Berlit

Spinal cord infarction (SCI) is rare, difficult to diagnose, and often fails to be detected by diffusion-weighted imaging (DWI) of spinal cord magnetic resonance imaging (MRI). Because the clinical features of SCI can vary widely, diagnosis during the acute phase of SCI is often challenging for clinicians. Although SCI shares similar etiologies with cerebral infarction, the characteristics of SCI without vessel dissection remain largely unknown. We present two older patients with mild neurological symptoms who each presented with a small, unilateral, upper cervical cord lesion, which was detected by thin-section, coronal DWI of brain MRI. Both unilateral small lesions were localized in the right lateral funiculus, and each patient showed good prognosis. The anatomical findings suggested that the pial collateral network surrounding the cervical cord contributed to lesion formation. Small and localized lesions have been associated with mild neurological symptoms and better short-term prognosis. The present report indicated that the use of thin-section coronal DWI when performing brain MRI may be helpful for the diagnosis of small, unilateral, upper cervical cord infarctions.

1. Introduction

Spinal cord infarction (SCI) is a rare disease that causes devastating neurological sequelae, such as paraplegia and incontinence [1–4]. SCI diagnosis during the acute phase is often challenging for clinicians because the clinical features of SCI can vary widely [1–4]. Numerous collateral systems, constructed by spinal cord vascular networks, may account for the rarity and clinical variations observed for SCI [1, 3, 4]. The most common etiologies of SCI include vascular risk factors, aortic disease, and vessel dissection; however, the mechanisms underlying spontaneous or nonsurgical SCI remain largely unclear [1, 3, 4].

A recent clinical study examining cervical cord infarctions in patients with and without vessel dissection showed that lesions were frequently located in the upper cervical cord among patients with dissection, whereas patients without dissection presented with an older mean age of onset and the lesions tended to be located in the lower cervical regions [2]. Owing to the rarity of SCI, the clinical characteristics and magnetic resonance imaging (MRI) findings associated with unilateral, upper cervical cord infarction without vascular dissection have been seldom discussed.

We present two cases of older patients with mild neurological symptoms and small, unilateral, upper cervical cord lesions that were detected by thin-section, coronal, diffusion-weighted imaging (DWI) of brain MRI.

2. Case Presentation

2.1. Case 1. An 84-year-old woman with a history of diabetes and hypertension experienced acute onset of severe right neck pain. Neurological examination showed no apparent abnormality. Brain MRI was performed, including thin-section, coronal DWI, and neither abnormal signal changes nor vertebral artery dissection were detected. Four days later, she noticed the impairment of temperature perception in her left foot while bathing. Subsequent neurological examination showed mild hypoalgesia of the left upper and lower limbs. No weakness, disturbance of vibration sense, or urinary incontinence was apparent. Brain MRI was performed again, and thin-section, coronal DWI showed a high-intensity lesion in the right lateral funiculus, within the cervical spinal cord, at the level of the C2/C3 intervertebral disc (Figure 1(a)). Subsequently, fast imaging employing steady-state acquisition sequences showed a small, hyperintense lesion in the right lateral funiculus (Figures 1(b) and 1(c)). Repeated magnetic resonance (MR) angiography showed mild atherosclerosis; however, no double-lumen signs, strings, or pearls signs were observed. Therefore, we concluded that the patient did not have any artery dissection (Figure 1(e)). She was able to walk without any assistance, but the temperature perception impairment in her limbs remained unchanged 4 weeks after onset. Follow-up MRI, examined 5 weeks after onset, showed a high-intensity lesion of the right lateral funiculus and anterior horn, within the cervical spinal cord (Figure 1(d)).

The settings used for the MRI protocols are summarized in the Table 1.

2.2. Case 2. A 74-year-old man with a history of prostate cancer, cholecystolithiasis, and hypertension experienced an unsteady gait 3 days after laparoscopic cholecystectomy. A neurological examination showed mild ataxia of his right lower limb, and tandem gait was impaired. No apparent weakness or sensory disturbance was found. Brain MRI was performed, and thin-section, coronal DWI showed a high-intensity lesion in the right lateral funiculus, within the cervical spinal cord, at the level of C1 (Figure 1(f)). Axial DWI showed a hyperintense lesion of the spinal cord (Figure 1(g)), and the corresponding T2-weighted images (Figure 1(h)) demonstrated a hyperintense area in the right lateral funiculus. MR angiography showed an occlusion in the right vertebral artery. Short-term prognosis was good, and he was able to walk without any assistance.

3. Discussion

Development of collateral circulation is associated with the rarity of SCI and variations in symptoms and lesion sizes: although the etiology of SCI is similar to that of cerebral infarction and systemic vascular disease, SCI is estimated to represent only 1% to 2% of all ischemic strokes [2, 5, 6]. The clinical features of SCI depend on the lesion location and the degree of arterial occlusion [3, 6]. Anatomically, the anterior two-thirds of the spinal cord and the anterior portion of the posterior column receive blood via the anterior spinal artery (ASA), whereas the posterior one-third of the spinal cord is supplied by the two posterior spinal arteries (PSAs) [7, 8]. These arteries construct collateral circulation networks, with individual variations, which may contribute to the rarity and clinical variations associated with the neurological symptoms that present in patients with SCI.

Associations between mild neurological symptoms and the locations of small cervical cord lesions in our patients: anatomically, the vasocorona that covers the cervical cord contributed to the formation of localized, unilateral, small-sized infarcts in our patients (Figure 2). The MRI findings in our patients showed high-intensity lesions in the lateral funiculus of the cervical cord on DWI and T2-weighted imaging in each patient. The surface layer of the lateral funiculus is supplied primarily by the coronary artery, which arises from the ASA. The medial region includes the gray matter, and the region of the lateral funiculus where the lesions were localized is supplied by the central artery [10]. A potential watershed zone has been hypothesized to exist between the regions supplied by the ASA and PSA, involving parts of the corticospinal and spinothalamic tracts [11], although little evidence has been presented to confirm its existence. In our patients, the unilateral, small-sized lesions were limited to the lateral funiculus and were associated with mild symptoms. We hypothesize that injuries to the spinothalamic tract may have contributed to the experience of neck pain and mild limb ataxia in our patients. Previous studies have indicated that central pain is likely to occur after the impairment of the spinothalamic tract, which is located in the lateral funiculus [4, 12].

Detection of small infarctions in the upper cervical cord using thin-section, coronal DWI of brain MRI: unilateral and small-sized SCI is exceedingly rare, and MRI sometimes fails to detect small ischemic lesions of the spinal cord. Kumral and colleagues have previously reported that in patients with SCI, spinal MRI was effective in only a portion of patients with unilateral ischemic lesions (57% in their series) [1]. The failure of spinal cord MRI to detect cervical lesions may be related to the phase of the illness or the size of the SCI [7]. In contrast to the mild neurological symptoms presented by our patients, most of the patients described by Kumral and colleagues showed moderate-to-severe neurological disturbances and required walking assistance or a wheelchair upon leaving the hospital [1].

Although DWI is the current gold-standard for the detection of acute ischemic stroke [13], DWI sometimes fails to detect very small ischemic lesions, especially those in the posterior fossa. Recent studies have shown that the performance of additional thin-section, coronal DWI of the posterior fossa can overcome this problem. Coronal plane slices in the upper cervical cord may be positioned perpendicular to sections of the coronary arteries associated with the ASA and the pial collateral network, allowing the capture and identification of even very small ischemic lesions in our patients.

Clinicians should be aware that hyperintense lesions on DWI may also be observed in the spinal cord during acute stage inflammatory diseases. In particular, "clinically isolated syndrome" sometimes shows an isolated lesion that is located peripherally and contacts the surface of the spinal cord [3]. A previous study indicated the importance of measuring apparent diffusion coefficient (ADC) values, which were found to be lower in spinal cord infarcts than in inflammatory spinal cord lesions [14]. Therefore, the measurement of ADC values may be useful for differentiating SCI from inflammatory myelopathies during the acute stages of these diseases.

The present study indicated that thin-section, coronal DWI can detect the presence of an upper cervical cord infarction.

Table 1: Summary of MRI protocols examined in our cases.

Parameters	Case 1				Case 2		
	DWI coronal	FIESTA axial	FIESTA sagittal	T2WI (spine)	DWI coronal	DWI axial	T2WI axial
Magnetic field strength		3.0 T				3.0 T	
Matrix size	288 × 288	512 × 512	1024 × 1024	512 × 512	282 × 282	320 × 320	704 × 704
Field of view	240 mm × 240 mm	160 mm × 160 mm	180 mm × 180 mm	180 mm × 180 mm	240 mm × 240 mm	240 mm × 240 mm	240 mm × 240 mm
Slice thickness (mm)	3	1.6	2	4	3	3	5
Repetition time (ms)	5000	1500	1500	3025	5000	5000	4000
Echo time (ms)	137	256	256	100	137	85	104
b values	1000				1000	1000	

DWI, diffusion-weighted image; FIESTA, 3D fast imaging employing steady-state acquisition; T2WI, T2-weighted image.

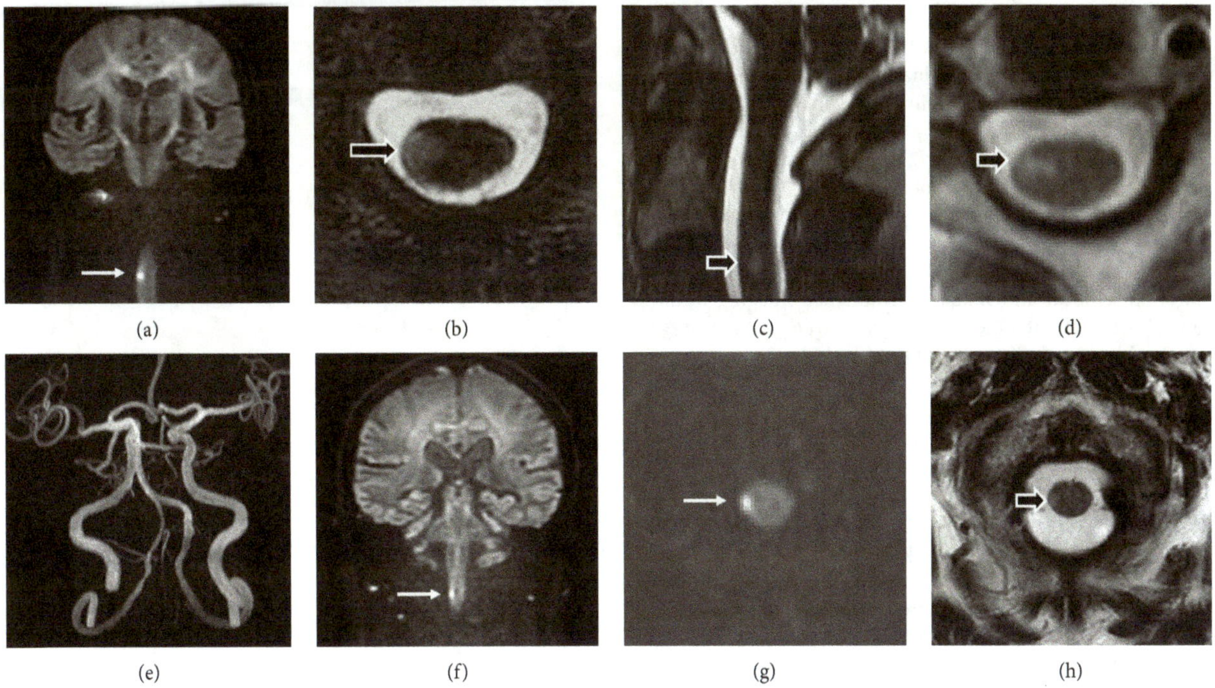

FIGURE 1: Magnetic resonance imaging (MRI) of spinal infarctions in two cases. The lesion for case 1 is presented in (a–e). (a) Thin-section coronal diffusion-weighted imaging (DWI), showing a high-intensity lesion of the cervical spine (arrow). (b and c) 3D fast imaging employing steady-state acquisition; MRI showing an upper cervical lesion. Axial (b) and sagittal (c); MRI showing a small, high-intensity lesion (arrows) at the level of the C2/3 intervertebral disc. (d) Axial, T2-weighted image of the cervical cord, examined 5 weeks after onset. (e) MR angiography of case 1, showing no apparent dissection of vertebral arteries. The MRI findings of case 2 are presented in (f–h). (f) Thin-section, coronal DWI and (g) axial DWI, demonstrating a high-intensity lesion (arrows) in the upper cervical cord. (h) T2-weighted axial image, showing a high-intensity lesion (arrow) in the right lateral funiculus at the level of the C1 vertebra.

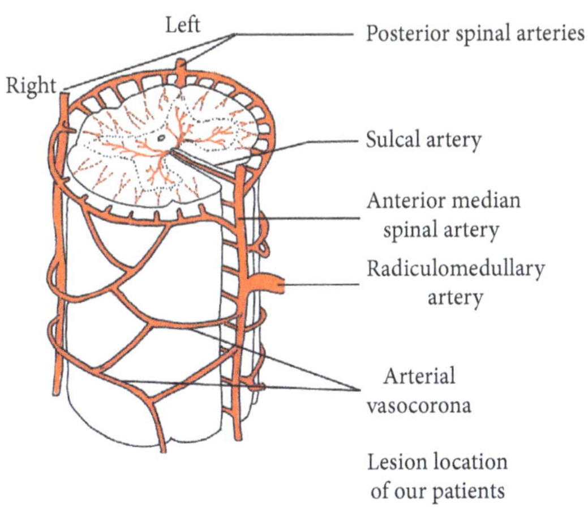

FIGURE 2: Schema showing the arterial supply to the cervical spinal cord (the figure is adapted from [9]).

However, the performance of coronal DWI for the detection of ischemic lesions in the upper cervical cord, relative to the performance of sagittal DWI, could not be evaluated. This is because we did not perform sagittal DWI during the spinal cord MRI in the acute phases of the disease in these patients.

4. Conclusion

We present two older patients, with unilateral, small-sized, cervical infarction, which were detected by thin-section, coronal DWI of brain MRI. Small and localized lesions may be related to good prognosis. Whether thin-section coronal DWI is superior to spinal cord sagittal DWI for the detection of upper cervical cord ischemic lesions remains uncertain. Further studies, using larger samples of patients with unilateral upper cervical cord infarctions, remain necessary to clarify the prognosis and advantages of thin-section, coronal DWI.

Acknowledgments

The authors thank Lisa Giles, PhD, from the Edanz Group (https://en-author-services.edanzgroup.com/ac) for editing a draft of this manuscript.

References

[1] E. Kumral, F. Polat, H. Güllüoglu, C. Uzunköprü, R. Tuncel, and S. Alpaydın, "Spinal ischaemic stroke: clinical and

radiological findings and short-term outcome," *European Journal of Neurology*, vol. 18, no. 2, pp. 232–239, 2011.
[2] J. L. Hsu, M.-Y. Cheng, M.-F. Liao et al., "The etiologies and prognosis associated with spinal cord infarction," *Annals of Clinical and Translational Neurology*, vol. 6, no. 8, pp. 1456–1464, 2019.
[3] S. Weidauer, M. Nichtweiß, E. Hattingen, and J. Berkefeld, "Spinal cord ischemia: aetiology, clinical syndromes and imaging features," *Neuroradiology*, vol. 57, no. 3, pp. 241–257, 2015.
[4] C. Masson, J. P. Pruvo, and J. F. Meder, "Spinal cord infarction: clinical and magnetic resonance imaging findings and short term outcome," *Journal of Neurology, Neurosurgery & Psychiatry*, vol. 75, no. 10, pp. 1431–1435, 2004.
[5] T. A. Sandson and J. H. Friedman, "Spinal cord infarction," *Medicine*, vol. 68, no. 5, pp. 282–292, 1989.
[6] J. Novy, A. Carruzzo, P. Maeder, and J. Bogousslavsky, "Spinal cord ischemia," *Archives of Neurology*, vol. 63, no. 8, pp. 1113–1120, 2006.
[7] M. I. Vargas, J. Gariani, R. Sztajzel et al., "Spinal cord ischemia: practical imaging tips, pearls, and pitfalls," *American Journal of Neuroradiology*, vol. 36, no. 5, pp. 825–830, 2015.
[8] B. G. Chakravorty, "Arterial supply of the cervical spinal cord and its relation to the cervical myelopathy in spondylosis," *The Annals of the Royal College of Surgeons of England*, vol. 45, no. 4, pp. 232–251, 1969.
[9] O. Benavente and H. J. M. Barnett, "Spinal cord ischemia," in Stroke, H. J. M. Barnet, J. P. Mohr, and B. A. Stein, Eds., pp. 751–765, Churchill Livingstone, New York, NY, USA.
[10] K. Ogawa, T. Akimoto, M. Hara et al., "Clinical study of thirteen patients with spinal cord infarction," *Journal of Stroke and Cerebrovascular Diseases*, vol. 28, no. 12, Article ID 104418, 2019.
[11] B. Crum, B. Mokri, and J. Fulgham, "Spinal manifestations of vertebral artery dissection," *Neurology*, vol. 55, no. 2, pp. 304–306, 2000.
[12] R. A. Davidoff, "The dorsal columns," *Neurology*, vol. 39, no. 10, p. 1377, 1989.
[13] P. Felfeli, H. Wenz, M. Al-Zghloul, C. Groden, and A. Förster, "Combination of standard axial and thin-section coronal diffusion-weighted imaging facilitates the diagnosis of brainstem infarction," *Brain and Behavior*, vol. 7, no. 4, Article ID e00666, 2017.
[14] C. Marcel, S. Kremer, J. Jeantroux, F. Blanc, J.-L. Dietemann, and J. Sèze, "Diffusion-weighted imaging in noncompressive myelopathies: a 33-patient prospective study," *Journal of Neurology*, vol. 257, no. 9, pp. 1438–1445, 2010.

5

A Reversible Cytotoxic Lesion of the Corpus Callosum Developing after a Rapid Alteration in Cerebrospinal Fluid Pressure/Volume in a Patient with New Daily Persistent Headache

Todd D. Rozen and Hector A. Robles

Department of Neurology and Neuroradiology, Mayo Clinic Florida, Jacksonville, USA

Correspondence should be addressed to Todd D. Rozen; rozen.todd@mayo.edu

Academic Editor: Jacqueline A. Pettersen

A case is presented of a woman with a history of daily persistent head pressure and dizziness who developed a cytotoxic lesion of the splenium of the corpus callosum after an acute withdrawal of chronic acetazolamide treatment and then, in quick succession, a CSF pressure/volume drop with a lumbar puncture. This is the first documentation that rapid alterations of CSF pressure/volume may trigger cytotoxic lesions in the central nervous system.

1. Introduction

Cytotoxic lesions of the corpus callosum have been associated with multiple conditions. In many cases, these lesions are reversible. The exact etiology for these lesions is unknown but may involve cytokine activation. A case is presented of a woman with a history of daily persistent head pressure and dizziness who developed a cytotoxic lesion of the splenium of the corpus callosum after an acute withdrawal of chronic acetazolamide treatment and then, in quick succession, a cerebrospinal fluid (CSF) pressure/volume drop with a lumbar puncture. This is the first documentation that rapid alterations of CSF pressure/volume may trigger the development of cytotoxic lesions in the central nervous system.

2. Case Presentation

A 48-year-old woman presented with a two-year history of persistent head pressure and dizziness. She awoke one day with the symptoms. She had no prior headache history. She described her symptoms as holocranial pressure with some pain along with persistent lightheadedness. She would also experience true episodes of intermittent vertigo. She did not recognize a triggering event for her headaches. She did have some migraine-associated symptoms with exacerbations of head pressure including nausea, photophobia, and phonophobia. She had consulted with multiple physicians without a true diagnosis or effective treatment. There was some consideration for vestibular migraine, but migraine preventives (topiramate, valproic acid, and nortriptyline) were ineffective. Prior imaging demonstrated a partial empty sella, with no Chiari malformation or tonsillar ectopia. She had no vessel imaging studies. Past medical history was significant for noninsulin-dependent type II diabetes mellitus and hyperlipidemia. Her BMI was slightly elevated at 28. Neurologic examination was nonfocal including no disc edema on fundus evaluation. Her head pressure, however, worsened in the Trendelenburg position (10 degree head-down tilt). MR angiography and venography were completed and were normal. Formal neuro-ophthalmologic evaluation was normal with no evidence of disc edema. She was started on acetazolamide and did extremely well with almost complete alleviation of all of her symptoms at a dose of 1,125 mg per day of the short-acting formulation. She was given a diagnosis of new daily persistent headache (NDPH) based on the International Classification of Headache Disorders criteria as her headache/pressure symptoms began one day out of the blue and lasted for longer than 3 months [1]. The underlying etiology was hypothesized to be an abnormal reset of CSF pressure/volume to an elevated state because of her worsening in the Trendelenburg position (which rapidly increases intracranial CSF pressure within seconds of head-down tilt) and her response to CSF pressure/volume-lowering medications. This subtype of NDPH has been previously described by one of the authors (TDR) [2, 3]. After trying to switch her to the extended release formulation of acetazolamide, she lost control of her headaches/head pressure. A lumbar puncture (LP) was carried out on a semiemergent basis, and thus, she was still on a tapering dose of short-acting acetazolamide (750 mg) at the time of the procedure. The LP was completed to help establish if CSF pressure/volume was indeed the cause of her head pressure syndrome and to hopefully alleviate her symptom exacerbation. Opening pressure in the prone position was 23 cm of H_2O, and closing pressure was 15 cm H_2O after 15 mL of CSF was removed. CSF analysis was negative. The patient felt immediately better after the LP, but a day after, she developed an orthostatic headache which did not respond to conservative measures including tapering off the acetazolamide. An epidural blood patch alleviated the post-LP headache, but this seemed to reset her CSF pressure high again as she was back to daily head pressure/pain and dizziness. Her opening pressure fell within the new guidelines of normal, but she was on acetazolamide at the time of the LP, and she improved with CSF removal [4]. Eventually, she stabilized again on chronic acetazolamide therapy (1,125 mg per day) and did well for one year. She then had a second exacerbation of head pressure that was unresponsive to an increased dosing of her medication. Therapeutic LP was arranged. One day prior to her LP, she acutely stopped acetazolamide on her own volition. Opening pressure was 22 cm H_2O, and closing pressure was 13 cm H_2O after 15 cc of CSF was removed. The patient felt remarkably better after the procedure. Her only neurologic symptom was a two-hour episode of facial numbness and contralateral hemibody numbness which occurred two days after the LP. She did not develop a post-LP headache. Her CSF analysis demonstrated no evidence of inflammation with only one nucleated cell and a normal total protein and glucose level. Her Gram stain and bacterial and fungal cultures were also negative. A brain MRI was completed 16 days after the LP to look for any secondary causes for her worsening head pressure, and this demonstrated a cytotoxic edematous lesion in the splenium of the corpus callosum (Figures 1(a)–1(c)). Laboratory studies (CBC and basic metabolic panel) were normal at the time of neuroimaging. Serum cytokine levels were not obtained. No additional neurologic testing (such as an EEG) was deemed necessary as the patient was having no neurologic symptoms at the time of the MRI, and her neurologic examination was normal. She clinically was still much improved in regard to her head pressure. Repeat imaging 2 weeks later noted near-to-complete resolution of the lesion (Figures 1(d) and 1(e)). In retrospect, it would have been helpful to obtain serum cytokine levels at the time of the abnormal MRI imaging to see if they were elevated. However, measuring cytokine levels in the CSF would have been even more sensitive to look for alterations within the central nervous system.

The patient provided written consent for the use of her images.

3. Discussion

The cytotoxic, typically reversible, lesions of the corpus callosum have an unknown etiology. One of the current theories is that a release of cytokines including tumor necrosis factor-alpha (TNF-α), interleukin-1 (IL-1), and interleukin-6 (IL-6) leads to a cascade of events which include microglial activation, increased glutamate synthesis with a rise in extracellular glutamine levels, mitochondrial dysfunction, and finally an influx of water into both glia and neurons causing cytotoxic edema [5, 6]. The splenium may be more susceptible to this process than the rest of the corpus callosum as it has a dual circulation and a higher abundance of cytokine and glutamate receptors [5]. Various triggers for the cytotoxic lesions including medications (typically antiepileptics: carbamazepine, lamotrigine, and phenytoin), infections (viruses: Epstein–Barr and adenovirus), CNS malignancies, subarachnoid hemorrhage, acute altitude sickness, metabolic disorders (acute renal failure, hypernatremia, hypoglycemia, and hepatic encephalopathy), and even several cases of migraine with aura have been reported [6, 7]. As our patient had none of these recognized factors, it can be theorized that a rapid alteration in CSF pressure/volume, first from acute withdrawal of chronic acetazolamide treatment with a presumed rise in CSF pressure/volume and then in quick succession a rapid CSF pressure/volume depletion with the LP, triggered cytokine release leading to various osmotic shifts resulting in the cytotoxic lesion.

Studies in the medical literature may help establish an association between rapid CSF pressure/volume alterations, cytokine activation, and cytotoxic lesions of the corpus callosum in patients with daily persistent headache from elevated CSF pressure. There are reports that patients with increased CSF pressure (idiopathic intracranial hypertension) have elevated levels of cytokines in their CSF including TNF-alpha and IL-6, but other studies have refuted this [8]. In addition, patients with NDPH have been shown to have elevated CSF TNF-alpha levels; thus, this could suggest that individuals with this unique headache syndrome are more susceptible to developing cytotoxic lesions of the corpus callosum from rapid alterations in CSF pressure/volume because they have cytokine activation at baseline [9]. Finally, after surgery to repair spinal fluid leaks, the levels of TNF-alpha, IL-6, and IL-10 dramatically increase in the CSF [10]. The cytokine release is suggested to be primarily secondary to the surgery itself, but a shift in

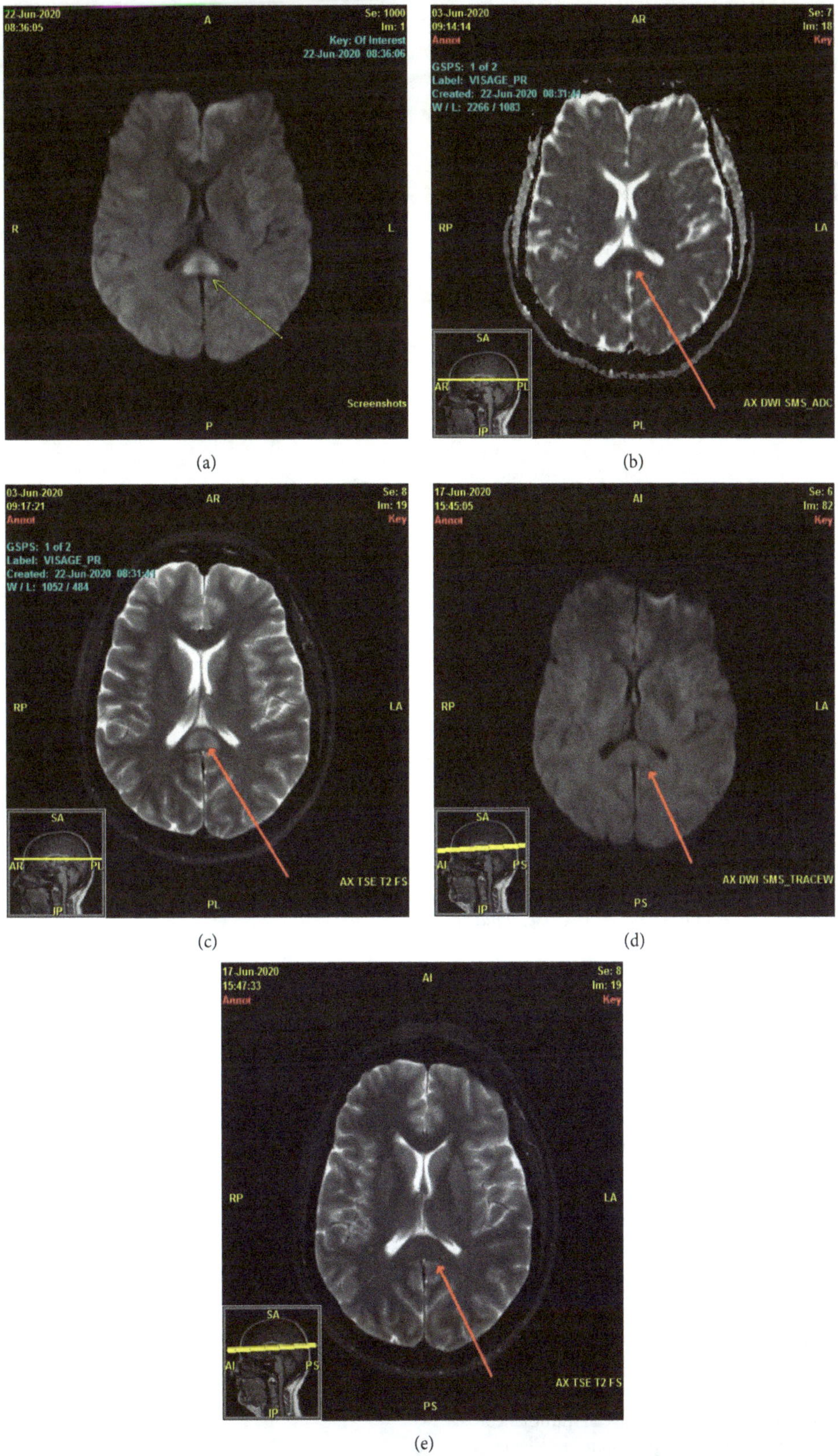

Figure 1: (a–c) MRI brain completed 16 days after lumbar puncture demonstrating an oval-shaped focus of abnormal unenhancing T2/FLAIR hyperintensity with restricted diffusion of the splenium of the corpus callosum (arrow). (a) Axial diffusion. (b) ADC mapping confirms true restricted diffusion. (c) Axial T2. (d, e) MRI brain completed 14 days after initial MRI with near-to-complete resolution of the corpus callosum lesion (arrow). (d) Axial diffusion. (e) Axial T2.

CSF pressure/volume may also be involved in the cytokine activation.

4. Conclusion

From the case presentation, it is suggested that CSF pressure/volume-modulating medications should be tapered slowly if there is chronic usage and to avoid a rapid reduction in CSF volume with lumbar puncture in the setting of acute withdrawal of these medications, as this may cause a cytotoxic insult to the corpus callosum. Our patient had minimal neurologic manifestations, but these lesions have been associated with a mild-to-severe encephalopathy, paresis/paresthesias, and severe headaches [6].

Consent

The patient provided written informed consent for the use of her images.

References

[1] Headache Classification Committee of the International Headache Society (IHS), "The international classification of headache disorders," *Cephalalgia*, vol. 38, pp. 1–211, 2018.

[2] T. D. Rozen, "A new subtype of chronic daily headache presenting in older women," *Journal of Women's Health*, vol. 27, no. 2, pp. 203–208, 2018.

[3] T. D. Rozen, "New daily persistent headache (NDPH) triggered by a single Valsalva event: a case series," *Cephalalgia*, vol. 39, pp. 785–791, 2019.

[4] D. I. Friedman, G. T. Liu, and K. B. Digre, "Revised diagnostic criteria for the pseudotumor cerebri syndrome in adults and children," *Neurology*, vol. 81, pp. 1159–1165, 2013.

[5] S. Tetsuka, "Reversible lesion in the splenium of the corpus callosum," *Brain Behaviour*, vol. 9, no. 11, Article ID e01440, 2019.

[6] J. Starkey, N. Kobayashi, Y. Numaguchi, and T. Moritani, "Cytotoxic lesions of the corpus callosum that show restricted diffusion: mechanisms, causes, and manifestations," *Radiographics*, vol. 37, pp. 562–576, 2017.

[7] F. Y. Lin and C. Y. Yang, "Reversible splenial lesion of the corpus callosum in migraine with aura," *Neurologist*, vol. 17, pp. 157–159, 2011.

[8] S. Dhungana, B. Sharrack, and N. Woodroofe, "IL-1β, TNF and IP-10 in the cerebrospinal fluid and serum are not altered in patients with idiopathic intracranial hypertension compared to controls," *Clinical Endocrinology (Oxf)*.vol. 71, pp. 896-897, 2009.

[9] T. Rozen and S. Z. Swidan, "Elevation of CSF tumor necrosis factor alpha levels in new daily persistent headache and treatment refractory chronic migraine," *Headache*, vol. 47, pp. 1050–1055, 2007.

[10] J. X. Tang, D. Baranov, M. Hammond, L. M. Shaw, M. F. Eckenhoff, and R. G. Eckenhoff, "Human alzheimer and inflammation biomarkers after anesthesia and surgery," *Anesthesiology*, vol. 115, pp. 727–732, 2011.

6

Cognitive Sequelae of Central-Variant Posterior Reversible Encephalopathy Syndrome (PRES)

Joseph Seemiller[1,2] and Muhammad Taimur Malik[1,2]

[1]Geisinger Neuroscience Institute, Danville, PA, USA
[2]Geisinger Commonwealth School of Medicine, Scranton, PA, USA

Correspondence should be addressed to Joseph Seemiller; me@josephseemiller.com

Academic Editor: Chao Jiang

Introduction. Although the posterior reversible encephalopathy syndrome (PRES) is often associated with headache and visual changes, central-variant PRES can be difficult to clinically diagnose in a patient with alteration of consciousness. Central-variant PRES has been previously described in the literature affecting subcortical white matter and the brainstem. *Case Presentation.* We describe a case presenting with hypertension (192/98) and altered level of consciousness requiring intubation. She was ultimately found to have extensive symmetric cortical and subcortical edema, with extensive involvement of bilateral thalami, consistent with central-variant PRES. Her mentation rapidly improved with blood pressure management. Confirmation of the diagnosis of central-variant PRES was made on repeat brain imaging. Our case is unique in demonstrating dramatic central white matter changes and their reversibility on repeat imaging six days later. Finally, persistent cognitive deficits at follow-up four months later are described. *Conclusion.* Atypical presentations of PRES, involving alterations in levels of consciousness, can be difficult to clinically diagnose. A thorough differential diagnosis is even more important in cases of PRES with atypical imaging. Recognition of the diagnostic patterns of PRES on brain imaging, with prompt reversal of the causative factors, is crucial for the appropriate care of these patients. The long-term sequelae, which could include cognitive deficits, are poorly studied and understood.

1. Introduction

Posterior reversible encephalopathy syndrome (PRES) refers to a reversible neurologic syndrome with symptoms including headache, changes in mental status, visual changes, and seizures. There are numerous causes of PRES including hypertension, immunosuppressive and antineoplastic medications, renal failure, autoimmune disorders, and many other causes [1–3]. Imaging shows subcortical and cortical white matter edema which is classically parieto-occipital predominant [4], however, less commonly can involve the brainstem, basal ganglia, and cerebellum [5].

We describe a case of central-variant PRES who presented atypically with alteration in level of consciousness. She had changes on magnetic resonance imaging (MRI) brain involving regions associated with atypical PRES, including changes in the subcortical white matter in the cerebellum and cerebrum, basal ganglia, and extensive involvement of bilateral thalami. The diagnosis was confirmed with an extensive workup including lumbar puncture, ultimately with confirmation of central-variant PRES diagnosis through repeat MRI brain. This case demonstrates the importance of prompt recognition of atypical or central-variant PRES and the differential diagnosis of atypical PRES, and further, provides impressive imaging findings consistent with central-variant PRES. Finally, the long-term cognitive deficits experienced by this patient demonstrate, with a discussion of literature, that the chronic sequelae of PRES are poorly understood and can include cognitive changes.

2. Case Report

A 59-year-old woman presented to a community hospital with two days of headache and vomiting followed by acute development of somnolence. On hospital presentation, late on day two after symptom onset, her initial blood pressure was 192/98 and temperature 38.0°C. Levetiracetam 500 mg twice daily was started despite no reported history of convulsions. She was then transferred to a tertiary care hospital in central Pennsylvania. Physical exam was remarkable for lower extremity hyper-reflexia and Babinski sign bilaterally and was otherwise nonfocal.

Empiric treatment for meningitis was initiated with ceftriaxone, vancomycin, acyclovir, and ampicillin. Antibiotics were stopped after lumbar puncture revealed 3 WBC/mm^3, 69 mg/dL protein, and 83 mg/dL glucose on day three after symptom onset.

On day four after symptom onset, MRI brain was obtained, showing bilateral subcortical FLAIR hyperintensities without diffusion restriction, consistent with vasogenic edema (Figure 1). Aggressive blood pressure control was initiated with a goal <140/90.

Low sensitivity C-reactive protein (CRP) was elevated at 22 mg/L and albumin was normal at 4.8 g/dL. Vitamin B12 was <150pg/mL, methylmalonic acid was elevated at 323 nmol/L, and homocysteine was elevated at 17.7 umol/L. Vitamin B12 supplementation was started with 1 mg intramuscular daily for seven days, followed by oral daily dosing of 1 mg on an ongoing basis. Thiamine was empirically supplemented with 500 mg intravenous daily for three days, after which 100 mg oral daily dosing was continued. However, whole-blood thiamine taken on admission was ultimately found to be normal at 105 nmol/L. Urine toxicology testing was significant for marijuana. Infectious studies including HIV antibody and antigen, lyme antibody, West Nile panel, arbovirus panel, anaplasma polymerase chain reaction (PCR), Babesia PCR and enterovirus PCR, and peripheral blood smear were negative. Additional studies including antinuclear antibody, antineutrophil cytoplasmic antibody, folate, copper, and peripheral blood smear were negative.

Ten days after symptom onset, repeat MRI brain showed significant improvement of white matter hyperintensities, and MRI cervical spine noted no myelopathy. Central-variant PRES was diagnosed based on rapid reversibility of white matter lesions with blood pressure control and lack of myelopathy to suggest symptomatic depletion of vitamin B12.

At follow-up four months after the initial hospitalization, the patient reported persistent cognitive impairments since her hospitalization, involving short-term memory and attention deficits. A Montreal Cognitive Assessment (MoCA) was 21/30 with errors including 1/30 for cube drawing (visuospatial), 1/30 for reading digits and 1/30 for tapping on a specified letter (attention), 2/30 for repetition and 1/30 for fluency (language), 2/30 for delayed recall, and 1/30 for orientation. She declined formal neuropsychological assessment.

3. Discussion

This patient's presentation, with an acute to subacute onset of headache, fever, and vomiting, with progression to somnolence, prompted an initially broad differential diagnosis. MRI brain was instrumental for the identification of central-variant PRES. The imaging features leading to this diagnosis included symmetric subcortical hyperintensity on fluid attenuated inversion recovery (FLAIR) sequences, without diffusion restriction or contrast enhancement.

3.1. Differential Diagnosis. A thorough differential diagnosis is important in evaluation for PRES, especially for PRES with atypical imaging characteristics, as the reversibility of the clinical and radiographic features of PRES requires time to confirm and might not even be entirely reversible. MRI brain imaging is vital for early workup of suspected PRES.

Vascular diagnostic considerations could include reversible cerebral vasoconstriction syndrome, cerebral venous sinus thrombosis, and central nervous system vasculitis, for which additional vascular imaging could be obtained if suspected. Infectious considerations should include encephalitis and meningitis. Autoimmune mimics could include ADEM, lupus cerebritis, or autoimmune encephalitis. Suspected infectious or autoimmune etiology should prompt CSF workup, and pleocytosis would support an underlying infection or inflammatory etiology. Toxic leukoencephalopathy, such as that caused by inhaled heroin, should be considered through correlate social history and urine drug toxicology testing. Acute hepatic encephalopathy could be considered with hepatic function serology. Neoplastic causes such as lymphoma and gliomatosis cerebri could be suggested with reported B-symptoms, weight loss, and presence of enhancement on MRI. Specific considerations for central PRES include osmotic demyelination syndrome, acute hepatic encephalopathy, and hypoxic ischemic injury.

Diagnosis of PRES is limited by the lack of specific diagnostic criteria, even though several criteria have been proposed based on retrospective cohort studies, and approaches have been proposed for evaluation of suspected PRES. Typical PRES can be evaluated through an algorithm in >90% of patients presenting with parieto-occipital or a posterior frontal cortical-subcortical pattern of vasogenic edema on FLAIR MRI sequences [6]. However, atypical PRES is not accounted for in this algorithm. A more recently proposed algorithm lists several differential diagnostic considerations for PRES, which should be carefully reviewed for all cases of atypical PRES imaging, or typical PRES imaging with poor reversibility of clinical or radiographic abnormalities [7].

In this patient, the possibility of myelopathy was considered given the patient's hyper-reflexia and vitamin B12 deficiency. However, cervical spine MRI was unremarkable, and ultimately, the patient's vitamin B12 deficiency was thought noncontributory to her presentation. Viral meningitis and tic-borne illness were also considered; however, lumbar puncture without pleocytosis made these possibilities unlikely. Ultimately, the patient rapidly improved clinically through her hospital course which, in conjunction with her repeat MRI showing resolved FLAIR hyperintensity, confirmed the diagnosis of central-variant PRES.

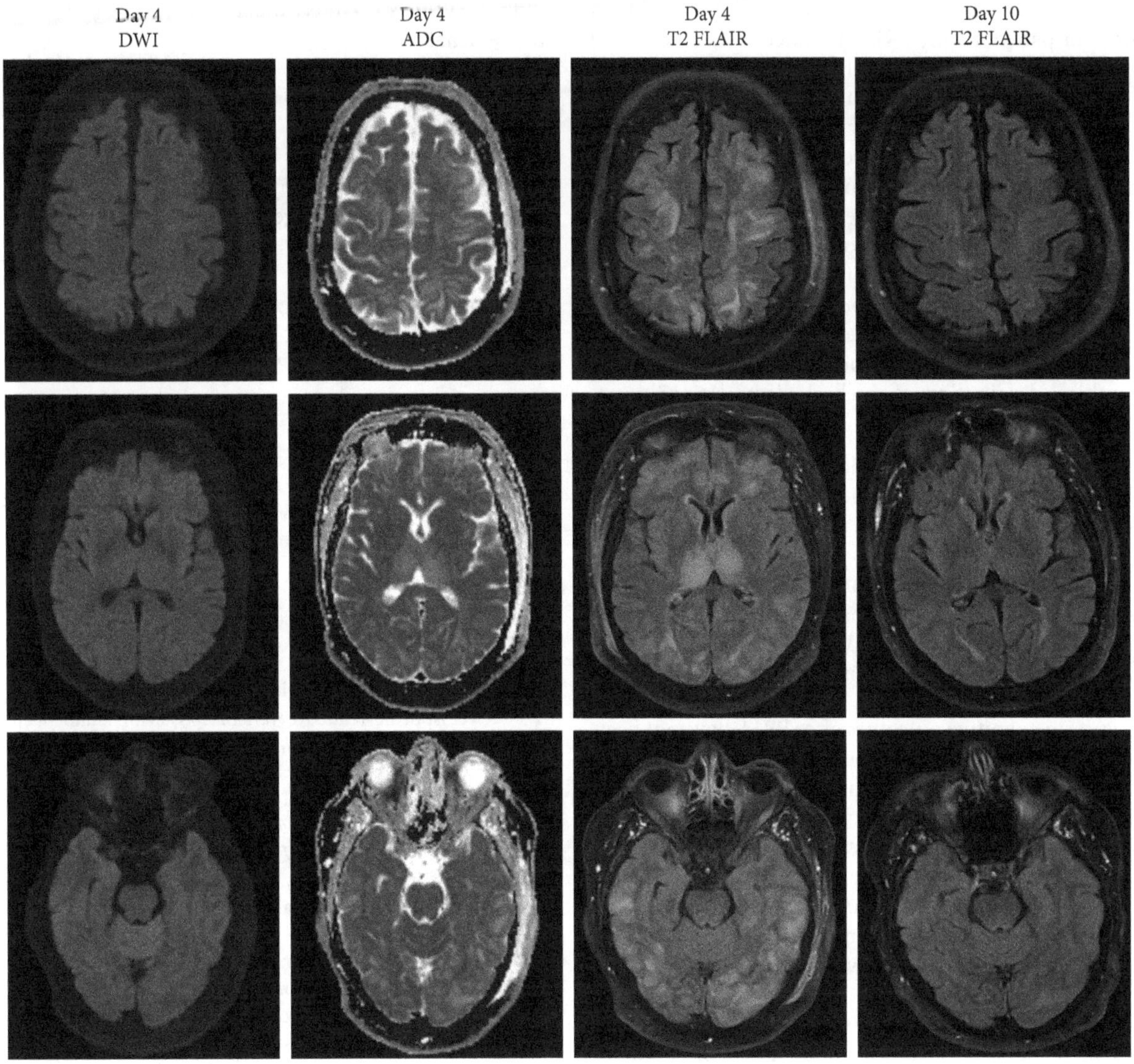

FIGURE 1: Sequences of MRI brain including DWI, ADC, initial FLAIR, and FLAIR on follow-up imaging, from left to right. Initial MRI (first three columns on the left) noted symmetric subcortical and cortical FLAIR hyperintensity involving the bilateral cerebral hemispheres including extensive involvement of the thalami and basal ganglia, without contrast enhancement. DWI was isointense, lacking diffusion restriction, and ADC was hyperintense, consistent with vasogenic edema. FLAIR sequence on repeat MRI (fourth column from the left) noted significant interval improvement, with mild residual hyperintensity in the parieto-occipital white matter.

3.2. Etiology of PRES. Originally, PRES was described by Hinchey in 1996 [3]. Typical imaging findings have been identified as symmetric hemispheric vasogenic edema in the white matter extending to the cortex, best seen on FLAIR with the absence of diffusion restriction [4].

Hypertension is one of the most common identified causes of PRES. There are multiple proposed theories explaining how hypertension enacts these effects. Traditionally, the vasogenic theory has maintained that severe hypertension exceeds the autoregulatory limits of the brain, resulting in extravasation of the fluid and edema [8–10]. However, this does not account for the findings of PRES in patients with normotension.

An alternative explanation for PRES pathogenesis is that cytotoxic insults from chemokines or exogenous toxins, or inflammatory insults from t-cell activation and cytokine release, can cause vasoconstriction. Vasoconstriction could also reduce perfusion, leading to ischemia and vasogenic edema. Supporting this theory are the findings of vasoconstriction and vasculopathy on angiography studies [11] as well as hypoperfusion [12] seen in PRES patients.

3.3. Imaging. The pattern of edema in PRES is known to occur in a posterior-to-anterior fashion, with involvement of the parieto-occipital region most commonly. However, central-variant PRES can involve the basal ganglia or brainstem and even spare the parieto-occipital region [5]. Our report demonstrates remarkable symmetric FLAIR hyperintensity involving cortical and subcortical regions, including the cerebellum and basal ganglia, notably with extensive involvement of bilateral thalami.

3.4. Serology. Serological markers have been associated with outcomes in patients with PRES. Elevated CRP levels have been associated with increased in-hospital mortality [13] The CRP level in this patient was elevated at 22, and although she survived the hospitalization, her morbidity could be reflected in her elevated CRP level; elevated CRP could reflect inflammation-related instability of the blood-brain barrier and associated endothelial damage [14]. Low serum albumin levels have been observed in 70% of patients with PRES [15]; however, albumin was normal in this patient. CSF albuminocytologic dissociation, without pleocytosis, was seen in this patient, which is a finding seen in 70% of patients with PRES. CSF protein is directly associated with the extent and topographical distribution of cerebral edema [16, 17].

3.5. Prognosis. Neurologic sequelae can persist in patients with PRES. In a study of 31 patients with PRES receiving chemotherapy, 84% of subjects returned to baseline, requiring a range of one to 167 days after symptom onset [18]. Another study with 111 cases reported 17 cases with ongoing neurologic sequelae [19]. There have also been suggestions that MRI severity could correlate with clinical outcome, but this relationship requires further study [6, 15, 20].

Long-term cognitive outcomes after PRES have not been well characterized in literature. One case series documented the long-term cognitive outcomes in two patients with typical PRES. Neuropsychological testing revealed predominantly spatial perception tasks, as well as milder impairments in attention and memory [21]. The deficits, primarily visuospatial, were thought consistent with posterior cortical involvement, seen in typical patterns of PRES. Similarly, in follow-up interviews of 210 women with a history of eclampsia, 22% reported decreased concentration or difficulty with recall [22]. However, neuropsychological assessment was unable to discern an attention or executive function impairment in patients with a history of eclampsia [23].

The cognitive deficits in this patient were limited by incomplete neuropsychological assessment; however, deficits were broad across domains tested in the MoCA. In the cases presented by [21], the visuospatial predominant deficits were thought related to the specific posterior cortical areas affected by PRES. In contrast, the extensive cortical involvement in our patient does not clearly localize. However, this case further supports existing evidence that the long-term sequelae of PRES are poorly understood. Long-term follow-up screening and neuropsychological testing in more patients with both typical and atypical PRES syndromes are needed to understand if its cognitive sequelae are less "reversible" than its imaging findings.

Consent

Written informed consent to publish the clinical details and photographs of this case was given by the patient. The copy of the written consent is available for review by the editor of this journal.

Disclosure

This study was prepared by J. S. and M. M. as part of their employment with Geisinger Medical Center.

Authors' Contributions

J. S. and M. M. both wrote and edited the manuscript.

Acknowledgments

The publication fee was paid by the office of Graduate Medical Education.

References

[1] J. M. Jarosz, D. C. Howlett, T. C. S. Cox, and J. B. Bingham, "Cyclosporine-related reversible posterior leukoencephalopathy: MRI," *Neuroradiology*, vol. 39, no. 10, pp. 711–715, 1997.

[2] R. B. Schwartz, S. K. Feske, J. F. Polak et al., "Preeclampsia-eclampsia: clinical and neuroradiographic correlates and insights into the pathogenesis of hypertensive encephalopathy," *Radiology*, vol. 217, no. 2, pp. 371–376, 2000.

[3] J. Hinchey, C. Chaves, B. Appignani et al., "A reversible posterior leukoencephalopathy syndrome," *New England Journal of Medicine*, vol. 334, no. 8, pp. 494–500, 1996.

[4] S. O. Casey, R. C. Sampaio, E. Michel, and C. L. Truwit, "Posterior reversible encephalopathy syndrome: utility of fluid-attenuated inversion recovery MR imaging in the detection of cortical and subcortical lesions," *AJNR. American Journal of Neuroradiology*, vol. 21, no. 7, pp. 1199–1206, 2000.

[5] A. M. McKinney, J. Short, C. L. Truwit et al., "Posterier reversible encephalopathy syndrome: incidence of atypical regions of involvement and imaging findings," *American Journal of Roentgenology*, vol. 189, no. 4, pp. 904–912, 2007.

[6] B. Kozak, C. Lyu, A. Lerner, and A. M. McKinney, "Controversy of posterior reversible encephalopathy syndrome: what have we learnt in the last 20 Years?" *Journal of Neurology, Neurosurgery & Psychiatry*, vol. 89, no. 1, pp. 14–20, 2018.

[7] S. Tetsuka and T. Ogawa, "Posterior reversible encephalopathy syndrome: a review with emphasis on neuroimaging characteristics," *Journal of the Neurological Sciences*, vol. 404, pp. 72–79, 2019.

[8] W. S. Bartynski, "Posterior reversible encephalopathy syndrome, Part 2: controversies surrounding pathophysiology of vasogenic edema," *American Journal of Neuroradiology*, vol. 29, no. 6, pp. 1043–1049, 2008.

[9] E. Ozkan, R. Gocmen, M. A. Topcuoglu, and E. M. Arsava, "Blood-retina-barrier disruption accompanying blood-brain-barrier dysfunction in posterior reversible encephalopathy syndrome," *Journal of the Neurological Sciences*, vol. 346, no. 1-2, pp. 315–317, 2014.

[10] G. Arsava, A. Greco, G. Iannella et al., "Posterior reversible encephalopathy syndrome-Insight into pathogenesis, clinical

variants and treatment approaches," *Autoimmunity Reviews*, vol. 14, no. 9, pp. 830–836, 2015.

[11] L. M. Brubaker, J. Smith, Y. Z. Lee, W. Lin, and M. Castillo, "Hemodynamic and permeability changes in posterior reversible encephalopathy syndrome measured by dynamic susceptibility perfusion-weighted MR imaging," *AJNR. American Journal of Neuroradiology*, vol. 26, no. 4, pp. 825–830, 2005.

[12] S. T. Engelter, J. R. Petrella, M. J. Alberts, and J. M. Provenzale, "Assessment of cerebral microcirculation in a patient with hypertensive encephalopathy using MR perfusion imaging," *American Journal of Roentgenology*, vol. 173, no. 6, pp. 1491–1493, 1999.

[13] E. Siebert, G. Bohner, T. Liebig, M. Endres, and T. G. Liman, "Factors associated with fatal outcome in posterior reversible encephalopathy syndrome: a retrospective analysis of the berlin PRES study," *Journal of Neurology*, vol. 264, no. 2, pp. 237–242, 2017.

[14] C. R. W. Kuhlmann, L. Librizzi, D. Closhen et al., "Mechanisms of C-reactive protein-induced blood-brain barrier disruption," *Stroke*, vol. 40, no. 4, pp. 1458–1466, 2009.

[15] B. Gao, B. X. Yu, R. S. Li et al., "Cytotoxic edema in posterior reversible encephalopathy syndrome: correlation of MRI features with serum albumin levels," *American Journal of Neuroradiology*, vol. 36, no. 10, pp. 1884–1889, 2015.

[16] S. Datar, T. D. Singh, J. E. Fugate, J. Mandrekar, A. A. Rabinstein, and S. Hocker, "Albuminocytologic dissociation in posterior reversible encephalopathy syndrome," *Mayo Clinic Proceedings*, vol. 90, no. 10, pp. 1366–1371, 2015.

[17] C. A. Ellis, A. C. McClelland, S. Mohan et al., "Cerebrospinal fluid in posterior reversible encephalopathy syndrome: implications of elevated protein and pleocytosis," *The Neurohospitalist*, vol. 9, no. 2, pp. 58–64, 2019.

[18] S. Singer, C. Grommes, A. S. Reiner, M. K. Rosenblum, and L. M. DeAngelis, "Posterior reversible encephalopathy syndrome in patients with cancer," *The Oncologist*, vol. 20, no. 7, pp. 806–811, 2015.

[19] N. Tambasco, E. Mastrodicasa, C. Salvatori et al., "Prognostic factors in children with PRES and hematologic diseases," *Acta Neurologica Scandinavica*, vol. 134, no. 6, pp. 474–483, 2016.

[20] A. M. McKinney, S. A. Kieffer, R. T. Paylor, K. S. SantaCruz, A. Kendi, and L. Lucato, "Acute toxic leukoencephalopathy: potential for reversibility clinically and on MRI with diffusion-weighted and FLAIR imaging," *American Journal of Roentgenology*, vol. 193, no. 1, pp. 192–206, 2009.

[21] I. Stroescu, C. M. Salinas, F. B. Nahab, and A. Y. Stringer, "Long-term neurocognitive and neuroimaging outcomes in posterior reversible encephalopathy syndrome: two case reports and implications," *The Clinical Neuropsychologist*, vol. 25, no. 8, pp. 1386–1402, 2011.

[22] A. B. Andersgaard, A. Herbst, M. Johansen, A. Borgström, A. G. Bille, and P. A. L. Øian, "Follow-up interviews after eclampsia," *Gynecologic and Obstetric Investigation*, vol. 67, no. 1, pp. 49–52, 2009.

[23] I. Postma, I. Wessel, J. Aarnoudse, and G. Zeeman, "Neurocognitive functioning in women with a history of eclampsia: executive functioning and sustained attention," *American Journal of Perinatology*, vol. 27, no. 9, pp. 685–690, 2010.

7

Carotid Dissection and Isolated Paralysis of Ipsilateral Half Tongue: Clinical Cases

Komi Igneza Agbotsou,[1,2] Damelan Kombate,[2] Christopher Mehri,[1] Kossivi Apetse,[2] Kpalma Duga Bakpatina-Batako,[2] Olivier Guerrier,[1] Albert Beschet,[1] Karine Blanc Lasserre,[1] Ludovic Breynaert,[1] and Victor Chan[1]

[1]*Neurology Department of Valence Hospital Center, Valence, France*
[2]*Neurology Department of Campus Teaching Hospital, Lome, Togo*

Correspondence should be addressed to Komi Igneza Agbotsou; oagbotsou2@gmail.com

Academic Editor: Peter Berlit

Objective. We report two cases of carotid dissection revealed by isolated paralysis of the ipsilateral half tongue. *Observations.* First patient, 52 years old, with no particular medical or surgical history, presented with isolated paralysis of the left half tongue preceded by two weeks of moderate-intensity cervicalgia and having been the subject to cervical manipulation. MRI revealed dissection of the left internal carotid artery in its prepetrous portion. The evolution after 6 weeks of platelet aggregating inhibitors treatment was favorable. The second patient, 74 years old, with no particular medical or chirurgical history, presented with a sudden onset of paralysis of the left half tongue preceded by unusual headaches associated with neck pain. Brain MRI showed aneurysmal ectasia of the left internal carotid with parietal irregularity suggestive of carotid dissection. The evolution after four weeks of treatment with anticoagulant was favorable. *Conclusion.* Carotid dissection revealed by isolated paralysis of the half tongue is rare. It is generally of good prognosis. However, in paralysis of half tongue, it must be urgently sought and treated to reduce the risk of a transient or constituted ischemic accident.

1. Introduction

Arterial dissection is defined by the formation of a hematoma within the lining of the artery, communicating or not with arterial light through a breach in the intima, cleaving the parietal leaflets. The result is an occlusion, stenosis, or aneurysmal dilation of the vessel [1]. A dissection of the internal carotid artery causes paralysis of the large hypoglossal nerve either by a compressive mechanism via the wall hematoma on the nerve or by a mechanism of vascular interruption of the vasa nervorum feeding the nerve [2].

Internal carotid artery dissections (ICA) are the most common dissections of the cervical end-brain arteries with cerebral infarction with an estimated incidence of 3/100,000 cases per year, affecting both sexes with an average age of 45 years [3, 4].

Carotid dissection may be responsible for the damage to the lower cranial nerves including the glossopharyngeal nerve (IX), the vagus nerve (X), the spinal nerve (XI), and the large hypoglossal nerve (XII). This is a very rare situation found in 8% of cases [5]. The damage to the hypoglossal nerve is most commonly found and is observed in 5% of patients [5].

Some cases of carotid dissection revealed by isolated paralysis of the half tongue have been described in the literature. We therefore set ourselves the goal of reporting two cases of carotid dissection revealed by isolated paralysis of the ipsilateral half tongue and literature review.

2. Patients and Methods

This was a retrospective and descriptive study of two cases of carotid dissection revealed by isolated paralysis of the ipsilateral half tongue. The study involved two patients, the first aged 52 and the second aged 74, who were admitted to the neurovascular unit of the neurology department of the Valencia Hospital Center. The diagnosis of carotid dissection was evoked before clinical signs suggestive of isolated paralysis of the large hypoglossal nerve. Diagnostic confirmation was performed by magnetic resonance imaging (MRI) of the neck vessels. Sociodemographic, clinical, radiological, therapeutic, and evolutionary data were studied.

3. Cases Presentation

3.1. Observation No. 1. Mr. L.D. born on July 20, 1965, a trader, right-handed, self-employed, with no cardiovascular risk factor or a personal or family pathological history, was admitted on December 30, 2017 for difficulties in moving his tongue. On December 29, 2017, he presented suddenly difficulties in mobilizing his tongue, at lunchtime with some difficulties in carrying the food bowl and chewing associated with articulatory difficulties. These symptoms were preceded 48 hours by left, unusual, and mild hemicranial headaches, partially relieved by paracetamol associated with cervicalgia and no vomiting. There was no infectious episode or traumatic context.

Mr. L.D.'s physical examination recorded normal hemodynamic constants with temperature at 37 degrees Celsius, blood pressure at 120/70 mmHg, pulse at 70 pulses per minute, and weight at 72 kilograms for a height of 175 cm (BMI at 23.51 kg/m^2). The general condition was good. The neurological examination had found a deviation of the tongue to the left when he pulled the tongue and vice versa when he returned it, a left lingual hemiatrophy. The consciousness was normal. The physical examination did not find any change in the taste or impairment of the other cranial pairs. Mr. L.D did not have a sensory deficit, nor a motor deficit with the limbs or the face. There was no osteotendon reflex disorder or Babinski sign. Cerebellar, proprioceptive, or vestibular ataxia was not found. The neck was flexible without the sign of Kernig or Brudzinski. The standing position with joined feet was correct when opening or closing eyes. The rest of the examination including cardiovascular, pleuropulmonary, and digestive was normal. Figure 1 shows Mr. L.D exhibiting an ipsilateral left deviation of the tongue when protracting, suggestive of a left carotid dissection.

Brain MRI (broadcast sequences, FLAIR, and ADC mapping) was normal. MRI of the neck vessels confirmed an aspect of wall hematoma in the left internal carotid artery in diffusion compatible with a dissection of the left internal carotid artery as shown in Figure 2. *C*-reactive protein was at 4 mg/l. At the blood formula count, the leukocyte level was 4500 cells/ml. Creatininemia was at 9 mg/l with a clearance at 105 ml/min. Retroviral serology was negative, as hepatitis and syphilis serologies. Total cholesterol was at 1.50 g/l, triglycerides at 1.10 g/l, HDL cholesterol at 0.50 g/l, and LDL cholesterol at 0.68 g/l. The autoimmune assessment was negative.

M. L.D. received treatment with a platelet aggregating inhibitor (acetyl salicylic acid 160 mg per day at meals) according to the cervical artery dissection in stroke study (CADISS), a level 1 analgesic treatment (paracetamol compressed one gram every 6 hours for headaches and cervicalgia) and speech therapy.

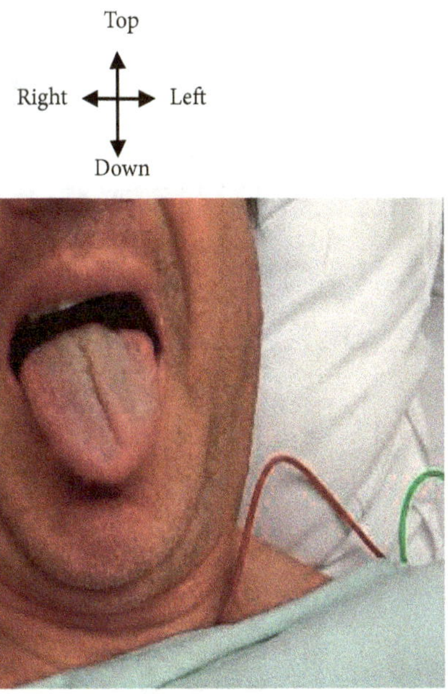

Figure 1: Left ipsilateral deviation of the tongue to protraction in Mr. L.D. in favor of a left carotid dissection.

The evolution was favorable marked by regression of headache, cervicalgia, and paralysis of the half tongue after six weeks.

3.2. Observation No. 2. Mr. C.E. born on September 28, 1942, right-handed, retired gendarme, married, autonomous, without cardiovascular risk factor, without a personal or familial pathological history, transferred by the emergency department of the Valencia Hospital to the neurology department on May 26, 2016, for the management of an isolated paralysis of the half tongue in a context of cervicalgia.

Fifteen days before his admission to the Valencia Hospital Center, he presented moderate-intensity mild neck pains that appeared without triggering factors or infectious contexts and that has increased on May 23, 2016. He then consulted his physiotherapist the next day who performed cervical manipulations on suspicion of cervical osteoarthritis. On May 25, 2016, he noticed a solid swallowing disorder. He consulted his physician who addressed him to the emergency department on May 26, 2016, where he was transferred to the neurology department.

In the neurology department, the general examination found normal hemodynamic constants with temperature at 37.1° Celsius, blood pressure at 110/60 mmHg, pulse at 75 pulses per minute, and weight at 70 kilograms for a height of 170 cm (BMI at 24.22 kg/m^2). The general condition was good. The consciousness was normal. Mr. C.E. had a mild neck pain. Examination of the cranial pairs had found paralysis of the left XII nerve with

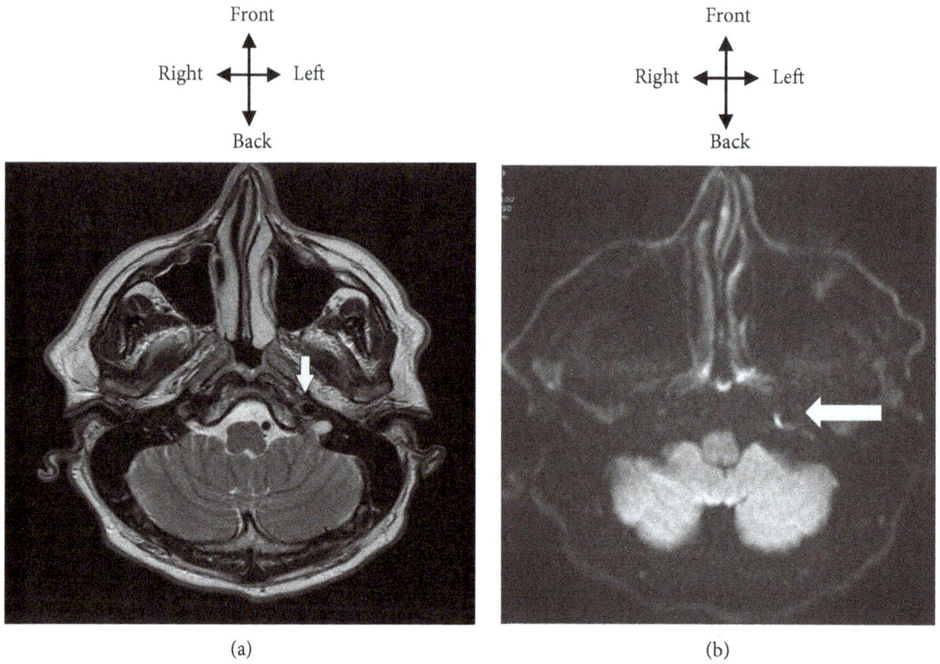

Figure 2: MRI of the neck vessels, T2 TSE axial (a) and diffusion axial (b), aneurysm ectasia of the left internal carotid with parietal irregularity.

deviation of the tongue to the left when tracting it out and vice versa when it enters it, a left lingual hemiatrophy and swallowing disorder. He had no sagging of the velum, and the nauseous reflex was present. There was no impairment of the other cranial pairs. Mr. C.E. did not have a sensitive or motor deficit at the limb and face. Osteotendon reflexes were present and normal, and the plantar skin reflex was in bilateral flexion. There was no cerebellar, proprioceptive, or vestibular ataxia. The neck was flexible without the sign of Kernig, nor the sign of Brudzinski. The rest of the examination including cardiovascular, pleuropulmonary, and digestive was normal. Figure 3 shows M.C.E. patient with a tongue ipsilateral deviation of the left suggesting a left carotid dissection. A brain MRI and neck vessels confirmed a subintimal hematoma of the left internal carotid artery in favor of a left carotid dissection as shown in Figure 4.

The *C*-reactive protein was at 4.5 mg/l. At the blood formula count, the leukocyte level was 5100 cells/ml. Creatininemia was 8.5 mg/l with clearance at 102 ml/min. Retroviral serology was negative, as hepatitis and syphilis serologies. Total cholesterol was at 1.40 g/l, triglycerides at 1.05 g/l, HDL cholesterol at 0.55 g/l, and LDL cholesterol at 0.60 g/l. The autoimmune assessment was negative.

The final diagnosis was an extracranial left carotid dissection in Mr. C.E. with no particular medical history with an isolated XII impairment. He benefited from a curative anticoagulation with unfractionate heparin, which was relayed by antivitamin K from day one according to the CADISS (cervical artery dissection in stroke study) with a target between goal of INR between 2 and 3, analgesic treatment level 1 (one gram tablet of paracetamol every 6 hours for headaches and cervicalgia).

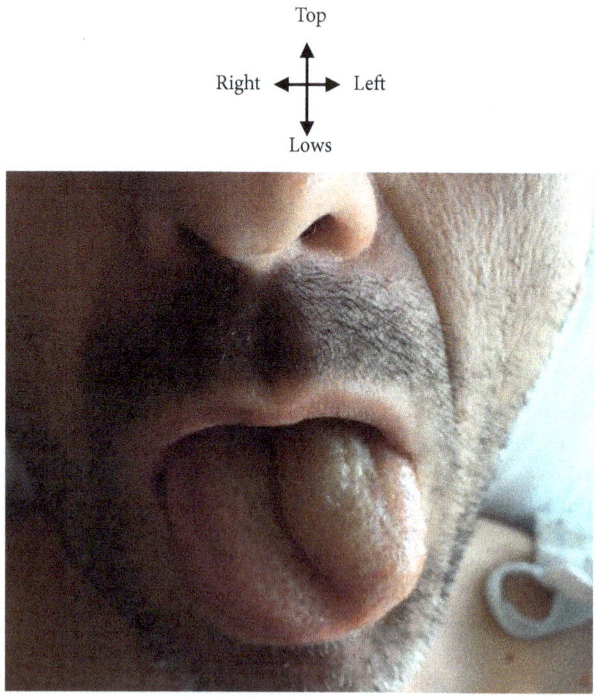

Figure 3: Left ipsilateral deviation of the tongue to protraction (arrow) in Mr. C.E. suggestive of a left carotid dissection.

The evolution in the service was favorable with a net improvement in cervicalgia after 72 hours. The failure to contract the left tongue associated with swallowing disorders had improved after four weeks without speech therapy. A mixed diet at the beginning and then gradually solid after a week of evolution had been introduced.

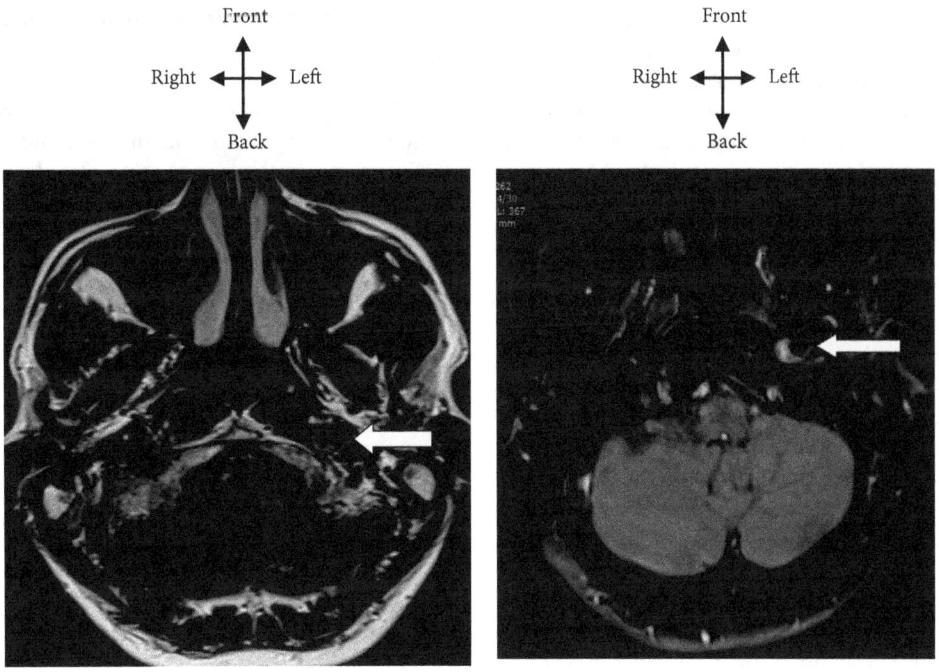

(a) (b)

FIGURE 4: MRI of the neck vessels, T2 FLAIR axial (a) and T1 FAT-SAT axial (b), hyperintense subintimal hematoma.

4. Discussion

Dissections of the cervicoencephalic arteries are responsible for about two percentages (2%) of all brain infarctions and 25% of heart attacks in people under 45 years [6–8]. The annual incidence is in the order of 3 per 100,000 [6]. This rate is underestimated because, based on stroke records, it only takes into account dissections diagnosed with cerebral ischemia and not benign forms, limited to local signs, or the severe forms that cause early death [6]. This incidence of dissections is also underestimated because a dissection may be overlooked because of its asymptomatic, paucisymptomatic (isolated local signs), or even atypical, as in our two patients with isolated paralysis of half tongue, sometimes not prompting a consultation, or a lack of means used to establish the diagnosis. Dissections of the internal carotid arteries (ICA) are the most common with an estimated incidence of 3/100,000 cases per year, affecting both sexes with an average age around 45 years [3, 4]. When the damage to the large hypoglossal nerve by carotid dissection is isolated as in our two patients, it may be unnoticed and delay the diagnosis of carotid dissection [5].

In our first patient, the neurological examination had found a deviation of the tongue to the left when he pulls the tongue and vice versa when he enters it, a left lingual hemiatrophy associated with swallowing disorders, and classic signs of paralysis of the half tongue. This had suggested an isolated paralysis of the half tongue. Our second patient also presented the same clinical picture as the first patient. Nevertheless, careful questioning remains the key to the etiological diagnosis of isolated half tongue paralysis [9]. The history of the disease is essential [9]. We should look for a triggering factor (cervical trauma and recent surgery) in the circumstances of occurence, a favorable background (cardiovascular history, arthropathy, system disease, and malignant tumor), and also associated signs [9]. This helps to guide the paraclinical assessment. However, no revealing context was found in two patients.

Paraclinical explorations of carotid dissection involve an echo-Doppler of neck vessels, a brain and angio-scanner scan of the neck vessels, and conventional arteriography with magnetic resonance imaging (MRI) and magnetic resonance angiography (MRA) of the neck vessels [10]. Arterial imaging is a primary part of investigations. Main exam is MRI, with in particular, the T1 fat suppression sequences (FAT-SAT) that allow to notice the wall hematoma, while the angiographic sequences (MRA) show stenosis, occlusion, or dissecting aneurysm and the diffusion sequence that is interesting for high dissection [10]. Sometimes, the hematoma can be visualized using other techniques such as the angioscanner or ultrasound [10, 11]. In both of our patients, MRI and cerebral and neck vessels MRA were performed to show the existence of carotid dissection and eliminated an ischemic stroke whose management differs from that of isolated paralysis of the hall tongue. Other diagnostic radiological check-ups including the echo-Doppler of the supraaortic trunks, the CT scan, and angioscanner of the supraaortic trunks were not carried out in our two patients because of the neurovascular emergency. Indeed, our two patients were admitted to the Valencia Hospital Center in a context of the neurovascular emergencies where the neurovascular emergency check-up to be performed was the brain and neck vessels MRI.

The treatment of isolated paralysis of the half tongue has two objectives: treat the mechanism of the lesion and restore nerve function [9]. The last objective is often secondary, on the one hand, because of the priority and emergency of the lesion process (dissection, metastases, and tumors of the base of the skull), and on the other hand, because of the discomfort with swallowing and phonation caused by paralysis that finally is little disabling, even in the absence of recovery [9] as in our two patients. In our two patients, the emergency lays in confirming carotid dissection and eliminating another, mostly cerebral impairment whose management differs from that of isolated paralysis of the half tongue.

The need for antithrombotic treatment to prevent a primary ischemic event or recurrence during arterial dissection is currently well established. This treatment includes anticoagulants or antiplatelets. At present, a superiority of one of the two therapies could not be demonstrated [12, 13]. A multicenter, randomized study, the cervical artery dissection in stroke study (CADISS), evaluated the efficacy of antiplatelet and anticoagulant therapies in extracranial spontaneous dissection [14]. The results of this study did not show any difference between the two treatments [14]. On the basis of this data, it is therefore lawful to use any of these agents in the presence of an extracranial dissection. Thus, our first patient benefited from platelet aggregating inhibitors treatment with acetylsalicylic acid unlike our second patient receiving low molecular weighted heparin anticoagulant treatment relayed by antivitamin K. Many centers offer routine aspirin in all cervical arterial dissections in view of the benefit and risk ratio including less side effects mainly less hemorrhagy risk, and it does not require biological follow-up unlike the antivitamin K. The duration of treatment depends primarily on the results of imaging performed during follow-up [15].

The prognosis of dissections of the internal carotid artery is generally good with a favorable evolution in more than 90% of cases [16]. Toko Djuidje et al., in France, in their observation on carotid dissection and isolated paralysis of the half tongue in a patient, noted the disappearance of symptoms including dysarthria and paresis of the tongue [2]. In both of our patients, the progression is also marked by the regression of the swallowing problem and paresis of the half tongue, four weeks after the introduction of platelet aggregating inhibitor treatment in our first patient and four weeks after the treatment of anticoagulant in our second patient.

5. Conclusion

Carotid dissection may be responsible for the damage to the lower cranial nerves. This is a very rare situation found in 8% of cases. The most commonly found damage to the hypoglossal nerve is observed in 5% of patients. When isolated, it can be unnoticed and delay the diagnosis of carotid dissection. Dissections of the cervical arteries and especially the carotid arteries are an important cause of stroke in young and middle-aged people accounting for 25% of strokes in this age group.

MRI, an main exam, must be performed as a matter of emergency in the face of diagnostic suspicion to confirm carotid dissection with a wall hematoma and its consequences on arterial flow in order to begin treatment.

The prognosis of dissections of the internal carotid artery is generally good with a favorable evolution in more than 90% of cases. In the face of any isolated paralysis of the half tongue, however, carotid dissection should be urgently sought and treated to reduce the risk of a transient or constituted ischemic accident.

Abbreviations

CADISS: Cervical artery dissection in stroke study
ICA: Internal carotid artery
INR: International normalized ratio
MRI: Magnetic resonance imaging.

Consent

Informed consent was obtained from the patient for publication of this case report and any accompanying images.

References

[1] B. Guillon and H. Desal, "Cervical arterial dissections: diagnostic and therapeutic modalities," *MT Cardio*, vol. 1, pp. 364–373, 2005.
[2] D. Toko Djuidje, F. Kenmogne Kamdem, and P. Le Coz, "Carotid dissection revealed by isolated paralysis of the large hypogloss," *Journal of Neurology*, vol. 170, pp. 73–94, 2014.
[3] S. Chabrier, P. Lasjaunias, B. Husson, P. Landrieu, and M. Tardieu, "Ischaemic stroke from dissection of the craniocervical arteriesin childhood: report of 12 patients," *European Journal of Paediatric Neurology*, vol. 7, no. 1, pp. 39–42, 2003.
[4] M. Arnold, L. Kappeler, D. Georgiadis et al., "Gender differences in spontaneous cervical artery dissection," *Neurology*, vol. 67, no. 6, pp. 1050–1052, 2006.
[5] R. Sztajzel, F. Perren, and P. Michel, "Spontaneous carotid and vertebral dissections," *Revue Médicale Suisse*, vol. 13, no. 560, pp. 900–906, 2017.
[6] C. Stapf, M. S. V. Elkind, and J. P. Mohr, "Carotid artery dissection," *Annual Review of Medicine*, vol. 51, no. 1, pp. 329–347, 2000.
[7] W. I. Schievink, "Spontaneous dissection of the carotid and vertebral arteries," *New England Journal of Medicine*, vol. 344, no. 12, pp. 899–906, 2001.
[8] K. Nedeltchev, T. Auf der Maur, D. Georgiadis et al., "Ischaemic stroke in young adults: predictors of outcome and recurrence," *Journal of Neurology, Neurosurgery & Psychiatry*, vol. 76, no. 2, pp. 191–195, 2005.
[9] V. Patron, P.-Y. Roudaut, J. Lerat, M. Vivent, J.-P. Bessède, and K. Aubry, "Paralysie isolée de l'hypoglosse par un ostéophyte cervical," *Annales Françaises d'Oto-Rhino-*

Laryngologie et de Pathologie Cervico-Faciale, vol. 129, no. 1, pp. 52–55, 2012.
[10] A. T. Vertinsky, N. E. Schwartz, N. J. Fischbein, J. Rosenberg, G. W. Albers, and G. Zaharchuk, "Comparison of multi-detector CT angiography and MR imaging of cervical artery dissection," *American Journal of Neuroradiology*, vol. 29, no. 9, pp. 1753–1760, 2008.
[11] D. H. Benninger, D. Georgiadis, J. Gandjour, and R. W. Baumgartner, "Accuracy of color duplex ultrasound diagnosis of spontaneous carotid dissection causing ischemia," *Stroke*, vol. 37, no. 2, pp. 377–381, 2006.
[12] P. Lyrer and S. Engelter, "Antithrombotic drugs for carotid artery dissection," *The Cochrane Database of Systematic Reviews*, vol. 4, p. 255, 2000.
[13] F. Kennedy, S. Lanfranconi, C. Hicks et al., "Antiplatelets vs anticoagulation for dissection: CADISS nonrandomized arm and meta-analysis," *Neurology*, vol. 79, no. 7, pp. 686–689, 2012.
[14] H. S. Markus, E. Hayter, C. Levi et al., "Antiplatelet treatment compared with anticoagulation treatment for cervical artery dissection: a randomised trial," *The Lancet Neurology*, vol. 14, pp. 361–367, 2015.
[15] S. T. Engelter, T. Brandt, S. Debette et al., "Antiplatelets versus anticoagulation in cervical artery dissection," *Stroke*, vol. 38, no. 9, pp. 2605–2611, 2007.
[16] F. Battaglia, L. Martini, C. Tannier et al., "Collet-sicard syndrome after carotid artery dissection," *Journal of Neurology*, vol. 165, no. 6-7, pp. 588–590, 2009.

8

Too Aggressive Drop in Blood Pressure in a Hypertensive Male Leading to "Man-in-the-Barrel Syndrome"

Chamara Dalugama[1] **Achila Jayasinghe,**[2] **Udaya Ralapanawa,**[1]
Shamali Abeygunawardena,[1] **and Thilak Jayalath**[1]

[1]*Department of Medicine, University of Peradeniya, Peradeniya, Sri Lanka*
[2]*Teaching Hospital, Peradeniya, Sri Lanka*

Correspondence should be addressed to Chamara Dalugama; chamaradalugama@yahoo.com

Academic Editor: Mathias Toft

Introduction. "Man-in-the-barrel syndrome" is a neurological phenotype with brachial diplegia, normal sensation, and preserved motor function of the lower limb. It has been described in various neuropathological conditions affecting the cerebral hemispheres, pons, upper spinal cord, and peripheral neurons. Severe hypotension leading to watershed infarctions leading to this phenotype has been reported. We describe the first case of "man-in-the-barrel syndrome" in a patient with a precipitous drop in blood pressure following oral antihypertensive medications. *Case Presentation.* A 75-year-old Sri Lankan male presented following a generalized tonic-clonic seizure to a tertiary care hospital. Upon recovery, he was noted to have severe brachia diplegia affecting shoulder movements with preserved hand muscle power and motor functions of the lower limb. The previous day, he was newly diagnosed with markedly elevated blood pressure without acute end organ involvement. Treatment with three antihypertensives had been initiated. Noncontrast CT of the brain revealed watershed infarctions affecting both cerebral hemispheres. *Conclusion.* It is generally unwise to lower blood pressure very rapidly, as ischemic damage can occur in vascular beds that are habituated to high levels of blood pressure in the brain. Ischemic damage caused by rapid lowering of blood pressure may rarely result in "man-in-the-barrel syndrome" leading to severe functional disability.

1. Introduction

Undiagnosed hypertension is a killer in disguise which can surface as hypertensive emergencies or urgencies and may cause hypertension-mediated end organ involvement [1–3]. Prompt but careful reduction of blood pressure is needed in a hypertensive emergency, whereas in markedly elevated blood pressure with end organ involvement, blood pressure needs to be brought down slowly over days to prevent cerebral, cardiac, or renal ischemia [4–6].

"Man-in-the-barrel syndrome" is a rare phenotype with severe brachial diplegia and intact motor functions of the lower limb, where the arms of the man appear to be confined to a "barrel" as the name implies [7, 8]. Multitudes of etiologies have been described to cause this phenotype, including severe and acute cerebral hypoperfusion leading to bilateral watershed infarctions [9].

We describe the first case where oral antihypertensive medications causing precipitous drop in blood pressure were leading to the "man-in-the-barrel" phenotype.

2. Case Presentation

We report a case of a 75-year-old Sri Lankan male who presented to a general practitioner for routine health checkup. A high blood pressure of 220/120 mmHg was found. His past medical record was unremarkable. At the time of presentation to the general practitioner, he did not have any symptoms or signs of new end organ involvement in the form of heart failure, aortic dissection, renal involvement, hypertensive encephalopathy, or retinal involvement. Treatment was initiated with losartan potassium 50 mg twice a day, hydrochlorothiazide 25 mg morning, and prazocin 1 mg three times daily at the same time by the general practitioner.

The next day morning, the patient was admitted to the Accident and Emergency department following a generalized tonic-clonic seizure. On admission, his blood pressure had been 80/50 mmHg. His blood sugar was 120 mg/dL. Urgent electrolyte profile revealed normal serum sodium, potassium, calcium, and magnesium. He was treated with intravenous fluids and the blood pressure improved.

After regaining consciousness after the seizure, the patient complained about difficulty in raising the arms above the head. Family members who witnessed the event assured that he did not have any trauma to the shoulder girdle during the seizure. His distal arm and finger movements were well preserved. He could walk without support and could get up on his own from a squatting position.

On neurological examination, we found a man who was fully conscious, rational, and oriented. His cranial nerve examination was normal with normal bilateral fundi.

Upper limb examination revealed reduced muscle power proximally with bilateral shoulder abduction 3/5, shoulder extension 4/5, and shoulder flexion 4/5. Shoulder adduction was in full strength. His power at the elbow flexion and extension was normal and distal hand motor functions were normal. Tone in the proximal muscle group was reduced. Reflexes of the upper limbs were normal with normal sensory examination. Lower limb examination was neurologically normal with bilateral flexor plantar response (Videos 1 and 2).

Noncontrast CT of the brain performed 24 hours after symptom onset revealed new bilateral hypodense areas involving parietal regions, suggestive of watershed infarctions and an occipital infarct (Figures 1 and 2) in comparison to the CT performed on admission. Shoulder joint X-rays excluded fractures or dislocations in the shoulder girdle. X-ray of the cervical spine did not show any evidence of cervical spondylosis. Electromyogram and nerve conduction studies excluded a myopathic disorder or cervical root pathology. Carotid artery duplex sonography was performed in bilateral carotid arteries and excluded carotid artery stenosis. 2D echocardiogram showed left ventricular hypertrophy without evidence of intracardiac thrombi or valvular dysfunction. Patient's resting ECG with a long rhythm strip was showing left ventricular strain without evidence of any arrhythmia and 24-hour holter monitoring did not show any clinically significant rhythm abnormality.

Biochemical blood measurements revealed hemoglobin of 14.6 g/dL with a platelet count of 340 $*$ 10^6/L. Serum creatinine was 90 mmol/L with blood urea of 6.5 mmol/L. Electrolyte profile revealed sodium of 138 mmol/L and potassium of 4.5 mmol/L. His coagulation profile was normal. EEG did not show evidence of seizure activity.

He was started on antiplatelets and statin. Physiotherapy and occupational therapy were arranged and the patient was started on phenytoin sodium for seizures. The blood pressure was monitored and controlled very cautiously with low doses of losartan potassium. He made a slow recovery with mild residual weakness in the shoulder abduction.

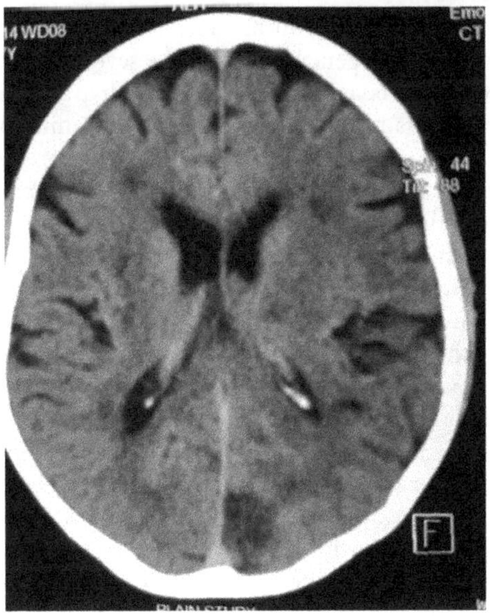

FIGURE 1: Noncontrast CT scan of the brain showing bilateral watershed infarctions in the fronto-parietal regions and a right-sided occipital infarction.

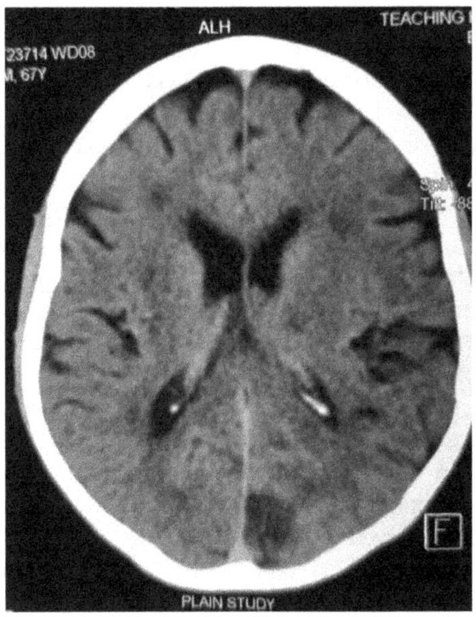

FIGURE 2: Noncontrast CT scan of the brain showing bilateral watershed infarctions in the fronto-parietal regions and a right-sided occipital infarction.

3. Discussion

Hypertension is a major killer in the world and is responsible for nearly nine million deaths a year according to the WHO [1]. Hypertension is defined as office systolic blood pressure values ≥140 mmHg and/or diastolic BP (DBP) values

≥90 mmHg by the European Society of Cardiology [2]. Hypertension emergency is defined as severe hypertension (grade 3) which is associated with acute hypertension-mediated organ damage. It may be life-threatening and immediate but careful reduction of blood pressure with intravenous antihypertensives is needed [3]. Severe hypertension (grade 3) without end organ involvement is defined as a hypertensive urgency where blood pressure needs to be reduced slowly over a period of 24–48 hours using oral medications [4]. Excessive reduction in blood pressure in a patient with markedly elevated blood pressure without target organ damage is not recommended as it can precipitate renal, cerebral, or coronary ischemia [5, 6]. In this case, our patient had markedly elevated blood pressure without evidence of end organ involvement and unfortunately his blood pressure was lowered over few hours using 3 potent antihypertensive medications.

Cerebral autoregulation is the ability to maintain stable perfusion to the brain tissue to meet the metabolic demands of the brain despite changes in blood pressure [7]. Myogenic, neurogenic, endothelial, and metabolic responses have been described in this autoregulatory process [8]. In longstanding untreated hypertension as in this case, it is well known that the static autoregulatory curve shifts rightward, placing patients at risk of impaired ability to tolerate hypotension [9]. Thus, too aggressive lowering of long standing blood pressure could have undesirable effects on brain function.

"Man-in-the-barrel syndrome" is a rare but well-reported syndrome of brachial diplegia. It was first described by Dide in 1917 [10]. Different terms were coined in medical literature to describe the same clinical presentation over the years such ascruciate paralysis [11], distal field infarction [12], and brachial amyotrophic diplegia syndrome [13]. The classic clinical presentation is paralysis of the upper extremity, more pronounced proximally than distally, with intact motor functions of the lower limbs. As the subject is unable to move his arms, it appears that the upper limbs are confined in a barrel [14]. In our case, the patient had marked weakness in the proximal upper limb muscles, but motor functions of the distal hand muscles and lower limb muscles were well preserved.

The phenotype of "man-in-the-barrel syndrome" has been described in many neuropathological conditions localizing to the cerebral cortex, pons, anterior horn cells of the cervical spinal cord, and peripheral nerves [15–18]. Acute systemic hypotension is the most commonly described aetiology leading to this syndrome. Several such cases have been described following cardiorespiratory arrest and postoperative hypotension [19–21]. We describe the first case of precipitous iatrogenic lowering of blood pressure using multiple antihypertensive drugs leading to this phenotype. Rapid lowering of blood pressure can result in ischemic lesions in the border zone between the middle and anterior cerebral artery territories. This is the location of the precentral gyrus, which is the motor region responsible for motor activity of the arm and the shoulder [22]. In our patient, CT scans of the brain revealed bilateral hypodense areas involving watershed zones. This suggested the development of ischemic lesion following rapid drop in blood pressure. His bilateral carotid arteries were normal indicating acute severe blood pressure drop is the sole cause for the bilateral watershed infarctions.

Many other etiologies have been described leading to a phenotypic presentation of "man-in-the-barrel syndrome." Multiple strokes [23] and metastases [24] involving bilateral cerebral cortices have been described with the syndrome. Telfer et al. described a case due to central pontine myelinolysis caused by hyponatremia [25]. Upper cervical cord lesions such as infarction or tumor have been found to cause similar phenotypes [26]. Amyotrophic lateral sclerosis (ALS) has also been described as a rare cause of "man-in-the-barrel syndrome" [13].

The prognosis of this condition is highly variable and it depends on the aetiology. Some case series with motor neuron disease reported mortality up to 90%. Other cases reported good recovery with minimum residual neurological deficits. Our patient's prognosis was good and his proximal weakness improved partially with physiotherapy.

4. Conclusion

In the absence of hypertension-mediated acute end organ damage, aggressive treatment of markedly elevated blood pressure should be avoided, as it can lead to grave consequences such as cerebral ischemia. "Man-in-the-barrel syndrome" is a rare phenotype that can be caused by multiple neuropathological processes localizing to the bilateral cerebral cortices, pons, upper spinal cord, or peripheral neurons. It can also be caused by watershed infarctions following cerebral ischemia, which may lead to severe functional impairment with a variable prognosis.

Consent

Explicit written consent to publish the clinical details and photographs as in the current form in the manuscript was given by the patient. The copy of the written consent is available for review by the Editor-in-Chief of this journal.

Authors' Contributions

CD, AJ, SA, TJ, and UR examined, assessed, and involved in the management of the patient. All authors involved in writing the manuscript. All authors read and approved the final manuscript.

References

[1] World Health Organization, *A Global Brief on Hypertension*, Report, Contract No.: WHO/DCO/WHD/2013.2, WHO, Geneva, Switzerland, 2013.

[2] B. Williams, "2018 ESC/ESH Guidelines for the management of arterial hypertension: the task force for the management of arterial hypertension of the European society of Cardiology (ESC) and the European society of hypertension (ESH)," *European Heart Journal*, vol. 39, no. 33, pp. 3021–3104, 2018.

[3] B.-J. H. van den Born, G. Y. H. Lip, J. Brguljan-Hitij et al., "ESC council on hypertension position document on the management of hypertensive emergencies," *European Heart Journal-Cardiovascular Pharmacotherapy*, vol. 5, no. 1, pp. 37–46, 2019.

[4] D. Grassi, M. O'Flaherty, M. Pellizzari et al., "Hypertensive urgencies in the emergency department: evaluating blood pressure response to rest and to antihypertensive drugs with different profiles," *The Journal of Clinical Hypertension*, vol. 10, no. 9, pp. 662–667, 2008.

[5] M. Sánchez, J. Sobrino, L. Ribera, M. J. Adrián, M. Torres, and A. Coca, "Long-acting Lacidipine versus short-acting nifedipine in the treatment of asymptomatic acute blood pressure increase," *Journal of Cardiovascular Pharmacology*, vol. 33, no. 3, pp. 479–484, 1999.

[6] M. M. Hirschl, D. Seidler, A. Zeiner et al., "Intravenous urapidil versus sublingual nifedipine in the treatment of hypertensive urgencies," *The American Journal of Emergency Medicine*, vol. 11, no. 6, pp. 653–656, 1993.

[7] K. P. Budohoski, M. Czosnyka, P. J. Kirkpatrick, P. Smielewski, L. A. Steiner, and J. D. Pickard, "Clinical relevance of cerebral autoregulation following subarachnoid haemorrhage," *Nature Reviews Neurology*, vol. 9, no. 3, pp. 152–163, 2013.

[8] A. Wang, S. Ortega-Gutierrez, and N. H. Petersen, "Autoregulation in the neuro ICU," *Current Treatment Options in Neurology*, vol. 20, no. 6, p. 20, 2018.

[9] Y.-C. Tzeng and P. N. Ainslie, "Blood pressure regulation IX: cerebral autoregulation under blood pressure challenges," *European Journal of Applied Physiology*, vol. 114, no. 3, pp. 545–559, 2014.

[10] M. Dide and J. Lhermite, "La diplegie brachiale spasmodique consecutive aux blessures par coups de feu de la region cervicale," *Progress in Preventive Medicine*, vol. 1, pp. 1–3, 1917.

[11] H. S. Bell, "Paralysis of both arms from injury of the upper portion of the pyramidal decussation: "cruciate paralysis"" *Journal of Neurosurgery*, vol. 33, no. 4, pp. 376–380, 1970.

[12] J. P. Mohr, "Distal field infarction," *Neurology*, vol. 19, p. 279, 1969.

[13] J. S. Katz, G. I. Wolfe, P. B. Andersson et al., "Brachial amyotrophic diplegia: a slowly progressive motor neuron disorder," *Neurology*, vol. 53, no. 5, p. 1071, 1999.

[14] C. C. Wahl, ""Man-in-the-Barrel" syndrome after endoscopic sinus surgery," *Anesthesia & Analgesia*, vol. 87, no. 5, pp. 1196–1198, 1998.

[15] E. A. Crisostomo and F. J. Suslavich, "Man-in-the-barrel syndrome associated with closed head injury," *Journal of Neuroimaging*, vol. 4, no. 2, pp. 116-117, 1994.

[16] E. J. Wilck, P. S. Gerard, M. Keilson, M. Bashevkin, and J. Lieberman, "Symmetrical cerebral metastasis presenting with bilateral upper extremity weakness," *Journal of Neuroimaging*, vol. 6, pp. 254–256, 1996.

[17] A. P. Moore and P. R. D. Humphrey, "Man-in-the-barrel syndrome caused by cerebral metastases," *Neurology*, vol. 39, no. 8, p. 1134, 1989.

[18] R. Alberca, L. M. Iriarte, P. Rasero, and F. Villalobos, "Brachial diplegia in central pontine myelinolysis," *Journal of Neurology*, vol. 231, no. 6, pp. 345-346, 1985.

[19] P. J. Shaw, S. Tharakaram, and S. K. Mandal, "Brachial diplegia as a sequel to cardio-respiratory arrest: "man-in-the-barrel syndrome"" *Postgraduate Medical Journal*, vol. 66, no. 779, p. 788, 1990.

[20] D. Georgiadis and W. J. Schulte-Mattler, "Cruciate paralysis or man-in-the-barrel syndrome? report of a case of Brachial Diplegia," *Acta Neurologica Scandinavica*, vol. 105, no. 4, pp. 337–340, 2002.

[21] J. Hurley and A. Wood, "Isolated man-in-the-barrel syndrome following cardiac surgery," *The Thoracic and Cardiovascular Surgeon*, vol. 41, no. 04, pp. 252–254, 1993.

[22] L. Jörgensen and A. Torvik, "Ischaemic cerebrovascular diseases in an autopsy series part 2. prevalence, location, pathogenesis, and clinical course of cerebral infarcts," *Journal of the Neurological Sciences*, vol. 9, no. 2, pp. 285–320, 1969.

[23] S. B. Sassi, "Man-in-the-barrel syndrome with combination of infarctions in the anterior spinal artery and posterior inferior cerebellar artery territories," *Cerebrovascular Diseases*, vol. 27, pp. 201-202, 2009.

[24] S. Kobayashi, H. Taniguchi, S. Murayama, M. Sakurai, and I. Kanazawa, "Man-in-the-barrel syndrome caused by bilateral intratumoral hemorrhage," *European Neurology*, vol. 54, no. 3, p. 164, 2005.

[25] R. B. Telfer and E. M. Miller, "Central pontine myelinolysis following hyponatremia, demonstrated by computerized tomography," *Annals of Neurology*, vol. 6, no. 5, pp. 455-456, 1979.

[26] D. Berg, W. Miillges, M. Koltzenburg, M. Bendszus, and K. Reiners, "Case report Man-in-the-barrel syndrome caused by cervical spinal cord infarction," *Acta Neurologica Scandinavica*, vol. 97, no. 6, pp. 417–419, 1998.

9

Negative Diffusion Weighted Imaging on Magnetic Resonance Imaging of the Brain in Creutzfeldt–Jakob Disease

Elijah Lackey, Deepal P. Shah-Zamora, Jodi Hawes, and Andy J. Liu

Duke University Department of Neurology, Duke University Medical Center 2905, 40 Medicine Circle, Durham, NC 27710, USA

Correspondence should be addressed to Andy J. Liu; andy.liu@duke.edu

Academic Editor: Fraser C. Henderson

A 76-year-old Caucasian woman initially presented to the Duke Memory Disorders clinic with a 9-month history of a rapid decline in cognitive, motor, and neuropsychiatric function. On initial presentation, the patient required assistance with activities of daily living. On neurological examination, she was found to have Gerstmann's syndrome along with appendicular apraxia. A positional tremor was noted without myoclonus or fasciculations. She had a paucity of speech and was unable to write her own name. Snout and grasp reflexes were present. Episodes of inappropriate laughter were noted during the exam. She was admitted to the inpatient neurology service for further evaluation. The Diffusion Weighted Imaging sequence on Magnetic Resonance Imaging of the brain was negative for restricted diffusion. An electroencephalogram was unremarkable. Cerebrospinal fluid analysis for Real-Time Quaking-Induced Conversion assay was positive along with an elevated 14-3-3 and increased total Tau protein levels. There was no family history of Creutzfeldt–Jakob disease. The cerebral spinal fluid results were consistent with a diagnosis of Creutzfeldt–Jakob disease, despite the negative MRI brain findings.

1. Introduction

Creutzfeldt–Jakob Disease (CJD) is commonly described as a rapidly progressive dementia with a subacute onset. The disease presents with a heterogeneous phenotype and may include progressive cognitive, behavioral, motor, and sensory deficits. Higher-order cortical deficits may be present in about 10–15% of cases as early symptoms and in about half of patients as the disease progresses [1]. A common biomarker of CJD is restricted diffusion on the Diffusion Weighted Imaging (DWI) sequence on Magnetic Resonance Imaging (MRI) brain localized to the neocortex, basal ganglia, and caudate [1–3]. A Fluid-Attenuated Inversion Recovery (FLAIR) or T2 sequence hyperintensity correlating with the neocortical restricted diffusion on DWI may also be seen [1, 3]. An electroencephalogram (EEG) may show 1-2 Hz periodic sharp wave complexes [1, 3]. Restricted diffusion on the DWI sequence has a sensitivity of 96% in patients with CJD [1–3]. This case report underscores the importance of pursuing a comprehensive evaluation including cerebrospinal fluid (CSF) analysis, MRI of the brain, and an EEG in all patients with subacute changes in behavior, motor function, or cognition.

2. Case Presentation

A 76-year-old female with a history of hypertension, hyperlipidemia, and coronary artery disease was referred to the Duke Memory Disorders clinic by her local neurologist for evaluation of a rapid decline in cognitive, behavioral, and motor symptoms over a 9-month period. She had no family history of neurodegenerative disease. Nine months prior to presentation, she experienced two myocardial infarctions that required two cardiac catheterization procedures. Before these procedures, family members stated that she lived independently. After her first cardiac catheterization, she began having progressive language difficulties. Evaluation by speech therapy was notable for difficulty in completing written assignments and a decrease in spontaneous speech. The patient was also noted to have executive dysfunction

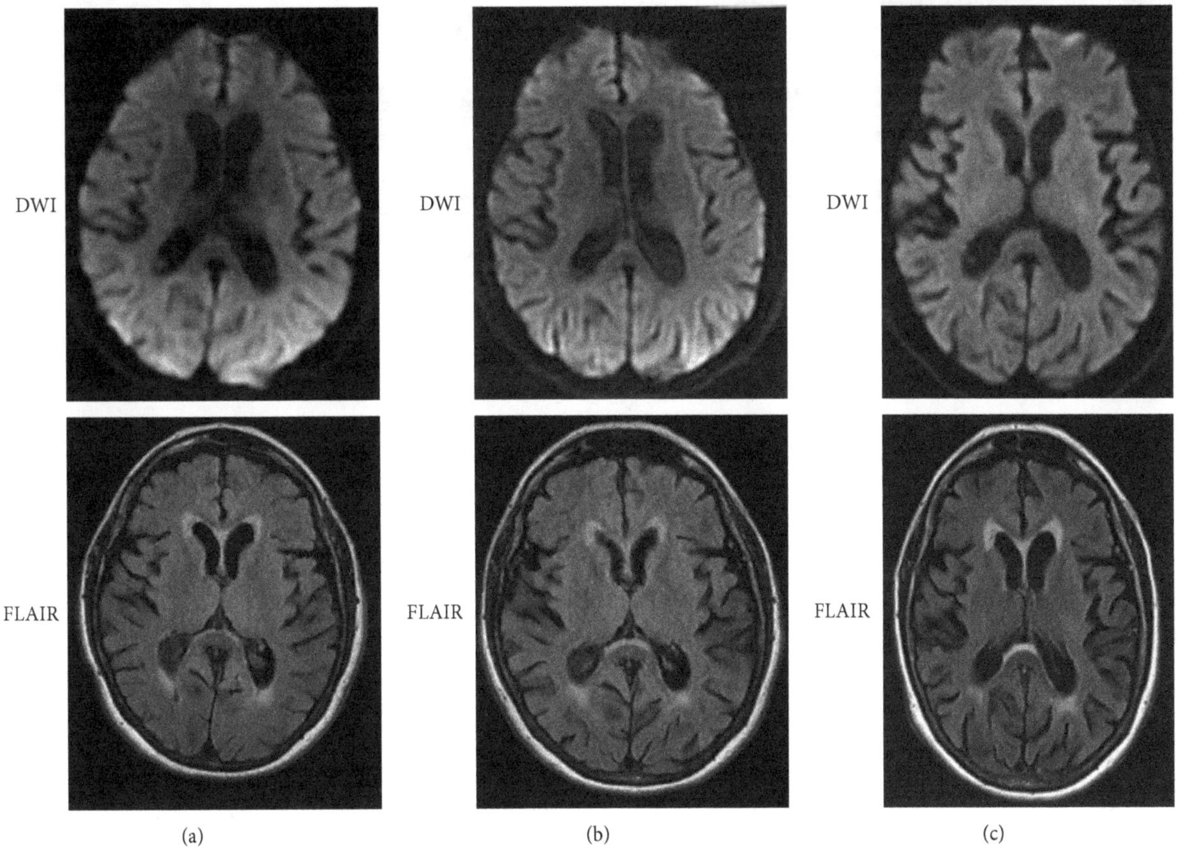

Figure 1: Axial MRI diffusion weighted images (top row) and fluid-attenuated inversion recovery images shown at about one month (a), four months (b), and nine months (c) from onset of symptoms. These images show no diffusion restriction on diffusion weighted images or hyperintensities on FLAIR that would support the diagnosis of Creutzfeldt–Jakob disease.

such as having challenges managing the family's finances or placing an empty pot on the stove with the burner on, which she could previously do independently. Behavioral changes were also appreciated by the family such as easily becoming upset and crying frequently, and she had become more agreeable after her cardiac procedures. She also became less energetic and spent more time sleeping. She then developed motor difficulties described as unsteadiness while walking, particularly going up stairs, and later had difficulty navigating her home.

On general examination in clinic, her vital signs were unremarkable. Mental status examination was notable for a paucity of speech and inability to write her own name. There were episodes of inappropriate laughter throughout the exam. Neurological examination revealed appendicular apraxia, an action tremor, along with snout and grasp reflexes. No myoclonus or fasciculations were noted. All elements of Gerstmann's syndrome were appreciated including finger agnosia, right-left confusion, agraphia, acalculia, and abulia.

MRI brain at one month after symptom onset showed no diffusion restriction (Figure 1). A Montreal Cognitive Assessment (MoCA) completed 3 months after her cardiac procedures was 18/30. The test was repeated 1 month later with a total score of 14/30. Three months after onset of symptoms, a routine EEG was ordered by the local neurologist which was unrevealing (Figure 2). Labwork including basic metabolic panel, complete blood count, urinalysis, and urine culture were normal. Four months after onset of symptoms, a repeat MRI showed no significant changes from the prior brain MRI.

Given concerns for CJD after the initial evaluation at our institution's memory disorders clinic, the patient was directly admitted to the inpatient neurology service for expedited evaluation. A repeat routine EEG and MRI brain were both unrevealing. CSF RT-QuiC assay and 14-3-3 protein was positive. The t-tau level was 1891 pg/ml. Collectively, the CSF results were consistent with a diagnosis of CJD (Table 1).

3. Discussion

CJD is difficult to diagnose because of its heterogeneous clinical phenotype. The heterogeneity is dependent on the anatomic area of involvement of the prion protein along with the histopathologic subtype. Histopathologic subtypes of spontaneous CJD are based on the polymorphism in the prion gene, PRNP, at codon 129 (methionine or valine) paired with the molecular weight of the PrP^{SC} protein as run on western blot [4, 5]. Subsequently, there are six possible combinations of polymorphisms paired with molecular weight (MM1, MV1, VV1, VV2, MM2, and MV2), which

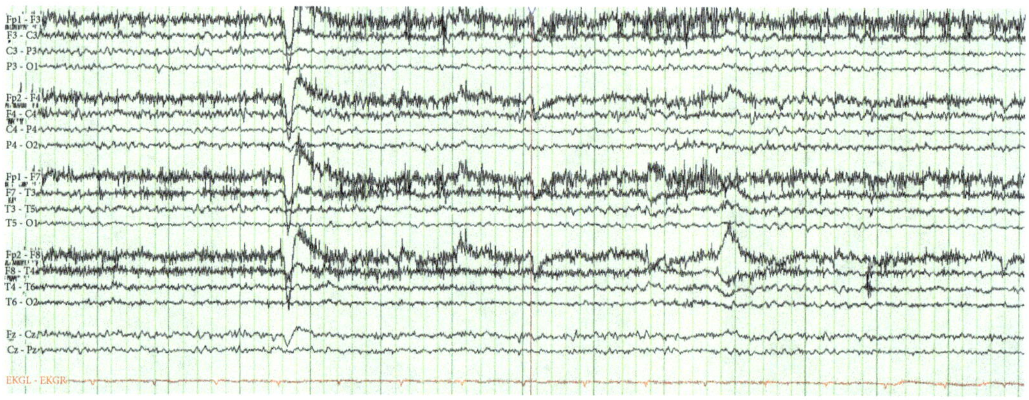

Figure 2: Electroencephalogram (EEG) completed at about nine months from the onset of symptoms. The occipital dominant rhythm was 9 Hz. EEG activity was reactive to stimulation. There were no 1-2 Hz periodic sharp wave complexes suggestive of Creutzfeldt-Jakob disease.

Table 1: Cerebrospinal fluid (CSF) studies sent approximately nine months from onset of symptoms along with serum studies completed throughout the clinical course.

Test (source)	Result	Normal reference range
RT-QuIC (CSF)	Positive	Negative
14-3-3 protein (CSF)	Positive	Negative
Total tau protein (CSF)	1891 pg/ml	0–1149 pg/ml
Nucleated cells (tube #4 CSF)	1/μL	0–5/μL
Red blood cells (tube #4 CSF)	13	<=0/μL
Glucose (CSF)	64 mg/dl	60% of plasma level (90 mg/dl)
Protein (CSF)	39 mg/dl	15–50 mg/dl
CSF and serum autoimmune panels	Negative for autoantibodies	Negative for autoantibodies
VDRL (CSF)	Negative	Negative
TSH (serum)	1.49 μLU/ml	0.358–3.74 μLU/ml
Vitamin B12 (serum)	625 pg/ml	211–911 pg/ml
Antithyroglobulin (TPG) antibody (serum)	<1	< or = 1 IU/mL
Antithyroperoxidase (TPO) antibody (serum)	<1	<9 IU/mL
Paraneoplastic panel (serum)	Negative for autoantibodies	Negative for autoantibodies

can be further subdivided based on location (MM2 cortical vs. MM2 thalamic), although sometimes both molecular weights may be present (MM1-2, MV1-2, and VV1-2). Comprehensive characterization of these subtypes has revealed stereotypical clinical phenotypes [6]. Nevertheless, histopathologic subtypes do not necessarily correlate with clinical phenotype, and diagnosis may not be straightforward [4]. Subsequently, a comprehensive evaluation including MRI of the brain, EEG, and CSF analysis are required for the diagnosis of CJD [7, 8]. Overall, MRI brain has 92–96% sensitivity for diagnosis of CJD although accuracy of the test depends on histopathologic subtype with striatal or cortical ribbon diffusion seen more often in common subtypes such as MM1 and MV1 [3, 4, 7, 9]. In contrast, the rare MM2 cortical and VV1 subtypes often do not show any MRI findings, and it is possible that our patient may have had one of these variants [10, 11]. The EEG has 60–80% sensitivity with higher sensitivity later in the disease course [12–14]. The RT-QuiC test combined with 14-3-3 has an estimated sensitivity of 77–92% and specificity of 99–100% making it highly useful as a diagnostic test if positive [15, 16]. Serologic codon 129 polymorphisms can now be identified with antemortem genetic testing which is useful for diagnostic confirmation and for assessing for inherited disease.

This case report highlights the importance of the clinical trajectory in patients with a rapidly progressive dementia. Three DWI sequences from the MRI brain studies were negative for restricted diffusion. Intriguingly, the CSF biomarkers supported the diagnosis of CJD. Based on the CSF RT-QuiC, t-tau, and 14-3-3 protein assays, the National Prion Disease Pathology Surveillance Center reported a likelihood of CJD of greater than 98%. Currently, the treatment for CJD is supportive.

Definitive diagnosis of CJD by WHO guidelines is made by postmortem autopsy. Genetic testing is performed on brain tissue obtained at biopsy. At this time, the patient is enrolled in Home Hospice; therefore, her histopathologic subtype and genotype of PRNP is unknown. Antemortem genetic testing was discussed with the daughter but deferred. In conclusion, if initial testing is discordant with the clinical presentation as was in this case, a comprehensive evaluation for a rapidly progressive dementia should be pursued.

Consent

Verbal consent was obtained from the patient's family member.

Disclosure

This research was performed while the authors were employed by Duke University Department of Neurology.

References

[1] M. D. Geschwind, "Prion diseases," *Continuum: Lifelong Learning in Neurology*, vol. 21, no. 6, pp. 1612–1638, 2015.

[2] P. Vitali, E. Maccagnano, E. Caverzasi et al., "Diffusion-weighted MRI hyperintensity patterns differentiate CJD from other rapid dementias," *Neurology*, vol. 76, no. 20, pp. 1711–1719, 2011.

[3] K. J. Baldwin and C. M. Correll, "Prion disease," *Seminars in Neurology*, vol. 39, no. 4, pp. 428–439, 2019.

[4] G. Puoti, A. Bizzi, G. Forloni, J. G. Safar, F. Tagliavini, and P. Gambetti, "Sporadic human prion diseases: molecular insights and diagnosis," *The Lancet Neurology*, vol. 11, no. 7, pp. 618–628, 2012.

[5] S. B. Prusiner, "Nobel lecture: prions," *Proceedings of the National Academy of Sciences*, vol. 95, no. 23, pp. 13363–13383, 1998.

[6] P. Parchi, A. Giese, S. Capellari et al., "Classification of sporadic Creutzfeldt-Jakob disease based on molecular and phenotypic analysis of 300 subjects," *Annals of Neurology*, vol. 46, no. 2, pp. 224–233, 1999.

[7] M. D. Geschwind, "Rapidly progressive dementia," *Continuum: Lifelong Learning in Neurology*, vol. 22, no. 2, pp. 510–537, 2016.

[8] I. Sala, M. Marquié, M. B. Sánchez-Saudinós et al., "Rapidly progressive dementia," *Alzheimer Disease & Associated Disorders*, vol. 26, no. 3, pp. 267–271, 2012.

[9] G. S. Young, M. D. Geschwind, N. J. Fischbein et al., "Diffusion-weighted and fluid-attenuated inversion recovery imaging in Creutzfeldt-Jakob disease: high sensitivity and specificity for diagnosis," *American Journal of Neuroradiology*, vol. 26, no. 6, pp. 1551–1562, 2005.

[10] A. Krasnianski, B. Meissner, W. Schulz-Schaeffer et al., "Clinical features and diagnosis of the MM2 cortical subtype of sporadic Creutzfeldt-Jakob disease," *Archives of Neurology*, vol. 63, no. 6, pp. 876–880, 2006.

[11] B. Meissner, I. M. Westner, K. Kallenberg et al., "Sporadic Creutzfeldt-Jakob disease clinical and diagnostic characteristics of the rare VV_1 type," *Neurology*, vol. 65, no. 10, pp. 1544–1550, 2020, http://www.neurology.org.

[12] B. J. Steinhoff, I. Zerr, M. Glatting, W. Schulz-Schaeffer, S. Poser, and H. A. Kretzschmar, "Diagnostic value of periodic complexes in Creutzfeldt-Jakob disease," *Annals of Neurology*, vol. 56, no. 5, pp. 702–708, 2004.

[13] H. Wieser, K. Schindler, and D. Zumsteg, "EEG in Creutzfeldt-Jakob disease," *Clinical Neurophysiology*, vol. 117, no. 5, pp. 935–951, 2006.

[14] S. J. Collins, P. Sanchez-Juan, C. L. Masters et al., "Determinants of diagnostic investigation sensitivities across the clinical spectrum of sporadic Creutzfeldt-Jakob disease," *Brain*, vol. 129, no. 9, pp. 2278–2287, 2006.

[15] L. I. McGuire, A. H. Peden, C. D. Orrú et al., "Real time quaking-induced conversion analysis of cerebrospinal fluid in sporadic Creutzfeldt-Jakob disease," *Annals of Neurology*, vol. 72, no. 2, pp. 278–285, 2012.

[16] R. Atarashi, K. Satoh, K. Sano et al., "Ultrasensitive human prion detection in cerebrospinal fluid by real-time quaking-induced conversion," *Nature Medicine*, vol. 17, no. 2, pp. 175–178, 2011.

10

Marchiafava–Bignami Disease Associated with Spinal Involvement

Jhon Perea,[1] **María Belén Luis**,[1] **Luciana Grimanesa Lázaro**,[1] **Sergio Scollo**,[1] **Agustina Tamargo**,[1] **José Crespo**,[1] **Maira Avalle**,[1] **Horacio Solarz**,[2] **Nora Fernández Liguori**,[1] **and Ricardo Alonso**[1]

[1]*Department of Neurology, Sanatorio Güemes—University Hospital, Buenos Aires, Argentina*
[2]*Anatomical Pathology, Sanatorio Güemes—University Hospital, Buenos Aires, Argentina*

Correspondence should be addressed to Jhon Perea; jhoper0289@hotmail.com

Academic Editor: Mehmet Turgut

Marchiafava–Bignami disease (MBD) is a rare disorder of unknown etiology, strongly associated with alcoholism and malnutrition. MBD causes primary involvement of the corpus callosum, leading to confusion, dysarthria, seizures, and frequent death. We report the case of a 54-year-old male without a history of alcoholism or known malabsorption disease, who presented with altered consciousness and neurologic impairment. Complex B deficiency was addressed. Magnetic resonance imaging (MRI) showed typical corpus callosum lesions. The clinical features and radiologic images suggested spinal cord involvement. Brain histopathologic findings were consistent with MBD. Despite vitamin replacement therapy, he had a poor outcome.

1. Introduction

Marchiafava–Bignami Disease (MBD) is a rare disorder that affects adults between 40 to 60 years of age, with a male predominance, and a history of chronic alcoholism and/or malnutrition. It has been associated with vitamin B complex deficiency, and its main feature is progressive demyelination and necrosis of the corpus callosum [1]. There is also involvement of other cerebral structures, such as hemispheric white matter, middle cerebellar peduncle, and basal ganglia. Few cases of spinal cord involvement were reported [2, 3]. Clinical features are heterogeneous and nonspecific. MBD can cause impairment of consciousness, neuropsychiatric symptoms, dysarthria, tetraparesis, hypertonia, ataxia, seizures, and symptoms of interhemispheric disconnection [4–6]. A clinical and radiologic classification proposed by Henrich divides patients into two types: *type A*, characterized by involvement of the entire corpus callosum, and *type B*, characterized by partial or focal callosal lesions [5, 7, 8]. Although the prognosis is variable, the mortality is high. Early thiamine replacement therapy is associated with a better outcome, whereas the effectiveness of steroids and other treatments remains hypothetical [9, 10]. Different etiologies (infectious, vascular, metabolic, demyelinating, or neoplastic) can cause corpus callosum signal abnormalities. Therefore, the exclusion of differential diagnoses is essential [11, 12]. We present the case of a 54-year-old man suffering from vitamin B complex deficiency and spinal cord involvement, with histopathologic examination consistent with MBD.

2. Case Report

A 53-year-old male was admitted to our hospital due to progressive weakness and impaired state of consciousness. He had a personal history of noninsulin-dependent diabetes, with no history of alcoholism or malnutrition. Two months before admission, he presented with lower limbs weakness, which rapidly progressed leading to severe gait impairment and wheel chair bound. Initial evaluation was performed at another medical center and was referred to our hospital one week later. On admission, he had signs of respiratory distress, which led to intubation and transfer to the intensive care unit. At the initial examination, the patient was in a spontaneous coma. Pupils were symmetric and reactive. There were no signs of cranial nerve impairment, and brainstem reflexes were normal. He had an abnormal extension posture of the upper limbs, with normal withdrawal of lower limbs to painful stimulus. Muscle tone and reflexes were normal, and no meningeal signs were found. A brain MRI showed hyper-intensities and extended T2-signal and fluid-attenuated inversion-recovery sequence (FLAIR) involving cerebral peduncles and middle cerebellar peduncles, parietal corpus callosum, and corona radiata (Figures 1(a)–1(d)).

On reviewing of diffusion-weighted imaging signal (DWI), there was homogenous and symmetrical hypersignal throughout the lesion and a corresponding decrease of apparent diffusion coefficient (ADC) values on the ADC maps diffusion restriction (Figures 2(a)–2(f)).

Furthermore, there was an abnormal focal enhancement in corona radiata of the right parietal lobe (Figures 1(e)–1(h)). Spinal cord MRI showed a longitudinally extensive, nonenhancing STIR-hyperintense lesion from C2-T1 with mild edema (Figures 3(a) and 3(b)).

Based on the clinical and image findings, MBD versus central nervous system demyelinating disorders (i.e., aggressive multiple sclerosis, acute disseminated encephalomyelitis, or neuromyelitis optica spectrum disorder) were suspected. Blood count showed severe pancytopenia with megaloblastic anemia. Serum vitamin B1 and B12 levels were very low. Levels of serum homocysteine were elevated, while malonic acid and serum folic acid were normal. CSF analysis revealed hyperproteinorrachia(468 mg/dl) and increased lactic acid (7 mmol/l). Oligoclonal bands, AQP4 IgG and anti-MOG IgG, were negative. Viral and bacterial infections were ruled out (viral PCR screen and bacterial cultures). Other laboratory tests are shown in Table 1.

Treatment with IV thiamine: high doses of parenteral B12 vitamin and methylprednisolone pulses (1000 mg/day for 5 days) were started. A brain biopsy was performed at the 20th day of hospitalization, revealing white matter necrosis, areas of demyelination, and gliosis, as well as macrophage infiltrates and perivascular lymphocytes (Figure 4).

These findings were also consistent with MBD. Although laboratory parameters improved with treatment (reaching normal values of both vitamins), there was no clinical improvement, as shown in Table 2. The patient died on day 125 of hospitalization.

3. Discussion

Marchiafava and Bignani were Italian pathologists who, in 1903, described a syndrome characterized by selective demyelination and necrosis of the corpus callosum. This entity affected consumers of large volumes of red wine [13]. Later on, this affection was also found in people with severe nutritional deficits [14]. It has been associated with vitamin B complex deficiency, primarily thiamine deficiency. In a few cases, low cyanocobalamin serum levels were also associated with spinal cord involvement [2, 3]. Even though our patient had no personal history of alcoholism or malnutrition, low serum levels of vitamins B1 and B12 were found. The pathophysiological mechanism of MBD remains unclear. Possible mechanisms include cytotoxic edema, the breakdown of the blood-brain barrier, demyelination, and necrosis. Cytotoxic edema is possibly the underlying mechanism involved in the early stages, while demyelination and necrosis take place in later stages. Morel's laminar sclerosis of cerebral cortex is seen [15].

MBD clinical manifestations vary and are nonspecific, posing a diagnostic challenge, and different clinical presentations were described [16]. Acute MBD causes seizures, altered consciousness, and limb hypertonia. Subacute MBD is characterized by confusion, dysarthria, behavioral abnormalities, visual disturbance, memory deficits, signs of interhemispheric disconnection, apraxia, tetraparesis, and gait disorders. The chronic clinical presentation of MBD is the least common and characterized by chronic dementia. Severe impairment of consciousness and neurocognitive deficits at the beginning appear to be indicators of a poor prognosis [1, 5, 15]. Clinical manifestation in our patient was consistent with an acute/subacute presentation. Typical MRI findings in patients with acute MBD include symmetric T2-signal and FLAIR hyperintensity of the corpus callosum, with low signal intensity in T1-signal sequences. DWI restriction of cerebral cortex, hemispheric white matter, middle cerebellar peduncles, and basal ganglia was also described. Contrast enhancement of the corpus callosum, which resolves in the subacute stage, has been reported. In some cases, the T2-signal of the corpus callosum normalizes, evolving into symmetric atrophy [5, 15]. Classifying our patient into *type A or B* was difficult, as he presented with clinic-radiological features of both types. *Type A* is characterized by severe impairment of consciousness, seizures, dysarthria, and hemiparesis. Imaging findings are swelling of the entire corpus callosum and extra callosal lesions. It has been associated with a poor outcome (death in up to 21% of cases). In contrast, *type B* presents with slight impairment of consciousness, focal callosal lesions on MRI, and a lower mortality rate [5, 17]. An interesting feature of our case was the extensive spinal cord involvement from C2 to T1. We thought that this finding could be associated with B12 hypovitaminosis. The combination of cerebral and spinal cord involvement has only been reported in two previous MBD cases [3, 18]. Histopathological findings of MBD showed demyelination (particularly of corpus callosum central fibers) with myelin breakdown products, foamy macrophages, perivascular lymphocytes, gliosis, and white matter necrosis [19, 20]. Most of the cases reported show postmortem examinations. In our case, a brain biopsy was performed, and the findings were consistent with MBD.

Regarding prognosis, MBD is usually associated with a high mortality, although some cases with a favorable outcome have been reported [9]. In a large published series, out of 250 patients, only 20 (8%) presented a favorable recovery [7]. Alcoholic MBD was associated with a less favorable outcome, and death was caused mainly by infectious complications [1, 21]. Related to vitamin B complex deficiency association, thiamine replacement has become a widespread treatment option, and better outcome was

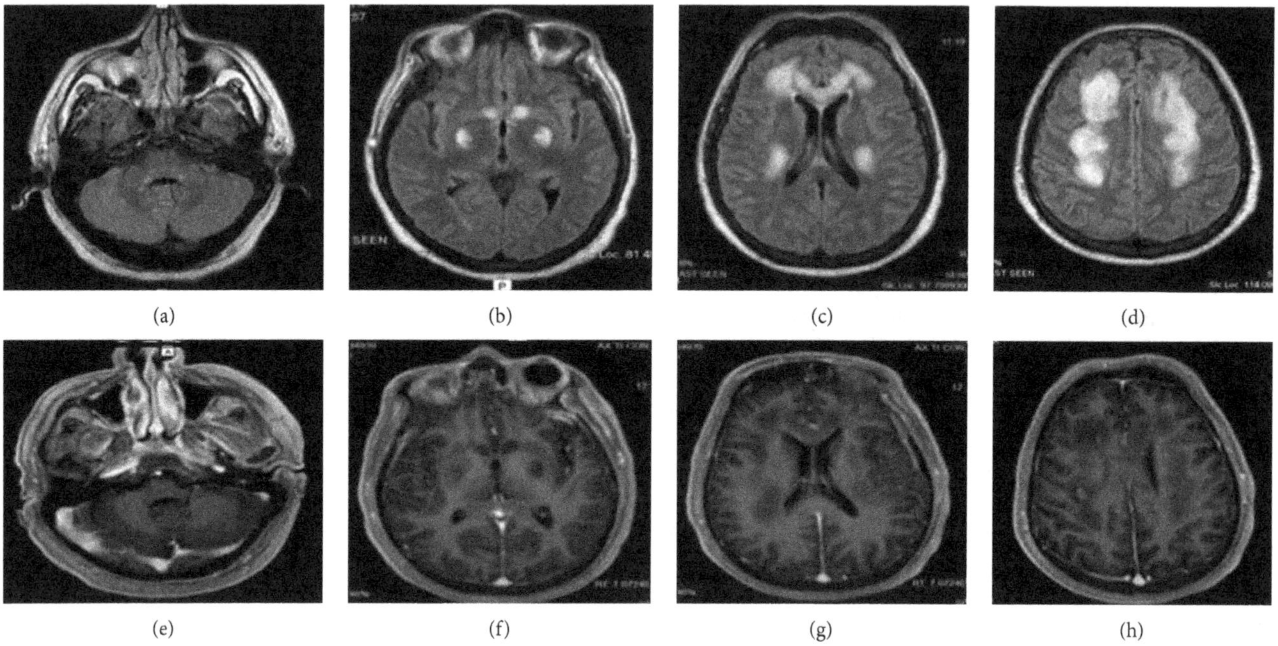

Figure 1: FLAIR brain MRI showing hyperintensity involving peduncles and middle cerebellar peduncles (a). Head of the caudate nucleus and both globus pallidus (b). Corpus callosum and corona radiata (c, d). Gadolinium T1 sequence (e–h) showing focal pathological enhancement in the right parietal lobe (h).

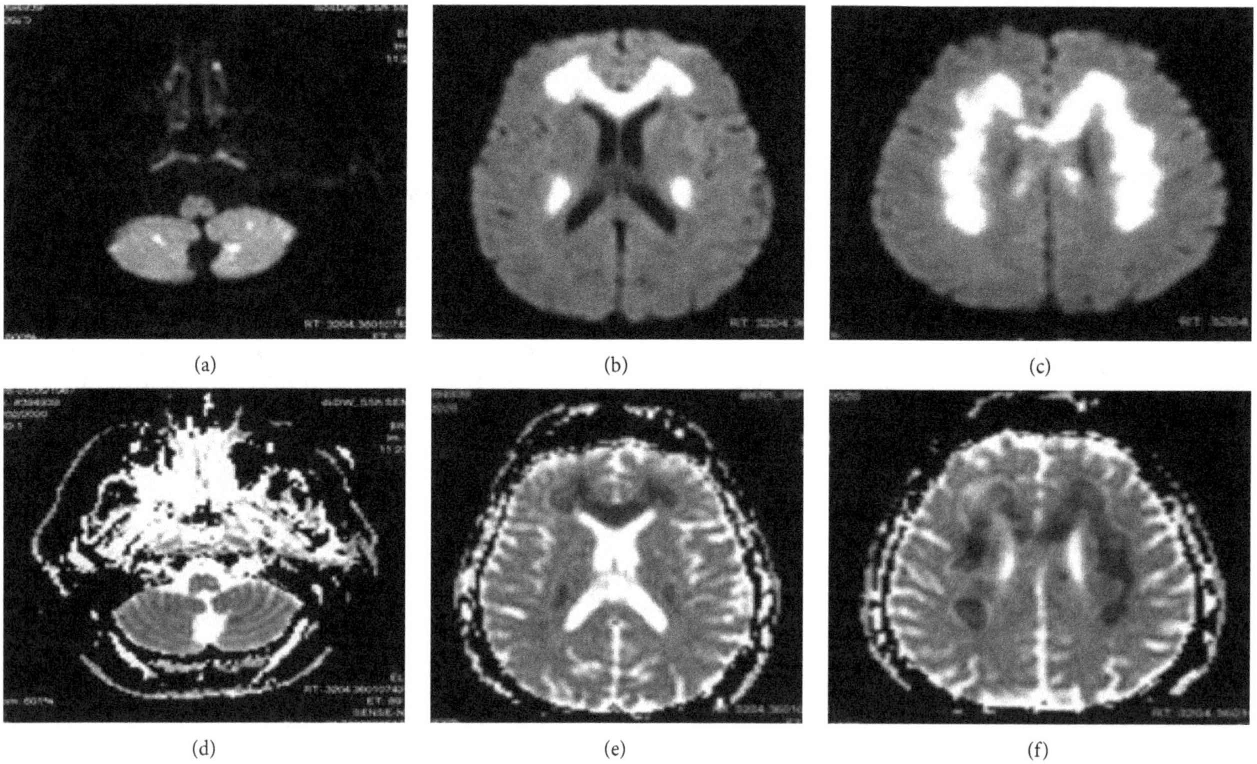

Figure 2: DWI brain MRI showing a hypersignal in the cerebellar hemisphere (a), corpus callosum (b, c), and corona radiata (c). There was a corresponding decrease of ADC values on the ADC map (d–f).

described in subjects treated in the acute stage. Corticosteroids may reduce brain edema, suppress demyelination, stabilize the blood-brain barrier, and reduce inflammation. Although some publications have reported an improvement with this therapy, its benefits are still doubtful and further research is required [12, 21].

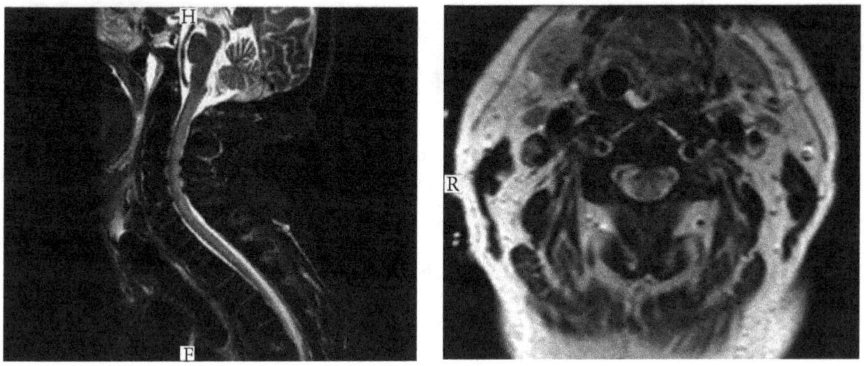

(a) (b)

Figure 3: Short-tau inversion-recovery (STIR) sequence and T2: sagittal and axial slice. (a, b) extensive medullar hyperintensity of the lateral and posterior cords at levels C2-T1.

Table 1: Blood chemical values.

Variable	Value	Reference values
Hematocrit (%)	25	40–50
Hemoglobin (g/dl)	8.8	13.9–17.2
Mean corpuscular volume (μm^3)	102.4	85–95
Medium corpuscular hemoglobin (pg)	35	27–33
White cells (per mm^3)	3100	4000–12000
Differential count (%)		
Neutrophils	61	50–65
Lymphocytes	30	25–45
Monocytes	3	2–8
Eosinophils	6	0–4
Platelets (per mm^3)	91000	15000–450000
Glucose (mg/dl)	164	60–110
Urea nitrogen (mg/dl)	54	18–45
Creatinine (mg/dl)	0.53	0.7–1.2
Sodium (mmol/liter)	148	138–150
Potassium (mmol/liter)	3.4	3.6–5
Chloride (mmol/liter)	116	98–105
Coagulogram		
TP	99	70–100
KPTT	30	30–45
Hepatogram		
Total bilirubin	1.2	0.4–1.4
ASAT	19.5	1–31
ALAT	19.8	1–34
Vitamin B1 (μg/l)	3.4	4.0–20
Vitamin B12 (pg/ml)	<50	180–900
Folic acid (ng/ml)	15	>5.3
Homocysteine (mmol/l)	>65	5–15
Malonic acid (nmol/l)	103	<0.4
TSH (mcμi/ml)	0.2	0.27–4.2
Serologies		
HIV	Negative	
Syphilis	Negative	
Hepatitis B	Negative	
Hepatitis C	Negative	
Erythrocyte sedimentation rate, mm	37	1–10
CSF flow cytometry	No immunophenotypic abnormalities were observed	
Oligoclonal bands	Type I	
Anti-MOG antibody IgG	Negative	
Aquaporin 4 IgG	Negative	

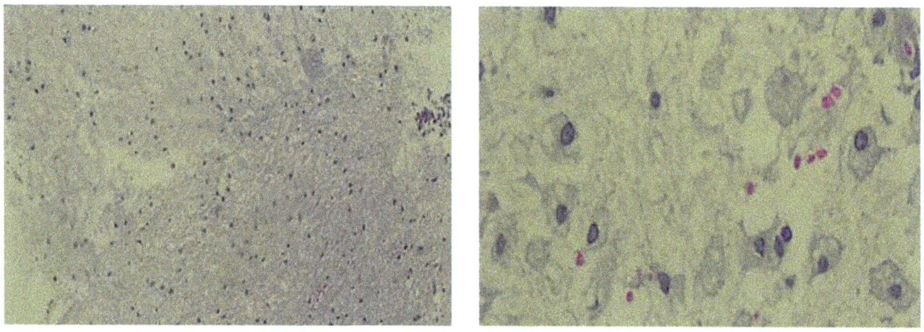

(a) (b)

Figure 4: Histopathology of a biopsied subcortical lesion of the right frontal lobe (hematoxylin and eosin staining). (a) The bottom of the image shows normal eosinophilic white matter and demyelinated tissue at the top. (b) Magnification of demyelination zones with macrophage infiltration.

Table 2: Blood chemical values after treatment.

Variable	Value	Reference values
Hematocrit (%)	35.5	40–50
Hemoglobin (g/dl)	11.1	13.9–17.2
Mean corpuscular volume (μm^3)	30.4 97.3	85–95 27–33
Medium corpuscular hemoglobin (pg)		
White cells (per mm^3)	10100	4000–12000
Differential count (%)		
Neutrophils	90	0–65
Lymphocytes	6	25–45
Monocytes	4	2–8
Eosinophils	0	0–4
Vitamin B1 (μg/l)	15.8	4.0–20
Vitamin B12 (pg/ml)	>2000	180–900

4. Conclusion

MBD is an uncommon entity, which represents a neurological emergency. It requires strict multidisciplinary care in the acute stage, due to its high morbimortality. Our patient had an atypical presentation with spinal cord involvement without typical comorbidities. His diagnosis was a real clinical challenge. Our hypothesis in this case was a double mechanism of neuronal degeneration due to nutritional deficiency of both vitamins B1 and B12.

Consent

Informed consent was signed by the patient's family member.

Acknowledgments

The authors thank their colleagues from Sanatorio Güemes University Hospital who provided expertise that greatly assisted the clinical case resolution, although they may not agree with all of the conclusions of this paper.

References

[1] P. E. Carrilho, M. B. Santos, L. Piasecki, and A. C. Jorge, "Marchiafava-Bignami disease: a rare entity with a poor outcome," *Rev Bras Ter Intensiva*, vol. 25, no. 1, pp. 68–72, 2013.

[2] C. Briani, C. Dalla Torre, V. Citton et al., "Cobalamin deficiency: clinical picture and radiological findings," *Nutrients*, vol. 5, no. 11, pp. 4521–4539, 2013.

[3] S. Kori, "Hyperintense splenium in vitamin B12 deficiency," *Neurology India*, vol. 53, no. 3, p. 377, 2005.

[4] M. B. Santosh, A. Jawaid, J. E. Bock, S. U. Qureshi, and J. E. Bock, "Marchiafava-bignami disease (MBD) in a non-alcoholic patient: a case report," *The Canadian Journal of Neurological Sciences. Le Journal Canadien des Sciences Neurologiques*, vol. 37, no. 1, pp. 138–140, 2010.

[5] W. Holger, E. Philipp, A. Dimitrios, A. Förster, and M. A. Brockmann, "Acute marchiafava-bignami disease with extensive diffusion restriction and early recovery: case report and review of the literature," *Journal of Neuroimaging*, vol. 24, no. 4, pp. 421–424, 2012.

[6] A. Rosa, M. Demiati, L. Cartz, and J. P Mizon, "Marchiafava-bignami disease, syndrome of interhemispheric disconnection, and right-handed agraphia in a left-hander," *Archives of Neurology*, vol. 48, no. 9, pp. 986–988, 1991.

[7] A. Heinrich, U. Runge, and A. V. Khaw, "Clinicoradiologic subtypes of Marchiafava-Bignami disease," *Journal of Neurology*, vol. 251, pp. 1050–1059, 2004.

[8] H. Parmanant, "Marchiafava-Bignami disease in chronic alcoholic patient," *Radiology Case Reports*, vol. 11, no. 3, pp. 234–237, 2016.

[9] J. Helenius, T. Tatlisumak, L. Soinne, L. Valanne, and M. Kaste, "Marchiafava-Bignami disease: two cases with favourable outcome," *European Journal of Neurology*, vol. 8, no. 3, pp. 269–272, 2001.

[10] M. Hillbom, P. Saloheimo, S. Fujioka, Z. K. Wszolek, S. Juvela, and M. A. Leone, "Diagnosis and management of Marchiafava-Bignami disease: a review of CT/MRI confirmed cases,"

Journal of Neurology, Neurosurgery & Psychiatry, vol. 85, no. 2, pp. 168–173, 2014.

[11] J. Staszewski, K. Macek, and A. Stepień, "Reversible demyelinisation of corpus callosum in the course of Marchiafava-Bignami disease," *Neurol Neurochir Pol*, vol. 40, pp. 156–161, 2006.

[12] J. Garcia-Monco, I. Escalza Cortina, E. Ferreira et al., "Reversible splenial lesion syndrome (RESLES): what's in a name?" *Journal of Neuroimaging*vol. 21, pp. 1–14, 2011.

[13] A. V. Canas, M. Rivas, R. G. Guerrero, and M. F. F. Caamano, "Marchiafava-Bignami's disease, as etiologic diagnosis of athetosis," *Annals of Neurosciences*, vol. 24, no. 1, pp. 57–60, 2017.

[14] G. Salazar, M. Fragoso, G. Español, and L. Cuadra, "Degeneración primaria del cuerpo calloso (Marchiafava-Bignami): 2 formas inusuales de presentación clínica," *Neurología*, vol. 28, no. 9, pp. 587–589, 2013.

[15] X. Dong, D. Bai, and J. Nao, "Clinical and radiological features of Marchiafava–Bignami disease," *Medicine*, vol. 97, no. 5, Article ID e9626, 2018.

[16] F. De Armas, R. Salamano, M. Martinez, O. Telis, and E. Meerovich, "Enfermedad de Marchiafava-Bignami, a propósito de un caso clínico e imagenològico," *The International Archives of Medicine*, vol. 35, no. 3, pp. 105–108, 2013.

[17] C. Franco Muccio, L. De Lipsis, R. Belmonte, and A. Cerase, "Reversible MR findings in marchiafava-bignami disease," *Case Reports in Neurological Medicine*, vol. 2019, Article ID 1951030, 3 pages, 2019.

[18] K. Takei, N. Motoyoshi, K. Sakamoto, and T. Kitamoto, "Marchiafava-Bignami disease with haemophagocytic lymphohistiocytosis as a postoperative complication of cardiac surgery," *BMJ Case Report*, vol. 12, no. 8, pp. 230–368, 2019.

[19] R. Ironside, F. D. Bosanquet, and W. H. Mcmenemey, "Central demyelination of the corpus callosum (Marchiafava-Bignami Disease)," *Brain*, vol. 84, no. 2, pp. 212–230, 1961.

[20] A. Al-Witri, A.-L. Vialatte, K. L. Tan, and M. A. J. Dexter, "Antemortem histopathology and imaging findings in a case of Marchiafava-Bignami disease," *Journal of Clinical Neuroscience*, vol. 66, pp. 273–275, 2019.

[21] S. Rodriguez-Fernández, J. Bravo Doviso, L. A. Ramos-Gómez, C. Martín-Delgado, R. Ortiz-López, and T. Puente-Domínguez, "Enfermedad de Marchiafava-Bignami en Cuidados Intensivos," *Medicina Intensiva*, vol. 29, no. 7, pp. 396–399, 2005.

11

Targeted Anterior Cervical Epidural Blood Patch in a Patient with Spontaneous Intracranial Hypotension

Ravindra Singh Shekhawat,[1,2] Ming Hui Yong,[1,2] Si Ying Julienne Keong,[2] Kunihiko Chen,[2] Chow Wei Too,[3] and Shahul Hameed[1,2]

[1]*Department of Neurology, National Neuroscience Institute-Singapore General Hospital, Singapore*
[2]*DUKE-NUS Medical School, Singapore*
[3]*Department of Vascular and Interventional Radiology, Singapore General Hospital, Singapore*

Correspondence should be addressed to Ming Hui Yong; yong.ming.hui@singhealth.com.sg

Academic Editor: Isabella Laura Simone

A 45-year-old male was admitted with severe orthostatic headache secondary to spontaneous intracranial hypotension. He had the site of cerebrospinal fluid (CSF) leakage identified at the anterolateral aspect of the C7-T1 spinal level. He first underwent a conventional posterior-approach cervical epidural blood patch (EBP) which provided immediate relief to the patient's symptoms; however, his symptoms recurred two days later. To better target the anterolateral leakage site, we employed an anterior-approach EBP under computed tomography (CT) guidance. After this attempt, the patient experienced complete relief of his symptoms, and the headache eventually resolved.

1. Background

Spontaneous intracranial hypotension (SIH) is a condition first described in 1938. SIH often occurs secondary to cerebrospinal fluid (CSF) leakage at the spinal level. Symptoms of SIH include orthostatic headaches, which can be associated with other symptoms including nausea, vomiting, photophobia, cranial nerve palsies, visual blurring, tinnitus, and neck stiffness [1]. On magnetic resonance imaging (MRI) of the brain, pachymeningeal enhancement, subdural hygroma, brain sagging with cerebellar tonsillar descent, pituitary enlargement, or venous sinus dilation is commonly visualized [1–3]. MRI of the spine, computed tomography (CT) or MRI myelogram, and radionuclide cisternography can also help to identify the site of leakage [3]. Treatment of SIH can be conservative with bed rest, hydration, caffeine, and analgesics. If symptoms persist or are severe, epidural blood patches (EBPs) are another treatment option. We present a case of a middle-aged male diagnosed with spontaneous intracranial hypotension, with an identified site of CSF leakage at the anterolateral aspect of the C7-T1 spinal level, who had no or minimal relief from conventional posterior-approach cervical EBP. He eventually underwent a more targeted anterior-approach cervical EBP approach. Our case demonstrates the feasibility and efficacy of an anterior-approach cervical EBP for SIH patients whose sites of CSF leak are anteriorly located.

2. Case Presentation

A 45-year-old Indian gentleman with a past medical history of hyperlipidemia and migraine presented to an inpatient Neurology ward of a tertiary hospital, complaining of a one-month history of headache that had begun after cervical manipulation during a neck massage. He complained of pain over the occipital region and over the vertex which radiated down the neck. This pain was shooting in nature at the occipital region and pressing in nature at the vertex. The onset was not thunderclap in nature. Most significantly, the pain had an orthostatic quality, worsening in intensity within a few minutes of sitting or standing and improving within a few minutes of lying down. Otherwise, the patient did not experience nausea, vomiting, limb weakness or numbness, or other focal neurological symptoms. He had no fever, photophobia, nor phonophobia. He had been treated previously with various analgesics which did not provide any relief. His last migraine headache had occurred more than ten years ago and differed in character from his current headache. A full neurological examination did not demonstrate any focal neurological deficits.

2.1. Investigations. The patient underwent extensive investigations to confirm the diagnosis of SIH and the site of the CSF leak. Contrast-enhanced MRI of the brain showed typical features of SIH (Figures 1(a)–1(c)): diffuse pachymeningeal enhancement, distension of the cerebral venous sinuses, bilateral subdural hygromas, reduced pre-pontine space, and slit-like ventricles. Contrast-enhanced MRI of the cervical spine showed supporting imaging features of intracranial hypotension, including a small thecal sac and prominent epidural veins in the cervical spine (Figure 2); no epidural CSF fluid collection was visualized.

To localize the CSF leak, the patient underwent radionuclide cisternography, which was more readily available in our institution compared to CT or MRI myelography. Intrathecal injection of technetium (Tc-99m) diethylenetriamine pentaacetic acid (DTPA) was administered, with serial static planar images acquired at 1.5-hour, 2-hour, and 3-hour intervals as per our institute's protocol. Within this time, the site of CSF leak was identified (and the study did not have to be prolonged up to 24 hours): his cisternogram showed tracer tracking out to the right of the upper cervical/lower thoracic vertebrae as early as 1.5 hours (Figure 3(a)). Supplementary single-photon emission computed tomography (SPECT) of the cervical and thoracic spine at the 2-hour interval showed focal extrathecal tracer accumulation at the right anterolateral aspect of the C7/T1 level, likely representing CSF tracking out from the right C7/T1 neural foramen (Figure 3(b)).

2.2. Treatment. Conventional treatment with bed rest, intravenous hydration, analgesia, and encouraged caffeine intake was initiated; however, this provided only minimal pain relief for the patient. Subsequently, the patient underwent a conventional posterior-approach cervical EBP performed by an experienced anaesthetist. At the right paramedian cervical region, 25 mL of autologous blood was injected into the epidural space at the C7/T1 level of the spine from the posterior approach, under fluoroscopy guidance (Figure 4). He was not on aspirin or anticoagulant therapy.

Following the procedure, the patient reported improvement of the headache by the next day and complete resolution of symptoms upon discharge. However, his headache later recurred 2 days after the initial EBP procedure and continued to increase in severity. He was rehospitalized 12 days after the EBP. A CT-brain performed showed persistent slit-like ventricles and increased size of bilateral subdural collections with iso-to-hyperdensity suggestive of interval bleeding and interval worsening of his SIH. At this point in time, the patient was extremely distressed by his symptoms—in addition to being severe and prolonged, they limited his activities greatly. While he agreed to a repeat EBP attempt, he found difficulty in accepting the possibility of yet another relapse after requiring further epidural blood patch attempts or even consideration of surgical intervention should his symptoms remain refractory to EBPs.

The patient underwent a second cervical EBP 20 days after the first EBP, which was now CT-guided and performed by an interventional radiologist who used an anterior approach to better target the right anterolateral site of the C7/T1 CSF leakage. The choice of the anterior transthyroid approach afforded the greatest precision to target the CSF leak site, and a 22G spinal needle was inserted via the transforaminal route followed by injection of a total of 7 mL of autologous blood around the C7/T1 epidural space under CT guidance (Figure 5).

2.3. Outcome and Follow-Up. The patient tolerated the procedure well with no neurological deficits or bleeding complications post-procedure. The patient experienced immediate and sustained improvement in his headache after the second EBP, and an interval MRI brain performed three weeks later showed partial resolution of the SIH changes. One month after the second EBP, the patient reported complete resolution of the headache and has returned to work since. More than a year after the targeted EBP procedure, the patient reported no headache recurrence, reflecting the successful outcome of this procedure.

3. Discussion

In this case report, we report a patient with SIH due to CSF leak after neck manipulation who needed two EBPs, the second being an anterior approach prior to of resolution of symptoms. The suspicion of SIH arises in patients with headaches that are exacerbated by upright posture and improved in the supine position [1]. Contrary to its name, SIH does not always occur spontaneously and may be classified as either primary SIH where no attributable cause is found or secondary SIH due to a provocative cause, such as spinal trauma, diagnostic/therapeutic spinal procedures like lumbar puncture, chiropractic manipulation, and degenerative spine disease [2]. The etiology of a spinal CSF leak can also be classified as resulting from a dural tear (type 1), meningeal diverticulum (type 2), or CSF-venous fistula (type 3) [4]. Our patient likely developed SIH from a dural tear following chiropractic manipulation of the cervical spine.

MRI brain generally has radiological features of low CSF pressure such as tonsillar herniation, flattening of the pons along the clivus, and displacement of the optic chiasm as primary features of SIH. It is postulated that the pachymeningeal enhancement and subdural effusion reported in few cases of SIH are secondary features that are due to dilated leaky meningeal vessels and rupture of bridging veins, respectively, which are thought to be due to the downward displacement of the brain due to low CSF pressure [3, 5, 6]. In SIH, CSF examination may be

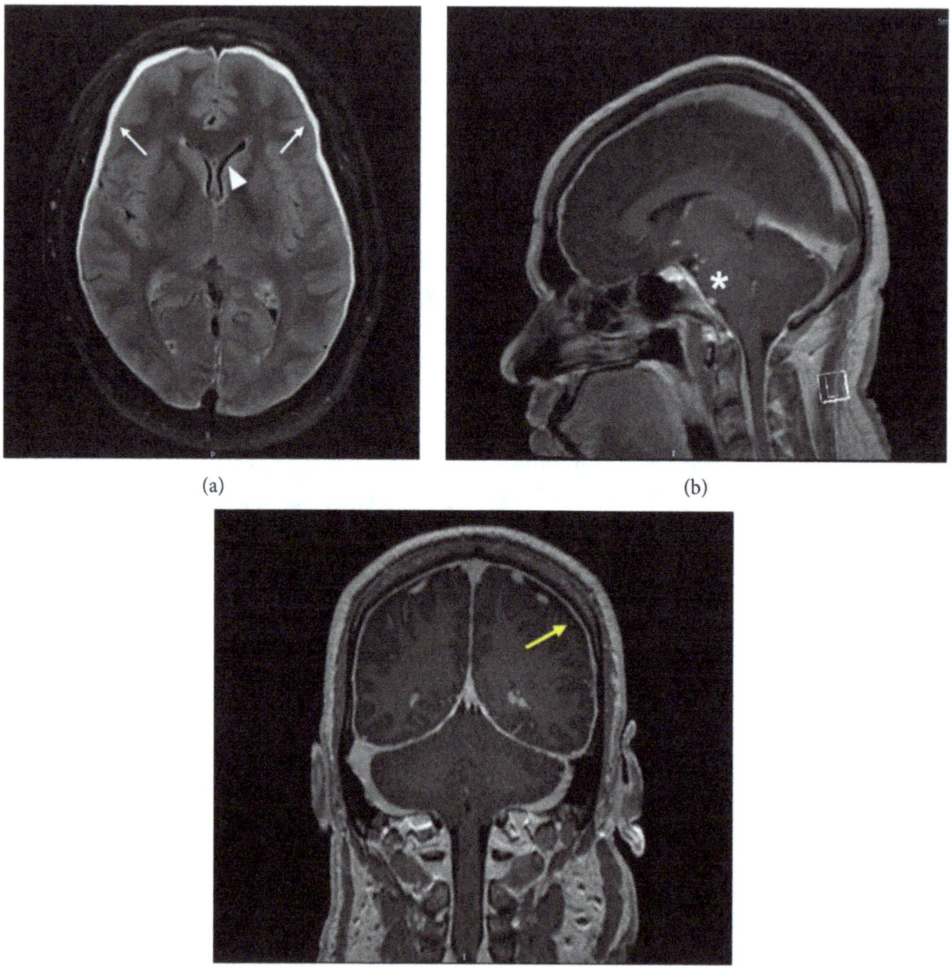

(a) (b) (c)

Figure 1: MRI of the brain showing features of intracranial hypotension. (a) FLAIR: bilateral subdural hygromas (white arrows) and slit-like ventricle (white arrowhead). (b, c) Post-contrast: reduced pre-pontine space (asterisk) and diffuse pachymeningeal enhancement (yellow arrow).

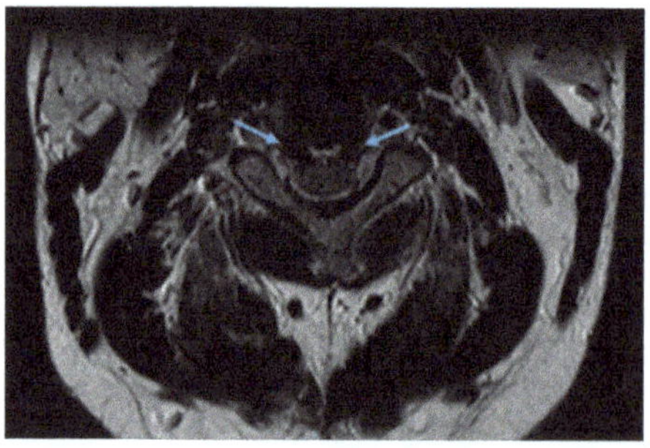

Figure 2: Contrast-enhanced MRI of the cervical spine, axial view. T2-weighted image: prominent epidural veins (blue arrows).

unremarkable or show mild pleocytosis (due to meningeal hyperemia associated with movement of cells into the subarachnoid space [7]) or mildly raised protein.

In patients with SIH, the lower cervical spine and upper thoracic spine are the most common sites of CSF leak [3]. Once SIH is suspected, imaging modalities such as CT/MRI myelography and radionuclide cisternography are often used to identify the site of CSF leak [3]. The characteristic finding is paradural extravasation of the radioisotope, as was observed in our patient. In some cases, often a slow cephalad extension of the radioisotope is noted, which indirectly signifies volume loss of CSF [8].

SIH can be conservatively managed by bed rest, analgesia, increased fluid intake, increased caffeine, or increased salt uptake. If conservative treatment fails, an EBP can be offered. EBP is thought to be effective in stopping the orthostatic headaches by the injected autologous blood in the epidural space forming a gelatinous seal at the site of leak and by increasing the intrathecal pressure which in turn can relieve the symptoms of CSF hypovolemia [9, 10].

For our patient with a clear right C7/T1 CSF leak, we had to decide between treating him upfront with a "blind" EBP or with an EBP targeted at the CSF leak site. Conventionally, "blind" EBP at the lumbar region was the first choice for patients who failed conservative treatment; however, lumbar EBPs may not be theoretically as

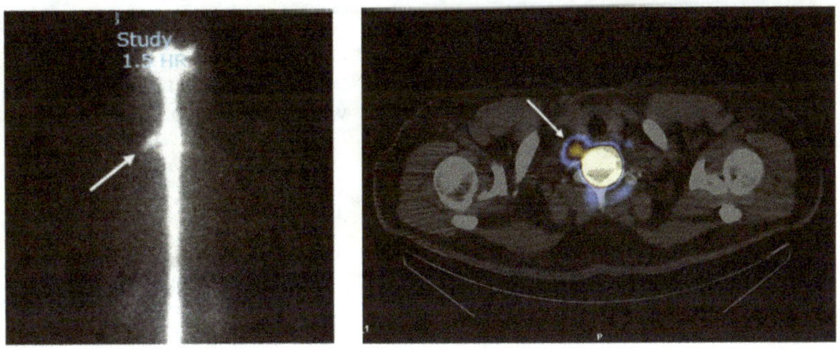

(a) (b)

FIGURE 3: (a) Radionuclide (Tc-99 DTPA) cisternogram at 3-hour interval showed Tc-99 DTPA tracking out at the right of the upper cervical/thoracic vertebrae (white arrow). (b) SPECT at 2-hour time interval, axial view, showed focal extrathecal tracer accumulating at the right anterolateral aspect of the C7/T1 level (white arrow).

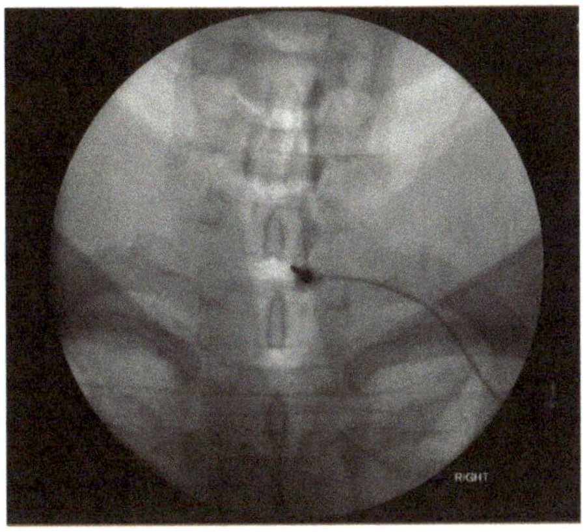

FIGURE 4: Posterior-approach cervical epidural blood patch under fluoroscopy.

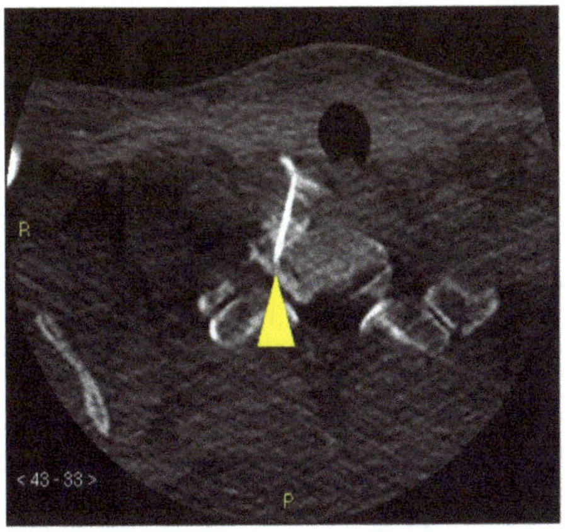

FIGURE 5: CT-guided injection. Axial section showing the tip of the 22G spinal needle at the right C7/T1 foramen. The contrast was injected to confirm flow centrally (yellow arrowhead).

effective if the site of leak is at the cervical or thoracic region. While no randomised controlled trials exist, observational and case series data suggest that targeted EBPs are more efficacious than blind EBPs [9, 11–13]. However, cervical epidural blood patch for our patient would be associated with increased risks, namely, injuries to the nerve roots or spinal cord, the possibility of blood and chemical meningitis, and the risk of injury to critical structures such as the carotid vessels, trachea, and esophagus [10, 14]. Despite these risks, given our patient's distress from severe symptoms, the presence of subdural collections with possibility of progression to developing worsening subdural hematoma and mass effect, and our concerns that a lumbar EBP would not be successful, we first attempted a targeted cervical EBP with a posterior approach by an experienced operator. However, while he had some relief, the relief was not sustained. Given the anterior position of his leak, the second cervical EBP was performed from an anterior approach with CT guidance, with a lower volume of autologous blood injected to minimize the risk of complications, and the procedure was successful in alleviating his symptoms without any side effects.

While targeted EBPs are common in established centers, they are usually from a posterior approach. Reports of anterior-approach cervical EBP for an anteriorly located cervical CSF leak are scarce. Park and Villblanca were the first to report an anterior-approach cervical EBP under fluoroscopic guidance for their patient with refractory severe SIH who had failed 2 prior lumbar EBPs in 2013 [14]. For our patient, CT rather than fluoroscopic guidance was utilized to allow better EBP placement at the exact site of CSF leak visualized on his previous SPECT-CT study and to minimize risk to other surrounding structures such as the thyroid gland that lay in the path of the spinal needle's planned approach. CT guidance can be considered in such cases where visualization of the neck structures is preferred or where a very focal location of the CSF leak to be targeted has been identified in prior CT or MRI spine imaging.

4. Conclusion

To the best of our knowledge, this is one of the few reports in the literature describing the successful use of an anterior-approach cervical epidural blood patch to treat a case of refractory SIH. Our report adds to the literature our experience and supports the feasibility of anterior-approach cervical EBP for effective treatment of SIH due to anterior cervical CSF spinal leaks.

Disclosure

An abstract with a similar title was presented as an E-poster at the 24th World Congress of Neurology 2019 in Dubai. However, our original manuscript and detailed images were not used in any other journal before. Ravindra Singh Shekhawat and Ming Hui Yong are co-first authors.

References

[1] D. G. Walker, "Refractory headache due to spontaneous intracranial hypotension from a CSF leak at C1-2," *Journal of Clinical Neuroscience*, vol. 10, no. 4, pp. 482–485, 2003.

[2] J. Inamasu and B. H. Guiot, "Intracranial hypotension with spinal pathology," *The Spine Journal*, vol. 6, no. 5, pp. 591–599, 2006.

[3] L. Spelle, A. Boulin, L. Pierot, P. Graveleau, and C. Tainturier, "Spontaneous intracranial hypotension: MRI and radionuclide cisternography findings," *Journal of Neurology, Neurosurgery & Psychiatry*, vol. 62, no. 3, pp. 291-292, 1997.

[4] W. I. Schievink, M. M. Maya, S. Jean-Pierre, M. Nuno, R. S. Prasad, and F. G. Moser, "A classification system of spontaneous spinal CSF leaks," *Neurology*, vol. 87, no. 7, pp. 673–679, 2016.

[5] S. Ishihara, S. Fukui, N. Otani et al., "Evaluation of spontaneous intracranial hypotension: assessment on ICP monitoring and radiological imaging," *British Journal of Neurosurgery*, vol. 15, no. 3, pp. 239–241, 2001.

[6] S. C. Pannullo, J. B. Reich, G. Krol, M. Deck, and J. B. Posner, "MRI changes in intracranial hypotension," *Neurology*, vol. 43, no. 5, pp. 919–926, 1993.

[7] S. A. Renowden, R. Gregory, N. Hyman, and D. Hilton-Jones, "Spontaneous intracranial hypotension," *Journal of Neurology, Neurosurgery & Psychiatry*, vol. 59, no. 5, pp. 511–515, 1995.

[8] B. Mokri, "Radioisotope cisternography in spontaneous CSF leaks: interpretations and misinterpretations," *Headache: The Journal of Head and Face Pain*, vol. 54, no. 8, pp. 1358–1368, 2014.

[9] D. Kantor and S. D. Silberstein, "Cervical epidural blood patch for low CSF pressure headaches," *Neurology*, vol. 65, no. 7, p. 1138, 2005.

[10] S. M. Hayek, M. Fattouh, T. Dews, L. Kapural, O. Malak, and N. Mekhail, "Successful treatment of spontaneous cerebrospinal fluid leak headache with fluoroscopically guided epidural blood patch: a report of four cases," *Pain Medicine*, vol. 4, no. 4, pp. 373–378, 2003.

[11] E. Wang and D. Wang, "Successful treatment of spontaneous intracranial hypotension due to prominent cervical cerebrospinal fluid leak with cervical epidural blood patch," *Pain Medicine*, vol. 16, no. 5, pp. 1013–1018, 2015.

[12] K. I. Cho, H. S. Moon, H. J. Jeon, K. Park, and D. S. Kong, "Spontaneous intracranial hypotension: efficacy of radiologic targeting vs. blind blood patch," *Neurology*, vol. 76, no. 13, pp. 1139–1144, 2011.

[13] K. A. Smith, "Spontaneous intracranial hypotension: targeted or blind blood patch," *Journal of Clinical Neuroscience*, vol. 25, pp. 10–12, 2016.

[14] J. K. Park and J. P. Villablanca, "Feasibility of placement of an anterior cervical epidural blood patch for spontaneous intracranial hypotension," *American Journal of Neuroradiology*, vol. 34, no. 8, pp. E84–E86, 2013.

12

Photosensitive Epilepsy and Polycystic Ovary Syndrome as Manifestations of MERRF

Josef Finsterer

Klinik Landstrasse, Vienna, Austria

Correspondence should be addressed to Josef Finsterer; fipaps@yahoo.de

Academic Editor: Peter Berlit

Objectives. Although endocrinologic involvement and epilepsy are frequent features of myoclonic epilepsy with ragged-red fibers (MERRF), polycystic ovary syndrome (PCOS) and photosensitive epilepsy have not been reported. *Case Report.* A 32-year-old female was diagnosed with MERRF at age 19 y upon presence of the four canonical features and the variant m.8344A > G in *MT-TK (tRNA (Lys))* (blood heteroplasmy rate: 50%). She experienced recurrent photosensitive focal and generalised seizures since age 19 y, which could be triggered by flickering light or by looking at small stones, leaves, or dirty snow on the ground. Since the last 42 months, she was seizure-free upon levetiracetam (4000 mg/d), clonazepam (1.5 mg/d), and topiramate (25 mg/d). Additionally, she suffered from secondary amenorrhoea since adolescence. She was married between ages 19 y and 25 y but did not get pregnant. PCOS was diagnosed and treated with desogestrel plus estradiol. Nonetheless, the course was progressive, particularly with regard to ataxia, myocloni, and myopathy. *Conclusions.* The phenotypic spectrum of MERRF is broader than anticipated and may additionally include PCOS and photosensitive epilepsy. PCOS in MERRF may respond to hormone substitution and photosensitive epilepsy to levetiracetam, clonazepam, and topiramate.

1. Introduction

Myoclonic epilepsy with ragged-red fibers (MERRF) is a rare syndromic mitochondrial disorder (MID) due to currently 26 mutations in 15 different genes [1]. The most frequent of these mutations is the variant m.8344A > G in *MT-TK* (*tRNA* (*Lys*)) [1]. Although MERRF is clinically characterised by the four canonical features, ataxia, epilepsy, myoclonus, and myopathy [1–3], it is a multisystem disorder with a much broader phenotypic spectrum (MERRF-plus) [1, 2]. Organs affected in addition to the brain and the muscle in MERRF-plus include the peripheral nerves, eyes, ears, heart, gastrointestinal tract, or the endocrine organs [1]. Although involvement of the brain and endocrine system in MERRF-plus is well appreciated [3, 4], polycystic ovary syndrome (PCOS) and photosensitive epilepsy have not been reported as a phenotypic manifestation of MERRF-plus.

2. Case Report

The patient is a 32-year-old Caucasian female, of height 166 cm and weight 50 kg, with uneventful early development who became noteworthy at age 7 y because of poor school performance due to impaired memory and concentration. She had nocturnal enuresis until age 14 y and menarche at age 13 y with normal periods thereafter. At age 17 y, recurrent, spontaneous myocloni of all four limbs began. A first generalised tonic-clonic seizure occurred at age 19 y. The postictal period was characterised by severe muscle weakness and muscle aching during 24 h. Electroencephalography (EEG) recording revealed epileptiform discharges in the frontocentral regions under hyperventilation and a decreased photoparoxysmal threshold. Valproic acid (VPA) was begun.

Despite VPA, seizures recurred with a frequency of 1-2 seizures/month. In addition to generalised seizures, she

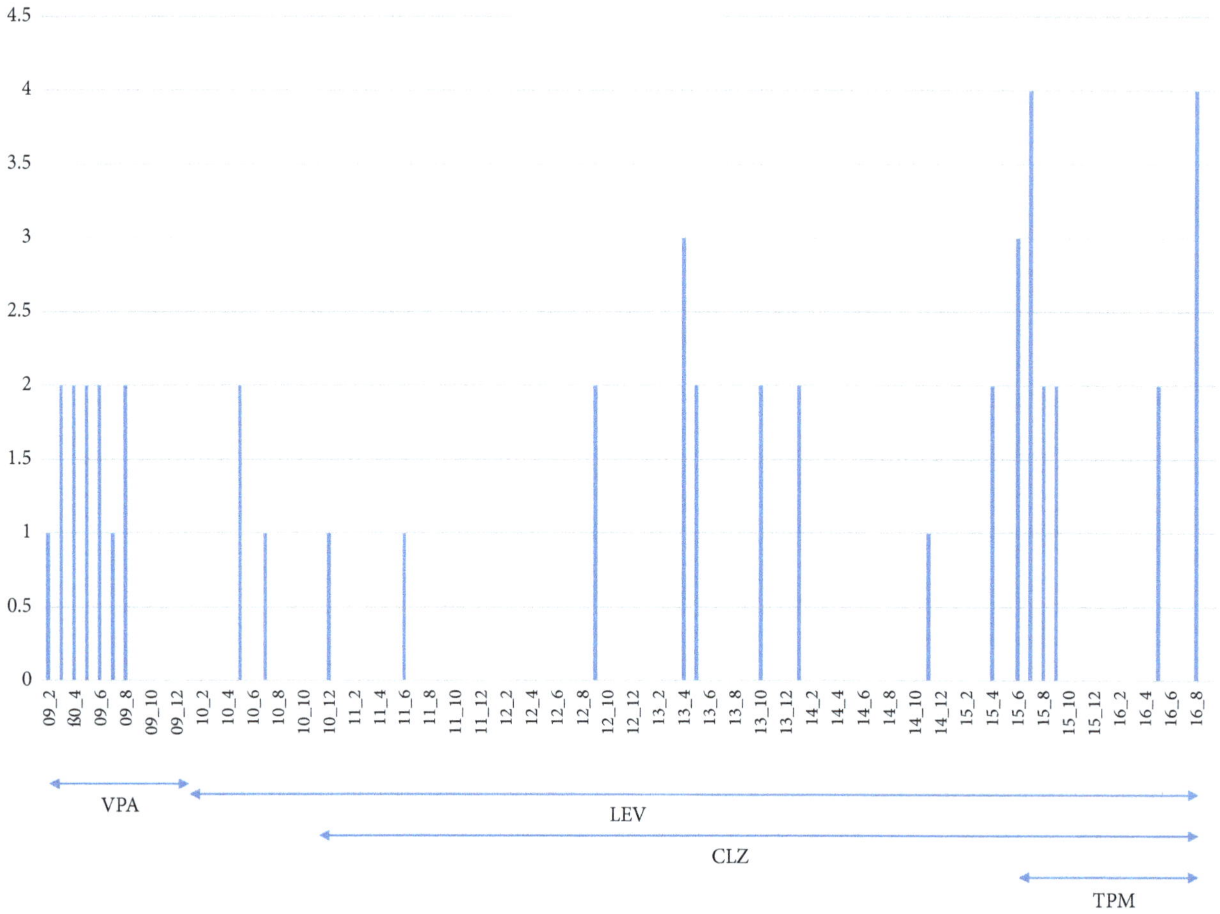

Figure 1: Frequency of focal and generalised seizures since onset at age 19 y in the index patient (1): focal seizure, (2): one generalised seizure, (3): two generalised seizures, (4): three generalised seizures per day).

rarely experienced focal seizures (Figure 1). Seizures could be triggered by flickering light or by looking at small stones, leaves, or dirty snow on the ground. Walking safely for 1 km with one stop was possible only after sunset. Nerve conduction studies revealed a mixed axonal/demyelinating neuropathy. Electromyography was myogenic. MRI of the brain at ages 19 y, 21 y, and 28 y revealed cerebellar atrophy exclusively. At age 20 y, VPA was replaced by levetiracetam (LEV) 3000 mg/d. Genetic work-up at age 21 y revealed the variant m.8344A > G with a heteroplasmy rate of 50% in blood lymphocytes. EEG at age 24 y revealed bilaterally synchronous spike-wave complexes in the occipital area. Flickering light triggered generalised, bilaterally synchronous spike-wave and polyspike-wave complexes (Figure 2). The patient had been married between ages 19 y and 25 y but never became pregnant. Work-up for infertility at age 20 y revealed a PCOS for which she received desogestrel (150 μg/d) + estradiol (20 μg/d) twice a year for three months since age 26 y. Since age 27 y, ataxic gait worsened such that she required support from another person for walking. Elevated serum lactate levels up to double the upper reference limits were noted for the first time. At age 27 y, topiramate (TPM) was added. Seizures had not recurred during 42 months prior to the last follow-up at age 32 y (Figure 1).

The family history was positive for easy fatigability (mother (48 yo), brother (26 yo), great aunt from mother's side), photosensitivity (mother, grandmother from mother's side, 2 great aunts from mother's side, 2 aunts and 1 uncle from mother's side), hand tremor (brother), myocloni (grandmother from mother's side, 2 aunts, 1 uncle, 2 cousins from the mother's side), seizures (1 great aunt from the mother's side, 1 cousin), Parkinsonism (1 great aunt from the mother's side, 1 uncle), ataxia (2 great aunts from the mother's side), and hypothyroidism (mother) (Figure 3). The mother felt unpleasant with flickering light and when looking at many stones, leaves, or dirty snow on the ground. Both mother and brother of the index patient carried the m.8344A > G variant, the mother had a heteroplasmy rate of 40% and the brother was homoplasmic. Clinical neurologic exam of the index patient at age 32 y revealed cognitive impairment, ataxia, photosensitivity, dysarthria, uncoordinated speech, myocloni of upper limbs, generalised wasting, absent tendon reflexes, and gait disturbance. The current medication included LEV (4000 mg/d), clonazepam (CLZ)

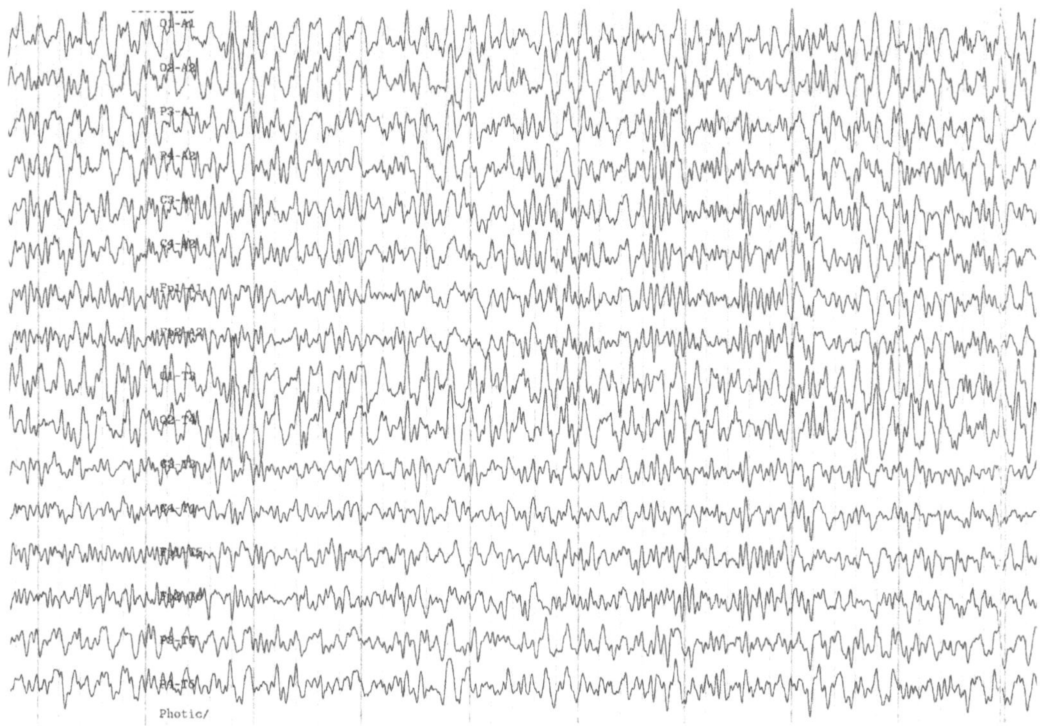

Figure 2: EEG under flickering light at age 24 y showing generalised, bilaterally synchronous spike-wave and polyspike-wave complexes.

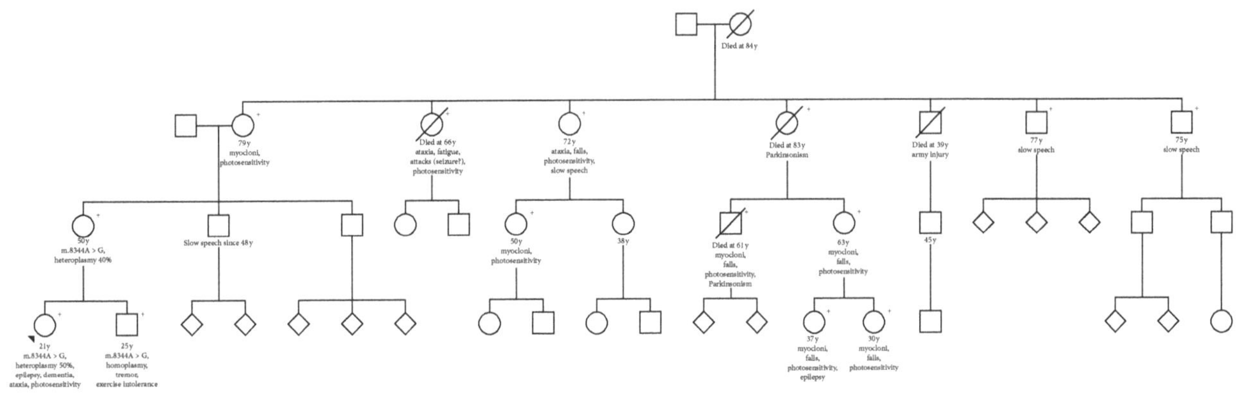

Figure 3: Pedigree of the index patient's family (the "+" indicates that the individual was clinically affected).

(1.5 mg/d), TPM (25 mg/d), coenzyme-Q (200 mg/d), L-carnitine (2 g/d), and vitamin-E (400 mg/d).

3. Discussion

The presented patient is interesting for the following aspects. First, the patient had MERRF, which is still a rare MID syndrome. MERRF was diagnosed upon presence of all four canonical features and the m.8344A > G variant. The index patient had inherited the disease from her mother who was only mildly affected. The low heteroplasmy rate of 50% does not exclude pathogenicity, as it had been determined only in blood.

Second, the patient had photosensitive epilepsy, which has not been reported in MERRF. It is characterised by the occurrence of seizures after exposure to certain visual stimuli. Many patients experience an aura prior to onset of the seizure or feel odd sensations before the seizure occurs [5]. Interestingly, the same triggers that induced epilepsy in the index patient induced only an unpleasant feeling in the mother. Although the mother had never recorded an EEG, it is conceivable that the unpleasant feeling actually represents focal seizures.

Third, the index patient had PCOS, which has not been reported in MERRF. PCOS was speculated to have been triggered by VPA, as has been previously reported [6], but the question if VPA truly causes PCOS is still under debate [7, 8]. A strong argument against VPA as the trigger of PCOS is that PCOS has been reported in MIDs other than MERRF and not under VPA [9, 10]. Thus, it is more likely that PCOS in the index patient was a manifestation of the underlying MID than a side effect of VPA. A further argument against VPA is that many MID patients received VPA without developing PCOS. Whether VPA enhanced the preexisting endocrine problem remains speculative.

Fourth, homoplasmy of the m.8344A > G variant has been only rarely reported [11, 12]. Whether patients carrying a homoplasmic m.8344A > G variant are more severely affected than heteroplasmic patients is unknown but the few cases available suggest that onset is earlier and the phenotype is more severe in homoplasmic than heteroplasmic patients.

Limitations of the study are that no muscle biopsy had been taken, that heteroplasmy was determined only in blood lymphocytes, that no prospective investigations for multisystem involvement had been carried out, that first-degree relatives were not systematically investigated, and that the progression of the disease had been only faultily monitored.

Overall, this case shows that the phenotypic spectrum of MERRF-plus is broader than anticipated and may additionally include PCOS and photosensitive epilepsy. PCOS in MERRF may respond to hormone substitution and photosensitive epilepsy to LEV, CLZ, and TPM.

Authors' Contributions

J. F. is responsible for design, literature search, discussion, writing of the first draft, and final approval.

References

[1] J. Finsterer, S. Zarrouk-Mahjoub, and J. M. Shoffner, "Merrf classification: implications for diagnosis and clinical trials," *Pediatric Neurology*, vol. 80, pp. 8–23, 2018.

[2] S. DiMauro and M. Hirano, *GeneReviews®*, University of Washington, Seattle, WA, USA, 2003, http://www.ncbi.nlm.nih.gov/books/NBK1520/.

[3] J. Finsterer, "Pharmacotherapeutic management of epilepsy in merrf syndrome," *Expert Opinion on Pharmacotherapy*, vol. 20, no. 10, pp. 1289–1297, 2019.

[4] N. Ohkoshi, A. Ishii, N. Shiraiwa, S. Shoji, and K. Yoshizawa, "Dysfunction of the hypothalamic-pituitary system in mitochondrial encephalomyopathies," *Journal of Medicine*, vol. 29, pp. 13–29, 1998.

[5] A. Martins Da Silva and B. Leal, "Photosensitivity and epilepsy: current concepts and perspectives-a narrative review," *Seizure*, vol. 50, pp. 209–218, 2017.

[6] Y. Kawakami, S. Fujii, G. Ishikawa, A. Sekiguchi, A. Nakai, and M. Takase, "Valproate-induced polycystic ovary syndrome in a girl with epilepsy: a case study," *Journal of Nippon Medical School*, vol. 85, no. 5, pp. 287–290, 2018.

[7] H. Goldberg-Stern, E. Yaacobi, M. Phillip, and L. De Vries, "Endocrine effects of valproic acid therapy in girls with epilepsy: a prospective study," *European Journal of Paediatric Neurology*, vol. 18, no. 6, pp. 759–765, 2014.

[8] D. Gotlib, R. Ramaswamy, J. E. Kurlander, A. DeRiggi, and M. Riba, "Valproic acid in women and girls of childbearing age," *Current Psychiatry Reports*, vol. 19, no. 9, p. 58, 2017.

[9] Y. Ding, B.-H. Xia, C.-J. Zhang, and G.-C. Zhuo, "Mitochondrial tRNALeu (UUR) C3275T, tRNAGln T4363C and tRNALys A8343G mutations may be associated with PCOS and metabolic syndrome," *Gene*, vol. 642, pp. 299–306, 2018.

[10] J. Finsterer and S. Zarrouk-Mahjoub, "Polycystic ovary syndrome in mitochondrial disorders due mtDNA or nDNA variants," *American Journal of Translational Research*, vol. 10, no. 1, pp. 13–15, 2018.

[11] P. Buda, D. Piekutowska-Abramczuk, A. Karkucińska-Więckowska et al., "Drop attacks as first clinical symptoms in a child carrying MTTK m.8344A > G mutation," *Folia Neuropathologica*, vol. 4, pp. 347–354, 2013.

[12] Y. Monden, M. Mori, M. Kuwajima, T. Goto, T. Yamagata, and M. Y. Momoi, "Late-onset leigh syndrome with myoclonic epilepsy with ragged-red fibers," *Brain and Development*, vol. 35, no. 6, pp. 582–585, 2013.

13

An Unusual Cause of Cranial Dural Thickening

Jing Ming Yeo,[1] **Donald MacArthur**,[2] **Jillian Davis**,[3] **Ian Scott**,[3] **and Bruno Gran**[4]

[1]*Department of Neurology, Queen's Medical Centre, Nottingham University Hospitals NHS Trust, Derby Road, Lenton, Nottingham NG7 2UH, UK*
[2]*Department of Neurosurgery, Nottingham University Hospitals NHS Trust, Nottingham NG7 2UH, UK*
[3]*Department of Pathology, Nottingham University Hospitals NHS Trust, Nottingham NG7 2UH, UK*
[4]*Department of Neurology, Nottingham University Hospitals NHS Trust, Nottingham NG7 2UH, UK*

Correspondence should be addressed to Bruno Gran; bruno.gran@nuh.nhs.uk

Academic Editor: Ritsuo Hashimoto

We describe an unusual cause of cranial dural thickening in an elderly female with a chronic meningeal inflammatory process. A 70-year-old ethnically Chinese, Singaporean female presented with a history of chronic daily headache with no other meningeal signs. Serial MRI brains showed progressive pachymeningeal and leptomeningeal enhancement in the left frontal region with underlying vasogenic oedema, similar appearances in the right frontal region to a lesser extent, and persistent inflammatory changes in her bilateral paranasal sinuses. Investigative work-up showed a chronically raised ESR with a normal CRP, negative ANCA, and a chronically raised serum IgA kappa paraprotein. Bone marrow trephine biopsy was suggestive of a low level plasma cell disorder. Olfactory cleft biopsy showed no evidence of IgG4-related disease or vasculitis and no significant plasma cell infiltrate. Histopathological examination from a meningeal biopsy revealed a diagnosis of an en-plaque meningioma (the WHO, 2016; Grade I) causing an unusual granulomatous reaction. We discuss the radiological and histological relations of this rare form of meningioma. Clinicians can consider en-plaque meningioma in the differential diagnosis of linear dural thickening and enhancement.

1. Introduction

Involvement of cranial dura mater often steers one to look for inflammatory causes such as granulomatosis with polyangiitis, neurosarcoidosis, rheumatoid, or IgG4-related disease; infective causes such as syphilis, mycobacterial or fungal pathology; or malignancy such as dural metastases or lymphoma [1]. Here, we describe a case of an elderly female with a slowly progressive cranial pachy- and leptomeningeal process revealed on meningeal biopsy to be an en-plaque meningioma causing an unusual granulomatous reaction.

2. Case Presentation

A 70-year-old ethnically Chinese female presented via the Emergency Department with a 2-week history of shortness of breath, productive cough, and confusion. A chest radiograph showed focal consolidation, and she was treated with antibiotics for community-acquired pneumonia and delirium. By day seven, her confusion had resolved. As part of the investigative work-up of her confusion, she received a CT head which showed a left frontal extra-axial lesion with patchy calcification (Figure 1). An outpatient MRI brain a month later demonstrated pachymeningeal and leptomeningeal enhancement bifrontally, with more marked changes on the left with underlying vasogenic oedema, and inflammatory opacification of the paranasal sinuses (Figure 2).

She was subsequently admitted to the neurology ward for further assessment. She reported a one year exacerbation in the intensity of her chronic left frontal headache which she has had since her 30 s. They were described as a left frontal ache with migrainous features of nausea and photophobia, with no raised pressure features. She also described a reduced sense of smell and taste for 20 years which transiently improves on receiving prednisolone for

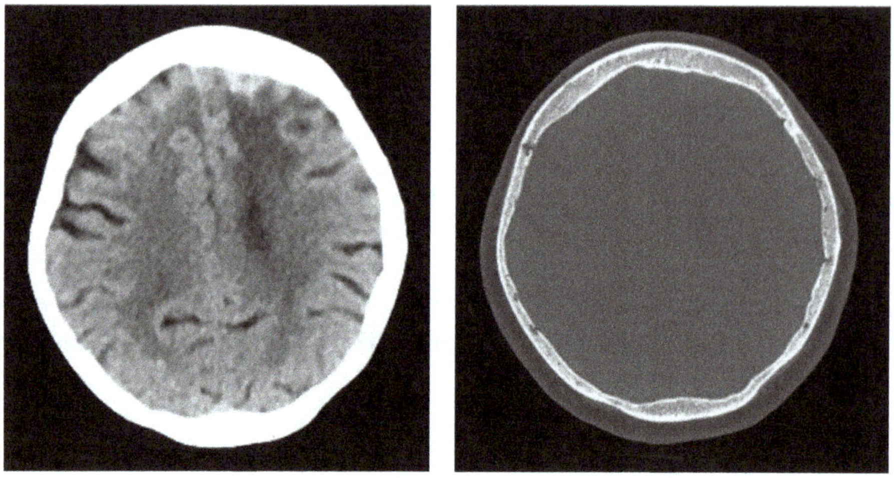

(a) (b)

Figure 1: CT head: (a) left frontal extra-axial lesion with patchy calcification and vasogenic oedema; (b) CT bone window setting showing osteopenia but no bony erosion or hyperostosis.

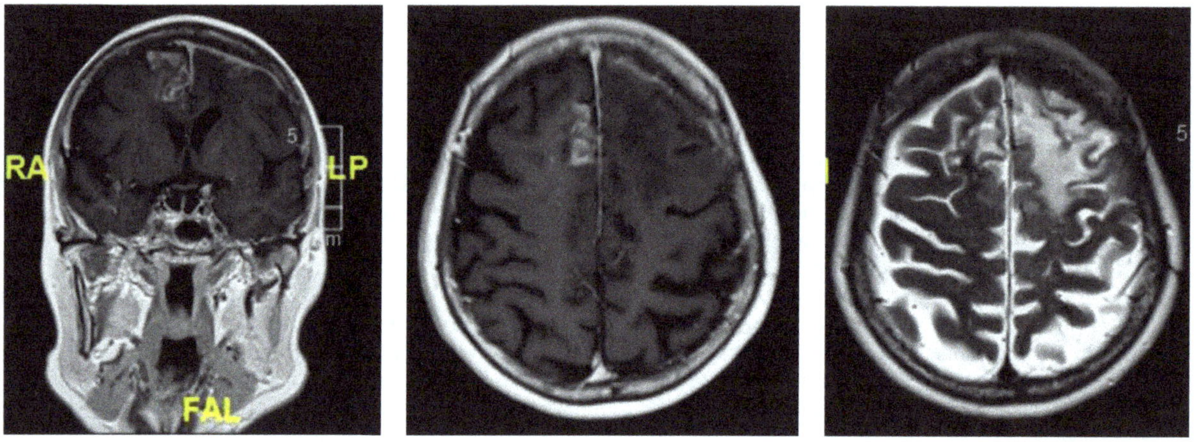

(a) (b) (c)

Figure 2: MRI brain. (a, b) Coronal and axial T1 postcontrast images showing pachymeningeal enhancement in the left frontal region and leptomeningeal enhancement in the left superior and middle frontal sulci, with vasogenic oedema. A nodular leptomeningeal enhancement is noted within the right parafalcine and superior frontal sulci with minimal underlying vasogenic oedema. There was no diffusion restriction. (c) Axial FLAIR image showing the extent of the vasogenic oedema.

exacerbation of asthma. There were no systemic features of arthralgia, weight loss, fevers, rash, or haemoptysis. Past medical history included childhood asthma, allergic contact dermatitis, and hypertension. Medication history included steroid and salbutamol inhalers, enalapril, and paracetamol. She was born in Singapore and has been a resident in the UK for 40 years. Neurological examination was normal with no nuchal rigidity, ophthalmic abnormalities, or cranial nerve signs.

Further investigations revealed a chronically raised ESR (35–63 mm/h) for the past eight years with a normal CRP. She also had a chronically raised serum total IgE (137 kU/L) with a normal eosinophil count. Serum ANA, ANCA, rheumatoid factor, double-stranded DNA, anti-Ro, La, Sm, RNP, Jo1, and Scl-70 were negative. She had a serum IgA kappa paraprotein band of 14 g/L with normal serum-free light-chain ratio, beta2-microglobulin, renal function, calcium, and albumin levels. Serum IgG subclasses including IgG4 were normal. Serum fungal and cerebrospinal fluid (CSF) tuberculosis cultures were negative. Two sets of CSF examination showed normal cell count, protein and glucose levels, negative PCR for herpes simplex, varicella zoster and enteroviruses, and no neoplastic cells. CT chest, abdomen, and pelvis were normal. CT sinus showed chronic rhinosinusitis, and an olfactory cleft biopsy showed inflammatory mucosal changes with no evidence of IgG4-related disease or vasculitis. Bone marrow biopsy showed 10% plasma cells on trephine biopsy and 7% plasma cells on aspirate, and borderline between monoclonal gammopathy of uncertain significance (MGUS) and myeloma. MRI whole body showed diffuse osteopenia but no active myelomatous lesions.

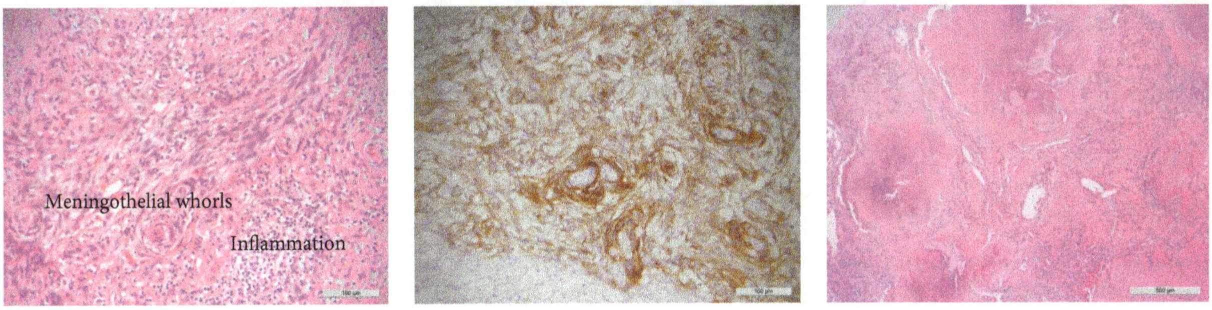

(a) (b) (c)

Figure 3: Histopathological examination from left frontal meningeal biopsy: (a) H&E stain demonstrating meningothelial whorls and associated chronic inflammation, (b) epithelial membrane antigen (EMA) stain confirming the meningothelial phenotype, and (c) H&E stain showing necrobiotic granulomata at the periphery of the lesion.

Serial MRI brains over two years showed a slow progression in the left frontal convexity pachymeningeal and leptomeningeal thickening and enhancement and bifrontal gliosis. She underwent an open left frontal meningeal biopsy two years into her initial presentation. Histopathological examination revealed a meningothelial neoplasm with a mitotic count of <4/10 high power fields and a low Ki67 labelling index (Figure 3). It also showed the presence of necrobiotic granulomata associated with elastotic degeneration. This was interpreted as an en-plaque meningioma (the WHO, 2016; Grade I) with associated granulomatous and fibroblastic reaction. Immunohistochemistry showed no tumoural expression of GFAP, CD34, STAT6, SMA, Desmin, MUC4, Cam5.2, or MNF116. Bacterial, fungal, and mycobacterial stains were negative.

It was discussed with the patient that she has a benign slow-growing growth within the meninges which occupies much of her left frontal lobe area and it would be difficult to safely remove the whole plaque. She remains under conservative management with serial radiological and clinical monitoring. If the meningeal areas were to grow more as a globular lump with associated symptoms, targeted resection or other forms of localised treatment may be considered.

3. Discussion

This is a case of an elderly female with a chronic meningeal inflammatory process. Her atopic tendency, paranasal sinus involvement, and chronically raised ESR initially raised the possibility of granulomatosis with polyangiitis; however, her serum ANCA was negative. The paranasal sinus inflammation was likely secondary to chronic rhinosinusitis unrelated to the meningeal process. Her IgA kappa paraprotein and bone marrow examination were suggestive of low level plasma cell disorder. However, meningeal involvement in plasma cell disorders often indicates advanced disease and this was inconsistent with the rest of her clinical presentation.

Meningiomas are classically morphologically globular with a rounded body growing inwards from the dura with a wide dural base and a dural tail. En-plaque meningioma constitutes 2–4% of all intracranial meningiomas and is characterised by its sheet-like growth along the meninges and invasion of the dura mater [2]. Due to the lack of an associated mass, they can present a diagnostic challenge. They are commonly found on the sphenoid wing, and only less than 1% grow on the frontal or temporal bones [3, 4]. On CT heads, a higher proportion of en-plaque meningiomas demonstrate hyperostosis compared to classical meningiomas (13 to 49% compared to 4.5%) [5]. Some are thought to be reactive, and others are thought to be due to true tumour growth within the bone inducing periosteal new bone formation [6]. They can also be associated with inward bulging of the skull vault and vasogenic oedema adjacent to the hyperostotic bone [7]. On MRIs, en-plaque meningiomas appear as linear dural thickening with homogenous contrast enhancement due to the presence of tumour cells and chronic inflammation [8].

Despite being locally invasive, en-plaque meningiomas are usually WHO Grade I [9]. Li et al. reported 2 out of 37 cases of sphenoid wing en-plaque meningiomas which turn out to be grade II [10]. Grade I meningiomas without clinical or functional limitations are usually managed conservatively. If there are atypical features, surgical resection of the involved areas including the bone, dura, muscle, intracranial, and intraorbital components is considered. Postoperative radiotherapy is used to reduce the risk of recurrence [11]. Goyal et al. reported that 79% of the 28 patients in his cohort who did not develop tumour recurrence were in the group who received radiotherapy [12]. Park et al. found that progression-free survival at 5 years was significantly higher in patients undergoing postoperative radiotherapy (58.7% versus 44.3%) [11]. Prognosis is generally favourable if excision is complete. However, total removal of sphenoid wing en-plaque meningioma is difficult due to extensive dural and bone involvement, and this corresponds to a high recurrence rate [13].

In cases of diagnostic uncertainty, a meningeal biopsy in consultation with the neurosurgery team can be pivotal in clinching the diagnosis. We suggest that clinicians consider en-plaque meningioma in the differential diagnosis of linear dural thickening and enhancement, particularly in the context of the described clinicoradiological features.

Acknowledgments

The authors would like to thank the patient whose case is reported in this manuscript.

References

[1] Y. C. Lee, Y. C. Chueng, S. W. Hsu, and C. C. Lui, "Idiopathic hypertrophic cranial pachymeningitis: case report with 7 years of imaging follow-up," *American Journal of Neuroradiology*, vol. 24, no. 1, pp. 119–123, 2003.

[2] A. Amirjamshidi, K. Abbasioun, R. S. Amiri, A. Ardalan, and S. M. R. Hashemi, "Lateral orbitotomy approach for removing hyperostosing en plaque sphenoid wing meningiomas. Description of surgical strategy and analysis of findings in a series of 88 patients with long-term follow up," *Surgical Neurology International*, vol. 6, no. 1, p. 79, 2015.

[3] O. De Jesús and M. M. Toledo, "Surgical management of meningioma en plaque of the sphenoid ridge," *Surgical Neurology*, vol. 55, no. 5, pp. 265–269, 2001.

[4] L. D. R. Thompson, J.-P. Bouffard, G. D. Sandberg, and H. Mena, "Primary ear and temporal bone meningiomas: a clinicopathologic study of 36 cases with a review of the literature," *Modern Pathology*, vol. 16, no. 3, pp. 236–245, 2003.

[5] W. F. Doyle and H. Rosegay, "Meningioma en plaque with hyperostosis: case report," *Military Medicine*, vol. 137, no. 5, pp. 196–198, 1972.

[6] D. R. Pieper, O. Al-Mefty, Y. Hanada, and D. Buechner, "Hyperostosis associated with meningioma of the cranial base: secondary changes or tumor invasion," *Neurosurgery*, vol. 44, no. 4, pp. 742–746, 1999.

[7] K. Kim, L. Rogers, and D. Goldblatt, "CT features of hyperostosing meningioma en plaque," *American Journal of Roentgenology*, vol. 149, no. 5, pp. 1017-1023, 1987.

[8] S. Kösling, K. Neumann, and S. Brandt, "CT and MRI of intrinsic space-occupying lesions of the bony skull base," *Radiologe*, vol. 49, no. 7, pp. 598–607, 2009.

[9] K. Basu, K. Majumdar, U. Chatterjee, M. Ganguli, and S. Chatterjee, "En plaque meningioma with angioinvasion," *Indian Journal of Pathology and Microbiology*, vol. 53, no. 2, pp. 319–321, 2010.

[10] Y. Li, J.-T. Shi, Y.-Z. An et al., "Sphenoid wing meningioma en plaque: report of 37 cases," *Chinese Medical Journal*, vol. 122, no. 20, pp. 2423–2427, 2009.

[11] H. J. Park, H.-C. Kang, I. H. Kim et al., "The role of adjuvant radiotherapy in atypical meningioma," *Journal of Neuro-Oncology*, vol. 115, no. 2, pp. 241–247, 2013.

[12] L. K. Goyal, J. H. Suh, D. S. Mohan, R. A. Prayson, J. Lee, and G. H. Barnett, "Local control and overall survival in atypical meningioma: a retrospective study," *International Journal of Radiation Oncology Biology Physics*, vol. 46, no. 1, pp. 57–61, 2000.

[13] N. J. Simas and J. P. Farias, "Sphenoid Wing en plaque meningiomas: surgical results and recurrence rates," *Surgical Neurology International*, vol. 4, no. 1, p. 86, 2013.

14

Longitudinally Extensive Transverse Myelitis: A Sub-Saharan Conundrum

Antonina Obayo,[1] Sylvia Mbugua,[2] and Sayed K. Ali[3]

[1]*Department of Medicine, Aga Khan University, Nairobi, Kenya*
[2]*Neurology, Department of Medicine, Aga Khan University, Nairobi, Kenya*
[3]*Internal Medicine, Department of Medicine, Aga Khan University, Nairobi, Kenya*

Correspondence should be addressed to Sayed K. Ali; sayed.karar@aku.edu

Academic Editor: Isabella Laura Simone

Spinal cord schistosomiasis is a rare, underdiagnosed manifestation of schistosomiasis. We present the case of a 36-year-old male who presented to our institution with a one-week history of low back pain with rapidly progressive lower limb weakness, loss of sensation, and flaccid paraparesis. An MRI of the spine showed a longitudinally extensive transverse myelitis from T6 to L1, with enhancement at the cauda equina region. Further review of the images and serological tests eventually led to diagnosis of spinal schistosomiasis. He was treated with praziquantel and high-dose steroids, with minimal improvement in his symptoms.

1. Introduction

According to the World Health Organization, in 2018, 229 million individuals were estimated to be suffering from schistosomiasis. Schistosomiasis is endemic in 78 countries worldwide. In Kenya, approximately 3 million individuals require preventive chemotherapy for schistosomiasis annually [1]. Schistosomiasis accounts for 1 to 4 percent of spinal cord lesions in sub-Saharan Africa. The prevalence of oviposition in the spinal cord varies among studies, ranging from 0.3% to 13% [2]. The clinical presentation of spinal cord schistosomiasis (SCS) is heterogeneous but often presents with low back pain and lower limb weakness sometimes affecting ambulation. Other symptoms include bladder dysfunction, lower limb paraesthesia, hypoesthesia or anaesthesia, deep tendon reflex abnormalities (hyper-, hypo-, or areflexia), constipation, and sexual impotence [2]. SCS usually presents acutely or subacutely and is classified into three clinical forms: medullary with a predominance of spinal cord involvement, myeloradicular, with mainly spinal cord and nerve root involvement, and conus-cauda equina syndrome, with predominantly conus or cauda equina involvement [2–4]. The diagnosis of SCS is based upon the presentation of neurological symptoms resulting from lesions of the spinal cord, the demonstration of schistosomal infection using microscopy and serological techniques, and the exclusion of other causes of myelopathy [4, 5]. Treatment usually includes antischistosomal drugs with corticosteroids [2, 4–6].

2. Case

A 36-year-old male from central region of Kenya presented to our institution with a 3-day history of back pain, followed by itching and numbness of the feet and ankles. On presentation, his symptoms had progressed to weakness of the lower limbs with inability to walk and he had developed urinary incontinence. He denied speech and swallowing difficulties and reported no weakness of the upper limbs. The patient reported no history of fevers, blurred vision, loss of consciousness, or seizure. He also denied a history of trauma, use of blood thinners, use of illicit drugs (including tobacco and alcohol use), a history of exposure to tuberculosis, or ingestion of raw milk. He did report swimming in a nearby pond for many years. His family history was unremarkable, and he was an only child.

On examination, he had normal vital signs and was conscious and alert. A neurological exam revealed normal cranial nerves. Visual field was also preserved. Examination of both his upper limbs was normal. He had tenderness of the lower back, power grade 4/5 on hip flexors and extensors bilaterally, grade 4/5 and 2/5 on the right and left knee extensors, respectively, and power grade 3/5 and 1/5 on the right and left knee flexors, respectively, and dorsiflexion was grade 1/5 bilaterally. A knee jerk reflex was present on his right lower extremity but reduced on the left. Ankle reflexes were absent bilaterally. Sensory level was present at L2.

His complete blood count and a comprehensive metabolic panel were within normal limits. A lumbar puncture revealed a protein count of 0.97 g/l (0.15–0.45 g/l), with a pleocytosis of 35 mm^3(normal <5). A differential count showed 30% of segmented neutrophils and 70% of lymphocytes. Monocytes, eosinophils, and basophils were absent. The glucose level was normal. Cultures of the cerebrospinal fluids, including for tuberculosis, were negative. Serological test for HIV, herpes virus, and syphilis was also negative. An autoimmune screen including ANA, anti-ds DNA, and ENA was negative. A vasculitis screen and serum angiotensin-converting enzyme were also reported as normal.

His thyroid stimulating hormone, vitamin B12, and folate level were all within normal limits.

An MRI of the spine showed longitudinally extensive transverse myelitis (T2 hyper intense intramedullary signal spanning T6-L1 with enhancement) (Figures 1–3).

Based on his MRI results and clinical symptoms, neuromyelitis optica (NMO) was high on the differential diagnosis. He was initiated on high-dose steroids, methylprednisone one gram intravenously for 5 days. However, his neurological status continued to decline. Five sessions of therapeutic plasma exchange were also attempted with no improvement in his symptoms. Serum and CSF neuromyelitis antibodies and oligoclonal bands as well as serum MOG antibodies (myelin oligodendrocyte glycoprotein) were later reported as negative.

A few days into his hospitalization, his Schistosoma antibody (IgG) titer was reported at at 1 : 80. A subsequent liver ultrasound was reported as normal. He was immediately started on praziquantel at 60 mg/kg/dose and high-dose steroids with minimal improvement in his overall symptoms. He was discharged home with recommendations for home care and aggressive physical therapy.

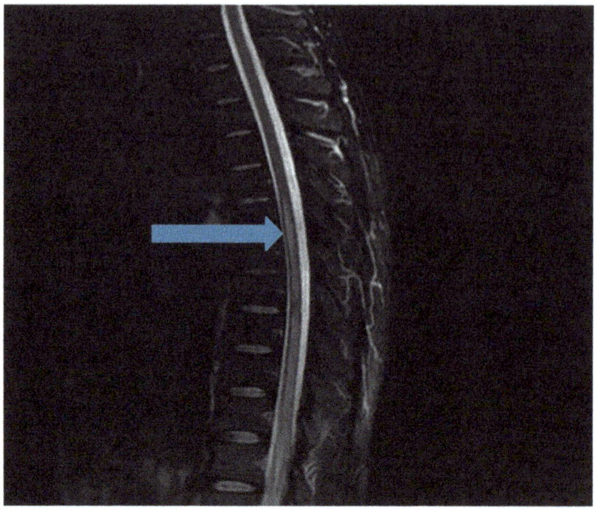

Figure 1: T2 lumbar sagittal, abnormal high signal at the cauda equina.

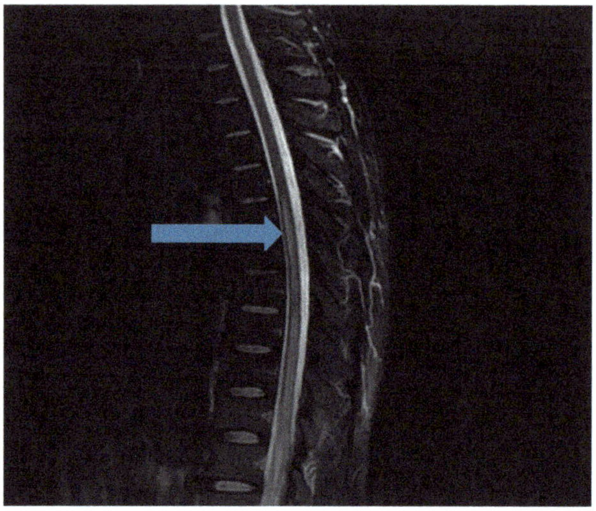

Figure 2: T2 sagittal hyperintense intramedullary signal from T6 to conus medullaris.

3. Discussion

Schistosoma mansoni and *Schistosoma haematobium* are the most common causes of spinal schistosomiasis [2]. Spinal schistosomiasis usually presents as symptoms of spinal cord compression, transverse myelopathy, and painful lumbosacral radiculopathy with low back pain or cauda equina or conus medullaris syndrome [4, 6–9].

Infections like tuberculosis or herpes viruses can present with conus lesions. Inflammatory, vascular, and demyelinating diseases such as multiple sclerosis and neuromyelitis optica can also present in a similar fashion, mostly affecting the cervical and mid-thoracic spine. Spinal cord schistosomiasis differs from the other conditions in that it predominantly affects the lower spinal cord.

In our patient, the diagnosis of spinal schistosomiasis was based on the prevalence of Schistosoma in Kenya, his neurological findings, imaging results, Schistosoma titers, and exclusion of other causes of spinal cord diseases [10]. Even though there was no evidence of hepatosplenic schistosomiasis nor any evidence of schistosomal eggs in urine and faecal samples, this is usually not sufficient to rule out schistosomiasis [2, 10].

Cerebrospinal fluid examination usually shows slight-to-moderate increases in both total protein concentration and lymphocytic count. Eosinophils can present in the CSF in about 50% of patients. A prospective study of 63 patients with schistosomal myeloradiculopathy done in Brazil revealed high total protein concentration in CSF and or

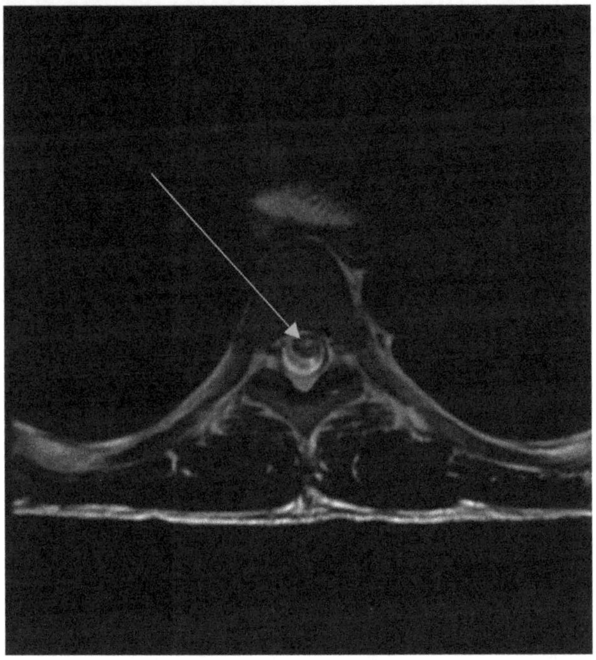

Figure 3: T2 sagittal and axial hyperintense lesion.

pleocytosis in the great majority (95.2%) of the cases [3]. A little more than half (57.4%) of the 63 cases presented with eosinophils in the CSF. In our patient, CSF analysis reflected an inflammatory pattern characterized by increase in the total protein concentration and pleocytosis. Eosinophils were not found.

Enlargement of the lower thoracic spinal cord, swelling of the conus medullaris, and thickening of spinal roots that form the cauda equina are some of the findings on an MRI. Furthermore, high-intensity signal on T2-weighted sequence and heterogeneous enhancement of gadolinium contrast on T1-weighted sequence can be observed in the acute spinal neuroschistosomiasis [2, 5, 10].

A definitive diagnosis of spinal schistosomiasis would require biopsy of the lesion which is associated with potential serious consequences like worsening of neurological signs and symptoms [2]. Due to the risks involved, our patient opted out of a biopsy.

No specific clinical picture is pathognomonic of spinal schistosomiasis. However, conus and cauda syndrome with intramedullary lesion in an endemic area should raise the suspicion of schistosomiasis [2, 3, 11].

Treatment with praziquantel and steroids is associated with clinical improvement, even when started late in the course of the disease [5]. Significant improvement was observed in lumbar and lower limb pain, urinary and intestinal dysfunction, lower limb strength, and ambulation within the first two months of therapy [5]. Some studies have shown that early treatment is better than late treatment [3]. Once treatment is initiated, the outcome of SCS is good [3, 5, 10].

Management of SCS is multidisciplinary and involves the participation of various professionals including nurses, physiotherapists, general clinicians, neurologists, psychologists, and occupational therapists. Physiotherapy remains key for patients with impaired motor functions and must be maintained even after the termination of corticosteroid therapy [10]. In our patient, a follow-up visit 3 months later showed improved bilateral plantar and dorsiflexion of his lower extremities with power grade 2/5 with plantar and dorsiflexion. However, he had power grade 2/5 on hip flexors and extensors bilaterally, grade 2/5 on the bilateral knee extensors respectively, and power grade 1/5 on the bilateral knee flexors.

4. Conclusion

Spinal schistosomiasis is a rare manifestation of schistosomiasis. Definitive diagnosis of spinal cord schistosomiasis is made by detection of the eggs in a spinal cord biopsy or at autopsy. However, a presumptive diagnosis can be made from involvement of the lower spinal cord especially the conus medullaris and cauda equina, suggestive clinical picture, and history or evidence of active schistosomiasis. Exclusion of other conditions is also essential for diagnosis.

References

[1] World Health Organization, *Schistosomiasis*, World Health Organization, 2013, https://www.who.int/en/news-%20room/fact-sheets/detail/schistosomiasis.

[2] T. C. A. Ferrari and P. R. R. Moreira, "Neuroschistosomiasis: clinical symptoms and pathogenesis," *The Lancet Neurology*, vol. 10, no. 9, pp. 853–864, 2011.

[3] T. C. A. Ferrari, P. R. R. Moreira, and A. S. Cunha, "Spinal cord schistosomiasis: a prospective study of 63 cases emphasizing clinical and therapeutic aspects," *Journal of Clinical Neuroscience*, vol. 11, no. 3, pp. 246–253, 2004.

[4] J. Al-Hashel, M. Ibrahim, J. John, I. Ismail, and E. Abdelnabi, "Neuroschistosomiasis presenting as Conus medullaris lesion; a case report," *Journal of Neurology and Neurological Disorders*, vol. 4, no. 2, p. 204, 2018.

[5] L. C. S. Silva, P. E. Maciel, J. G. R. Ribas, S. R. Souza-Pereira, C. M. Antunes, and J. R. Lambertucci, "Treatment of schistosomal myeloradiculopathy with praziquantel and corticosteroids and evaluation by magnetic resonance imaging: a longitudinal study," *Clinical Infectious Diseases*, vol. 39, no. 11, pp. 1618–1624, 2004.

[6] M. S. Palin, R. Mathew, and G. Towns, "Spinal neuroschistosomiasis," *British Journal of Neurosurgery*, vol. 29, no. 4, pp. 582–584, 2015.

[7] F. J. C. Artal, "Cerebral and spinal schistosomiasis," *Current Neurology and Neuroscience Reports*, vol. 12, no. 6, pp. 666–674, 2012.

[8] C. Szekeres, P. Galletout, S. Jaureguiberry et al., "Neurological presentation of schistosomiasis," *The Lancet*, vol. 381, no. 9879, p. 1788, 2013.

[9] J. V. Salgado, I. A. d. S. C. Salgado, L. L. Braga Júnior et al., "Myeloradicular form of neuroschistosomiasis in a six-year-old

boy infected with schistosoma mansoni," *The Pediatric Infectious Disease Journal*, vol. 34, no. 12, pp. 1409–1411, 2015.
[10] J. R. Lambertucci, L. C. Silva, and R. S. Amaral, "Orientações sobre o diagnóstico e tratamento da mielorradiculopatia associada à esquistossomose," *Revista da Sociedade Brasileira de Medicina Tropical*, vol. 40, no. 5, pp. 574–581, 2007.
[11] P. Nepal, V. Ojili, S. Songmen, P. Batchala, D. Kumar, and A. M. Nagar, "Multisystem imaging review of human schistosomiasis: characteristic imaging findings," *Clinical Imaging*, vol. 54, pp. 163–171, 2019.

15

Development of Neuroleptic Malignant Syndrome in a Patient with Lewy Body Dementia after Intramuscular Administration of Paliperidone

Ho-Man Yeung,[1] Sarah Schmitz,[1] Nino Kvantaliani,[2] and Christina Martin[2]

[1]*Department of Medicine, Lewis Katz School of Medicine at Temple University, Philadelphia, PA, USA*
[2]*Department of Neurology, Lewis Katz School of Medicine at Temple University, Philadelphia, PA, USA*

Correspondence should be addressed to Ho-Man Yeung; ho-man.yeung@tuhs.temple.edu

Academic Editor: Roberto Massa

Neuroleptic malignant syndrome (NMS) is a potentially fatal diagnosis composed of hyperpyrexia, muscle rigidity, altered mental status, and autonomic instability. This syndrome has significant systemic complications including acute renal failure, rhabdomyolysis, hyperkalemia, and seizure. It is associated with the use of both typical and atypical antipsychotics. Due to the extensive neurodegenerative destruction of dopaminergic and acetylcholinergic pathways, patients with Lewy body dementia (LBD) are particularly sensitive to antidopaminergic and anticholinergic medications, making them more susceptible to extrapyramidal side effects and NMS. We present a case of a 72-year-old female with LBD who developed muscular rigidity, vital sign instability, and altered mental status after receiving one dose of paliperidone palmitate injection two weeks prior to admission. Initial blood work was unrevealing. Extensive workup including EEG, lumbar puncture with cerebrospinal fluid analysis, and brain MRI was unremarkable. She was treated with seven days of bromocriptine and a lorazepam taper with improvement in muscle rigidity. However, her mental status never improved, and she remained comatose. She was later intubated for airway protection after an aspiration event that led to hypoxia. Her respiratory status never recovered, and she was transitioned to comfort care. This case demonstrates the complexity and potential fatality of NMS. Clinicians should be aware of this dangerous complication of antipsychotic use in patients with LBD as these patients may be more susceptible to this complication.

1. Introduction

Neuroleptic malignant syndrome (NMS) is a rare complication of antipsychotic use, with an incidence of 1 to 2 cases per 10,000 patients treated with antipsychotics [1]. It is characterized by the tetrad of altered mental status, muscle rigidity, fever, and autonomic instability. The rigidity is typically described as cogwheel and lead-pipe rigidity. It usually occurs shortly after initiation of therapy or after a dose adjustment, often over a period of 1 to 3 days [1]. Common laboratory abnormalities include elevated creatine kinase and leukocytosis; however, neither are specific for the syndrome. NMS is associated with all typical antipsychotics and most atypical antipsychotics including aripiprazole, clozapine, olanzapine, risperidone, and ziprasidone. Notably, fever and autonomic instability have less commonly been reported as features of NMS associated with atypical antipsychotics [1].

Risk factors for the development of NMS are the initiation or increased dosing of an antipsychotic medication, the potency of the drug, and the route of administration of the drug. The use of high-dose, high-potency, or long-acting or intramuscular forms of antipsychotics increases the risk of developing NMS [2]. Other risk factors identified in epidemiological and case studies of NMS include the presence of a structural or functional brain disorder such as tumor, encephalitis, delirium, or dementia [3].

Lewy body dementia (LBD) is characterized by Parkinsonism with visual hallucinations and fluctuating alertness. On microscopic review, Lewy bodies are seen throughout the cerebral cortex, which are often also associated with Alzheimer disease pathology. The prevalence is likely underestimated given the difficulty in making the neuropathologic diagnosis; however, LBD represents about 15% of dementias seen at autopsy [4]. Patients with LBD are highly sensitive to metabolic disturbances, and in some patients, the first manifestation of illness is delirium precipitated by a new medication, infection, or other systemic disturbances. The mainstay of treatment for LBD is cholinesterase inhibitors. If psychosis is a prominent symptom, an atypical antipsychotic can be used. However, they may worsen extrapyramidal symptoms, even at low doses. These medications are associated with an increased risk of death; therefore, they should be used cautiously, especially because patients with LBD are very sensitive to dopaminergic medications [5]. Although there is a significant overlap between the physical findings of Parkinsonism due to LBD and NMS, the two entities can be distinguished by the acuity and severity of rigidity. Furthermore, those with NMS will often experience autonomic instability and hyperthermia.

We present a case of a 72-year-old Puerto Rican female with LBD, hypertension, and type 2 diabetes mellitus who received 1 dose of paliperidone palmitate intramuscular injection and later presented with clinical features of NMS, complicated by aspiration and pneumonia, requiring mechanical ventilation. This case demonstrates the caution that should be taken when treating LBD with atypical antipsychotics, especially in the long-acting injectable form.

2. Case Presentation

A 72-year-old Puerto Rican female with a past medical history of advanced dementia with Lewy bodies, type 2 diabetes mellitus, and essential hypertension was brought to the emergency department by her granddaughter with acute change in mental status. At baseline, the patient was nonverbal, but could typically eat, use the restroom independently, and walk without significant assistance. For the past two weeks, she was unable to perform any tasks without full dependence, and she was unable to recognize her family. There was no history of drug or alcohol use. Her home medications included aspirin 81 mg daily, donepezil 10 mg daily, docusate sodium 100 mg daily, losartan 50 mg daily, linaclotide 72 mcg daily, metformin 500 mg twice daily, ranitidine 150 mg twice daily, and simvastatin 40 mg daily. Review of systems per family was negative for fevers, chills, cough, diarrhea, change in urinary frequency, or dysuria.

Lewy body dementia was diagnosed several years prior by a neurologist and had been progressive with urinary incontinence, hallucinations and paranoia, and speech difficulty. Due to her hallucinations and behavioral challenges, her primary care physician had initiated low-dose oral haloperidol. Medication adherence was difficult given her dementia, and she continued oral haloperidol inconsistently for several months. Two weeks prior to admission, her PCP initiated paliperidone palmitate extended-release intramuscular injection of 156 mg, as the patient had been off antipsychotic therapy for three months.

On admission, the patient had a temperature of 97.4°F (36.3°C), a heart rate of 102 bpm, a blood pressure of 130/67 mmHg, and an oxygen saturation of 97% on room air. On examination, the patient responded only to painful stimuli by grimacing. Pupils were equal but sluggishly reactive to light. Her head was deviated to the left and stiff when moved toward the midline. She did not follow any commands or demonstrate any voluntary movements. She had muscular rigidity of her upper extremities and lower extremities bilaterally. Her patellar and brachial reflexes were brisk at 3+, and her toes were mute bilaterally. The following day, she became hyperthermic to 101.8°F (38.8°C) with a blood pressure of 149/88 mmHg. On hospital day 3, her temperature continued to fluctuate between 97.6 and 100.7°F (36.4–38.2°C) with heart rate ranging 89–110 bpm, and her blood pressures ranged 130–172/61–93 mmHg. She was seen by toxicology, psychiatry, and neurology on hospital day 2 and was transferred to the ICU. She was started on dantrolene, bromocriptine, and benzodiazepines for symptomatic management of suspected neuroleptic malignant syndrome.

Basic laboratory workup showed no leukocytosis and no electrolyte abnormalities. See Table 1 for a summary of the workup. Total creatine kinase (CK) was 276 U/L (lab reference range: 26–192 U/L) on admission, which subsequently decreased to 222 U/L and later 205 U/L. Head CT was unremarkable, and EEG showed diffuse slowing. MRI brain without contrast revealed no acute findings. Urinalysis had 0–2 WBCs/HPF and was negative for leukocyte esterase; however, urine culture grew >100k cfu *Enterococcus faecalis*. Given her critical condition, she was initiated on vancomycin and piperacillin/tazobactam without clinical improvement.

Lumbar puncture was performed with normal opening pressure. Cerebrospinal fluid (CSF) was clear in color with 2 WBCs/mm^3, glucose 92 mg/dL, and protein 27 mg/dL, which was not suggestive of meningitis or encephalitis. CSF smear showed no organisms, and cultures grew no organisms. CSF VDRL was nonreactive. Acid-fast stain and smear showed no acid-fast bacilli. CSF cryptococcus antigen was negative. CSF anti-NMDA receptor antibody was negative. Cytology analysis of the CSF showed no malignant cells. Antibiotics were discontinued on hospital day 5 as blood cultures had no growth.

The patient remained unresponsive, but her rigidity and vital signs improved on hospital day 4. She was afebrile and normotensive. Two days later, the patient became tachypneic and hypoxic, saturating 87% on room air, with suspicion for aspiration. She was intubated for airway protection. A postintubation chest X-ray showed right lower lobe infiltrative changes, for which ampicillin/sulbactam was started. She was also started on amantadine and was titrated off all sedating medications. Unfortunately, she did not have any significant improvement in her mental status and remained mechanically ventilated. She completed a 7-day course of antibiotics for aspiration pneumonia; however, she continued to be apneic on spontaneous breathing trials.

After an ongoing discussion about the patient's grim prognosis, the family decided on palliative extubation and transition to comfort care. The patient was ultimately discharged to inpatient hospice on hospital day 15.

TABLE 1: Laboratory and radiographic workup.

Laboratory data	Culture data
Hemoglobin 14.3 g/dL	Blood cultures NGTD
WBC $9.0 \times 1000/mm^3$	CSF cultures NGTD
Sodium 139 mEq/L	Urine culture > 100k *E. faecalis*
Potassium 5.2 mEq/L	Sputum culture < 10k *S. aureus*
BUN 19 mg/dL	**Imaging findings**
Creatinine 0.89 mg/dL	Normal CT head
Glucose 193 mg/dL	Normal MRI brain without contrast
LFTs wnl	No seizure activity on EEG
Lactate 1.2 mmol/L	**CSF fluid analysis**
Creatine kinase 276 μ/L	Clear color
Ammonia wnl	2 WBCs/μL
TSH 0.970 mU/L	Glucose 92 mg/dL
UDS negative	Protein 27 mg/dL
RPR nonreactive	VDRL nonreactive
Hepatitis C Ab nonreactive	Cryptococcal Ag negative
HIV nonreactive	AFB stain negative
B12 wnl	NMDA receptor Ab negative

WBC: white blood cell; BUN: blood urea nitrogen; LFT: liver function test; TSH: thyroid-stimulating hormone; UDS: urine drug screen; RPR: rapid plasma reagin; NGTD: no growth to date; VDRL: venereal disease research laboratory; AFB: acid-fast bacillus; NMDA: N-methyl-D-aspartate; wnl: within normal limits.

3. Discussion

The case described here is the first known case in the English literature of a patient with Lewy body dementia that suffered from neuroleptic malignant syndrome after receiving an intramuscular injection of paliperidone palmitate. Prior to making a diagnosis of NMS, other diagnoses should be excluded. The differential diagnosis includes metabolic, toxicologic, infectious, and endocrine disorders. Neuroleptic malignant syndrome may be difficult to distinguish clinically from serotonin syndrome. Serotonin syndrome generally has a more rapid onset of 2–24 hours, hyperreflexia, myoclonus, nausea, vomiting, diarrhea, and less intense muscle rigidity and fever [1].

Our patient was diagnosed with NMS as she experienced the tetrad of a change in mental status progressing to coma, muscular rigidity, hyperthermia >38°C, and autonomic instability in the setting of recent administration of a long-acting injection of an antipsychotic [6]. There are several confounders in this case. She may have had worsening Parkinsonism from LBD, which may explain the rigidity and elevated CK; however, it would not completely explain the patient's coma, hyperthermia, or autonomic instability. Her urine culture was concerning for a urinary tract infection; however, her urine had very few WBCs on microscopy, contrary to what one would expect from an active infection leading to critical illness. This would suggest colonization rather than infection, especially when the patient did not improve despite broad-spectrum antibiotics. Lastly, the patient's serum CK was mildly elevated. Although the serum CK is typically >1000 U/L in NMS, it is nonspecific for NMS, and normal to mildly elevated CK levels have been reported if the rigidity is nonsevere, in early onset of the disease, or in patients with muscle wasting [7–9].

The mainstay of treatment for NMS is discontinuation of the offending agent and supportive care. External cooling can be utilized to reduce the patient's temperature; however, antipyretics such as acetaminophen have not been shown to be beneficial. Sedation with benzodiazepines is recommended to decrease agitation and sympathetic activity. Those with fever and rigidity may require intubation because neuromuscular paralysis reduces muscle contraction and therefore can reduce fever. Nonpolarizing agents are preferred over depolarizing agents for intubation [1].

Most deaths due to NMS are related to profound muscle rigidity resulting in complications including respiratory failure, rhabdomyolysis, renal failure, disseminated intravascular coagulation, and cardiovascular collapse. No treatment has been shown to be superior to supportive care; however, reported cases have described the use of dantrolene, bromocriptine, benzodiazepines, and amantadine [1]. The mortality rate is around 10%; however, most patients completely recover in 2 to 14 days if NMS is recognized early and treated aggressively. If diagnosis and treatment are delayed, then those who survive may have residual catatonia or Parkinsonism [10].

Paliperidone palmitate is a long-acting formulation of paliperidone, an active metabolite of risperidone. It is an antagonist of brain dopamine D_2 and serotonin (5-hydroxytryptamine) receptors. Effects are usually seen about 8 days after injection, and peak plasma level is reached about 13 days after injection. The half-life ranges from 25 to 49 days [11]. Intramuscular administration of a neuroleptic may result in higher peak levels and abrupt dopamine blockade. Therefore, paliperidone palmitate should be used with caution in those with LBD as these patients have been reported to have marked sensitivity to this class of medications [2]. Patients with LBD have poor adherence to medications; therefore, accurate supervision by caretakers is crucial for medication optimization [12], before deciding to switch to a different medication or escalate doses. Prior to administering long-acting intramuscular antipsychotic in any patients, the risk-to-benefit ratio with oral agents should be considered first, as their response may be difficult to predict and may be severe, particularly those with LBD. As potential adverse effects from long-acting intramuscular antipsychotics may not be easily reversed, oral medications such as clozapine or quetiapine at a low dose may be appropriate choices to minimize potential extrapyramidal symptoms [13, 14]. Relative to other NMS cases seen with oral agents [15–17], one may speculate that long-acting injections may have longer onset time and have long-lasting side effects due to their delayed peak plasma concentration and long half-lives. Kane et al. reported the incidence of NMS associated with paliperidone palmitate as 4/10,000 patient-years using the Janssen database. Of the 5008 patients enrolled, only 1 case of NMS was identified. Although that patient did not carry a diagnosis of dementia, he received a 50 mg injection of paliperidone palmitate and subsequently suffered NMS on day 14 with full recovery after 32 days [18]. Our case is the first reported case of NMS in a patient with LBD following the administration of paliperidone palmitate. As the use of novel long-acting antipsychotics is still in its nascency, clinicians should be aware of this serious and potentially fatal complication of paliperidone palmitate use, especially in those with underlying dopamine sensitivity.

Disclosure

This case was presented as a poster at the Annual Sol Sherry Symposium at Temple University on June 5, 2019, and orally at the Department of Neurology Annual Matthew T. Moore Conference at Temple University Hospital in June 2020.

Authors' Contributions

NK, CM, SS, and HY contributed to the writing and editing of the entire manuscript and approved the submitted version of the manuscript.

References

[1] M. R. Ware, D. B. Feller, and K. L. Hall, "Neuroleptic malignant syndrome: diagnosis and management," *Prim Care Companion CNS Disord*, vol. 20, no. 1, Article ID 17r02185, 2018.

[2] R. Oruch, I. Pryme, B. Engelsen, and A. Lund, "Neuroleptic malignant syndrome: an easily overlooked neurologic emergency," *Neuropsychiatric Disease and Treatment*, vol. 13, pp. 161–175, 2017.

[3] B. D. Berman, "Neuroleptic malignant syndrome: a review for neurohospitalists," *The Neurohospitalist*, vol. 1, no. 1, pp. 41–47, 2011.

[4] W. Petrie and H. S. Kirshner, "Neurocognitive disorders," in *Current Diagnosis & Treatment: Psychiatry*McGraw-Hill Education, New York, NY, USA, 2019, http://accessmedicine.mhmedical.com/content.aspx?aid=1158259019.

[5] W. W. Seeley, C. M. Tanner, and B. L. Miller, "Dementia with Lewy bodies," in *Harrison's Principles of Internal Medicine*McGraw-Hill Education, New York, NY, USA, 2018, http://accessmedicine.mhmedical.com/content.aspx?aid=1155958612.

[6] R. J. Gurrera, S. N. Caroff, A. Cohen et al., "An international consensus study of neuroleptic malignant syndrome diagnostic criteria using the delphi method," *The Journal of Clinical Psychiatry*, vol. 72, no. 9, pp. 1222–1228, 2011.

[7] K. Nisijima and K. Shioda, "A rare case of neuroleptic malignant syndrome without elevated serum creatine kinase," *Neuropsychiatric Disease and Treatment*, vol. 10, pp. 403–407, 2014.

[8] J. Nielsen and A. M. Bruhn, "Atypical neuroleptic malignant syndrome caused by olanzapine," *Acta Psychiatrica Scandinavica*, vol. 112, no. 3, pp. 238–240, 2005.

[9] R. Singh and D. Hassanally, "Neuroleptic malignant syndrome with normal creatine kinase," *Postgraduate Medical Journal*, vol. 72, no. 845, p. 187, 1996.

[10] A. Shalev, H. Hermesh, and H. Munitz, "Mortality from neuroleptic malignant syndrome," *The Journal of Clinical Psychiatry*, vol. 50, pp. 18–25, 1989.

[11] M. T. Morris and S. P. Tarpada, "Long-acting injectable paliperidone palmitate: a review of efficacy and safety," *Psychopharmacology Bulletin*, vol. 47, no. 2, pp. 42–52, 2017.

[12] M. H. Connors, L. Quinto, I. McKeith et al., "Non-pharmacological interventions for Lewy body dementia: a systematic review," *Psychological Medicine*, vol. 48, no. 11, pp. 1749–1758, 2018.

[13] R. B. Mortimer and A. R. Mortimer, "Antipsychotic use in patients with dementia with Lewy bodies," *American Family Physician*, vol. 96, no. 10, p. 629, 2017.

[14] L. A. Hershey and R. Coleman-Jackson, "Pharmacological management of dementia with Lewy bodies," *Drugs & Aging*, vol. 36, no. 4, pp. 309–319, 2019.

[15] Y. F. Shea and L.-W. Chu, "Neuroleptic malignant syndrome caused by quetiapine in an elderly man with Lewy body dementia," *Journal of the American Geriatrics Society*, vol. 64, no. 9, pp. e55–e56, 2016.

[16] G. Sechi, V. Agnetti, R. Masuri et al., "Risperidone, neuroleptic malignant syndrome and probable dementia with Lewy bodies," *Progress in Neuro-Psychopharmacology and Biological Psychiatry*, vol. 24, no. 6, pp. 1043–1051, 2000.

[17] P.-R. Teng, C.-H. Yeh, C.-Y. Lin, and T.-J. Lai, "Olanzapine-induced neuroleptic malignant syndrome in a patient with probable dementia with Lewy bodies," *The Journal of Neuropsychiatry and Clinical Neurosciences*, vol. 24, no. 4, pp. E01–E02, 2012.

[18] J. M. Kane, C. U. Correll, N. Delva, S. Gopal, A. Savitz, and M. Mathews, "Low incidence of neuroleptic malignant syndrome associated with paliperidone palmitate long-acting injectable: a database report and case study," *Journal of Clinical Psychopharmacology*, vol. 39, no. 2, pp. 180–182, 2019.

16

Tolosa–Hunt Syndrome: A Painful Ophthalmoplegia

Marcellin Bugeme,[1] **Ousmane Cissé**,[2] **Olivier Mukuku**,[3] **and Amadou Gallo Diop**[2]

[1]*Faculty of Medicine, University of Lubumbashi, Lubumbashi, Democratic Republic of the Congo*
[2]*Université Cheikh Anta Diop, Dakar, Senegal*
[3]*Institut Supérieur des Techniques Médicales de Lubumbashi, Lubumbashi, Democratic Republic of the Congo*

Correspondence should be addressed to Olivier Mukuku; oliviermukuku@yahoo.fr

Academic Editor: Peter Berlit

Tolosa–Hunt syndrome is a painful ophthalmoplegia characterized by recurrent unilateral orbital pain, ipsilateral oculomotor paralysis, and a rapid response to steroids. Our report describes a 37-year-old young woman who presented with right ptosis, ipsilateral ophthalmoplegia, and painful headache with no other neurological deficits in which all biological and neuroimaging investigations were normal. Complete recovery within one week of corticosteroid therapy was observed. This is probably the first case of Tolosa–Hunt syndrome reported in Dakar, Senegal.

1. Introduction

Tolosa–Hunt Syndrome (THS) is a rare neurological condition of unknown etiopathogenesis, characterized by unilateral pain and ipsilateral oculomotor paralysis [1]. This disease is caused by an unspecific inflammation (of unknown origin) in the region of the cavernous sinus and the sphenoid cleft. Its evolution is considerably shortened by corticosteroid therapy correctly within 72 hours [2]. In 1954, Tolosa reported the first patient with this syndrome, who presented with left orbital pain, ipsilateral progressive visual loss, total left ophthalmoplegia, and reduced sensation over the first division of the trigeminal nerve. After 7 years of this, in 1961, Hunt described this clinical entity, on the basis of six patients [3].

We report a case of a patient admitted with a right droopy eyelid and right orbital headache evolving for two months before her consultation. Neurological examination revealed a right ptosis and an ipsilateral oculomotor paralysis. The additional examinations performed had returned to normal. After a week of corticosteroid therapy, all the symptoms had completely subsided.

2. Case Report

A 37-year-old Senegalese woman with hypertension history, presented with right, excruciating, permanent, intense, nonpulsatile orbital headache associated with right ptosis without visual loss. The onset of symptoms dated back to two months before her arrival at the hospital with headache that had appeared about 11 days before a right drooping eyelid, associated with ipsilateral orbital pain. The patient had not yet received any treatment.

Medical examination showed the patient in good general state, the mucosa were well colored, there were no folds of dehydration or malnutrition, no edema of the lower limbs, and the calves were flexible. The vital parameters were within the norms.

Neurological examination found a paralysis of the right oculomotor nerves (III, IV, and VI) associated with a homolateral ptosis (Figure 1). The rest of the exam was unremarkable. Brain magnetic resonance imaging (MRI) with contrast was performed and was unremarkable (Figure 2).

Laboratory investigations including complete blood count, erythrocyte sedimentation rate, fasting blood sugar, renal and liver functions, angiotensin-converting enzyme, antinuclear antibody, serum protein electrophoresis, anti-neutrophil cytoplasmic antibody, C-reactive protein, and viral serologies (hepatitis A, B, and C, human immunodeficiency virus, and venereal disease research laboratory) testing were either normal or negative. The cerebrospinal fluid analysis was within normal ranges with normal glucose and protein and negative cytology. Intradermal tuberculin test was negative.

The patient had received a treatment with oral corticosteroids (prednisone 60 mg daily) combined with adjuvant therapy (calcium 500 mg per day orally and potassium 600 mg per day orally). After a week of treatment, complete remission of oculomotor disorders and other symptoms was noted (Figure 3).

The probable diagnosis of Tolosa–Hunt Syndrome was retained in the face of the negativity of all investigations carried out as well as spectacular response to treatment.

3. Discussion

Tolosa–Hunt syndrome is a painful ophthalmoplegia due to nonspecific inflammation of the cavernous sinus. Existence of this syndrome has long been debated, and its nosological framework was discussed [2].

Pathophysiological and etiopathogenic mechanisms of THS remain controversial. It is a diagnosis of exclusion retained after eliminating other etiologies of painful ophthalmoplegia [4, 5]. Following essentially clinical criteria has been established by Hunt [5, 6]: one or more episodes of unilateral orbital pain persisting for weeks without treatment; paresis of the third, fourth, and/or sixth cranial nerve and/or detection of granulomas by MRI or by biopsy; paresis in conjunction with sudden onset of eye pain or pain within 2 weeks of ocular dysfunction; pain and paresis disappear within 72 hours if treatment with corticosteroids is adequate; other etiologies have been excluded by appropriate investigations.

Age of patients varies between 4 and 75 years [7], but THS can affect people of any age, without predominance of sex. In general, it is unilateral, but cases of bilaterality have been reported [8]. Our patient was 38 years old, and she presented with unilateral symptoms. The diagnosis of this syndrome was retained in the face of the negativity of all the investigations carried out as well as the response to treatment. Extensive diagnosis tests to exclude other common etiologies of painful ophthalmoplegia were not found in our patient.

Many studies have looked at THS and the contribution of MRI, an examination essential for the diagnosis of this syndrome, because it allows [9] to eliminate a specific inflammatory process (sarcoidosis) or tumor and to show the existence of an isosignal zone in T1 and T2 and the deformation of cavernous sinus which are suggestive signs. However, it seems possible that MRI techniques can be faulted and do not detect minimal infiltrates (as is certainly the case with our patient). Failure to visualize these infiltrates by MRI would indicate an early stage of the disease and therefore a better response to treatment [10].

Recently, diagnostic criteria for THS have been published by the International Headache Society in the 3rd edition of International Classification of Headache Disorders (ICHD-3) which places the THS in position 13.8 [11]. This ICHD-3 classification reinforces the important role of MRI in the diagnosis of THS. MRI also allows the exclusion of other similar causes such as lymphoma, meningioma, and sarcoidosis [12]. The MRI was normal in our patient, and patients with THS with normal MRI have already been reported in the literature [2, 12–14]. In addition, in this category, the use of biopsy is considered to highlight a granulomatous inflammation of the cavernous sinus, superior orbital fissure, or orbit [2]. In our context, where optimal conditions are not easily met, a biopsy of a patient suspected of THS with an excellent response to corticosteroid therapy to confirm the diagnosis should not be necessary because it carries a risk of complications. Thus, exposing patients to a risky procedure such as a biopsy should not be a necessity for diagnosis. Kóbor et al. [13] recommend a repeat of the MRI in a patient with an initially normal MRI to reveal new inflammatory signs which could appear months after the initial presentation. Mainly because of costs, our patient did not have MRI in the follow-up, and she was monitored by clinical visits only. The lack of follow-up MRI in our case reflects the day-to-day reality in our settings. Health insurance systems are almost nonexistent, and the population has to take care of itself for medical care.

Zhang et al. [2] proposed introduction of categories of definitive, probable, and possible since it is highly doubtful whether the diagnostic criteria for ICHD-3 are so completely based on it (or on a biopsy). Patients with normal MRI or with a time interval between the onset of pain and ophthalmoplegia of more than 2 weeks or whose diagnosis is dependent on pain and paresis resolving within 72 hours of starting corticosteroid therapy cannot be diagnosed as definitive TSH and is not better explained by another ICHD-3 diagnosis. This is how probable or possible THS are working alternatives. We believe this is reasonable and may be helpful in reducing the financial burden and complications of unnecessary investigations to confirm the diagnosis of THS. In addition, in agreement with Zhang et al. [2], we also believe that the response to steroids is probably still important to support the diagnosis of THS in clinical practice, in the absence of other specific and reliable criteria.

The spectacular efficacy of corticosteroid therapy is suggestive but not specific. Hence it is necessary to conduct prolonged monitoring of several months to retain this diagnosis definitively. Treatment consists of a high dose of oral prednisone for 4 weeks. Significant improvement is often evident from the first 24 hours of treatment [12]. Our patient received a dose of prednisone 60 mg per day, and after a week, a complete dramatic regression of the symptoms was observed. After more than six months of monitoring, no

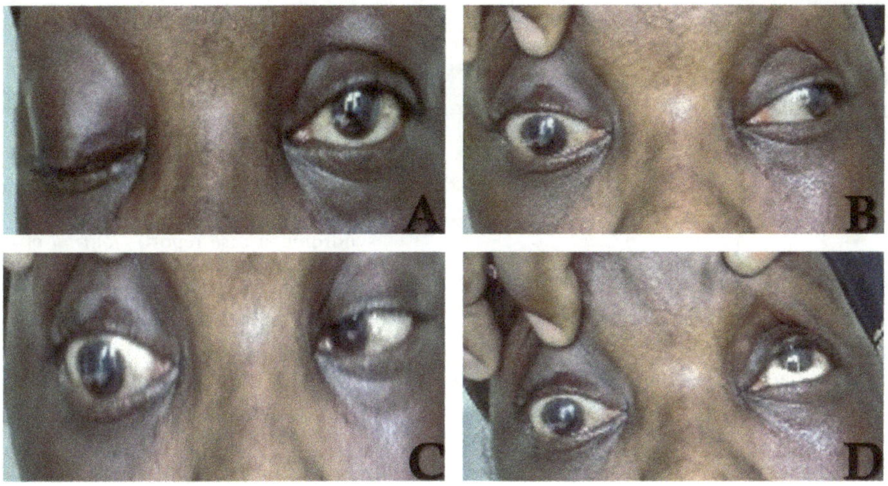

FIGURE 1: (a) Right ptosis. (b) Paresis of the third cranial nerve. (c) Paresis of the sixth cranial nerve. (d) Paresis of the fourth cranial nerve.

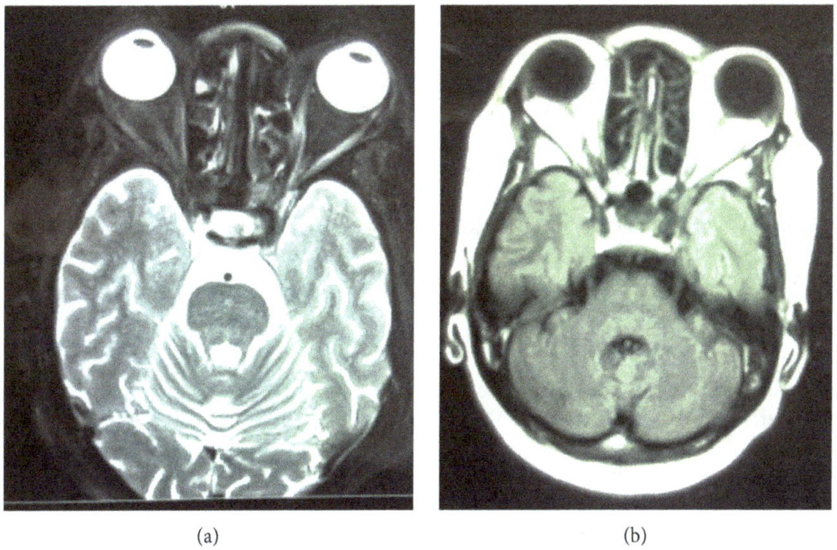

FIGURE 2: MRI axial slice of the brain in (a) T2 sequence and (b) T2-FLAIR sequence after contrast injection showing no abnormalities in the cavernous sinus.

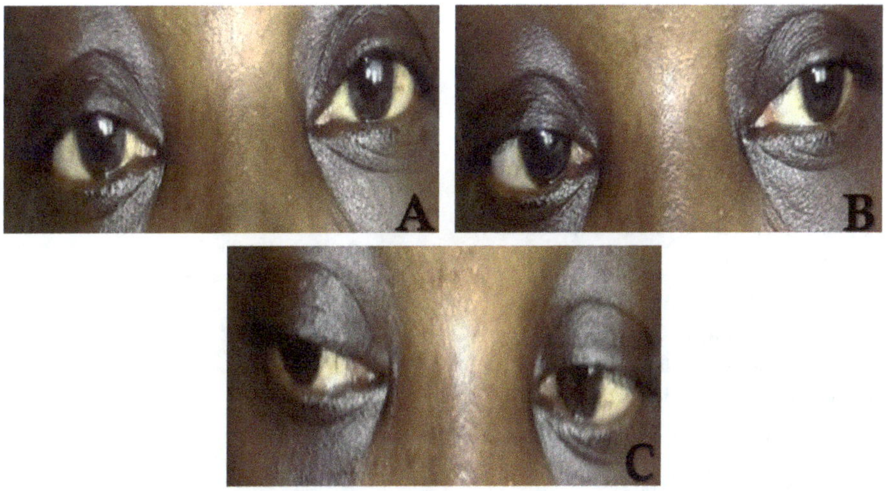

FIGURE 3: (a) Regression of right ptosis. (b) Complete remission of the third cranial nerve. (c) Complete remission of the sixth cranial nerve.

clinical abnormality was observed in our patient. Zhang et al. [2] reported that 77.5% of patients obtained complete relief of orbital pain within a week after the start of steroid treatment. This spectacular efficacy of corticosteroid therapy has been observed in several other studies [3, 5, 15, 16].

4. Conclusion

Tolosa–Hunt syndrome is a rare entity well-defined clinically but of unknown etiopathogenesis. It remains a diagnosis of exclusion. In our case, the negativity of investigations and spectacular response to corticosteroids allowed us to retain the diagnosis.

References

[1] L. L. Mantia, M. Curone, A. Rapoport, and G. Bussone, "Tolosa-hunt syndrome: critical literature review based on IHS 2004 criteria," *Cephalalgia*, vol. 26, no. 7, pp. 772–781, 2006.

[2] X. Zhang, Z. Zhou, T. J. Steiner et al., "Validation of ICHD-3 beta diagnostic criteria for 13.7 Tolosa-Hunt syndrome: analysis of 77 cases of painful ophthalmoplegia," *Cephalalgia*, vol. 34, no. 8, pp. 624–632, 2014.

[3] V. Chaudhary, S. Venu, and J. Deswal, "Painful ophthalmoplegia due to Tolosa-Hunt syndrome: a case report," *International Journal of Medical Science and Public Health*, vol. 5, no. 5, pp. 1045–1049, 2016.

[4] M. A. Mnaili, Y. Benmoh, N. Abida et al., "Syndrome de Tolosa-Hunt," *Revue Neurologique*, vol. 172, pp. A33-A34, 2016.

[5] M. K. Singh, B. Marshall, and J. Hawley, "Painful ophthalmoplegia: a case of tolosa-hunt syndrome," *Military Medicine*, vol. 179, no. 11, pp. e1409-e1410, 2014.

[6] P. Rousseaux, P. Perruzi, and M. Schaiso-cusin, "Should Tolosa-Hunt syndrome still be an exclusion diagnosis?" *Rev Neurol*, vol. 149, pp. 315–319, 1993.

[7] J. Mandrioli, G. Frank, P. Sola et al., "Tolosa-hunt syndrome due to actinomycosis of the cavernous sinus: the infectious hypothesis revisited," *Headache: The Journal of Head and Face Pain*, vol. 44, no. 8, pp. 806–811, 2004.

[8] L. B. Kline and W. F. Hoyt, "Nosological entities?: the Tolosa-Hunt syndrome," *Journal of Neurology, Neurosurgery & Psychiatry*, vol. 71, no. 5, pp. 577–582, 2001.

[9] X. Drouot, C. Brosset, E. Sagui, and M. Bregigeon, "Le syndrome de Tolosa-Hunt: apport de l'imagerie actuelle," *La Revue de Médecine Interne*, vol. 23, no. 5, pp. 479–481, 2002.

[10] S. Aktan, C. Aykut, and C. Erzen, "Computed tomography and magnetic resonance imaging in three patients with Tolosa-Hunt syndrome," *European Neurology*, vol. 33, no. 5, pp. 393–396, 1993.

[11] Headache Classification Committee of the International Headache Society (IHS), "The international classification of headache disorders," *Cephalalgia*, vol. 38, 2018.

[12] S. Çakirer, "MRI findings in Tolosa-Hunt syndrome before and after systemic corticosteroid therapy," *European Journal of Radiology*, vol. 45, no. 2, pp. 83–90, 2003.

[13] J. Kóbor, E. Vörös, and A. Deák, "Magnetic resonance imaging in Tolosa-Hunt syndrome," *European Journal of Pediatrics*, vol. 163, no. 12, p. 753, 2004.

[14] M. Abdelghany, D. Orozco, W. Fink, and C. Begley, "Probable Tolosa-Hunt syndrome with a normal MRI," *Cephalalgia*, vol. 35, no. 5, pp. 449–452, 2015.

[15] K. Okabe, R. Kaneko, T. Kawai, D. Mochizuki, S. Tsuchiya, and H. HIbi, "Ophthalmoplegia considered to be Tolosa-Hunt syndrome: a case report," *Journal of Oral and Maxillofacial Surgery, Medicine, and Pathology*, vol. 30, no. 5, pp. 461–465, 2018.

[16] J. Paovic, P. Paovic, I. Bojkovic, M. Nagulic, and V. Sredovic, "Tolosa-Hunt syndrome-diagnostic problem of painful ophthalmoplegia," *Vojnosanitetski Pregled*, vol. 69, no. 7, pp. 627–630, 2012.

17

A Case of Invasive *Aspergillus* Rhinosinusitis Presenting with Unilateral Visual Loss and Subsequently Associated with Meningitis, Subarachnoid Hemorrhage, and Cerebral Infarction

Koji Tsuzaki,[1,2] Kenji Murakata,[1,3] Mayu Kamei,[1] Akihiro Kikuya,[1] Yuwa Oka,[1,2] and Toshiaki Hamano[1,2]

[1]*Department of Neurology, Kansai Electric Power Hospital, Osaka, Japan*
[2]*Division of Clinical Neurology, Kansai Electric Power Medical Research Institute, Osaka, Japan*
[3]*Department of Neurology, Nakatsu Hospital, Osaka, Japan*

Correspondence should be addressed to Koji Tsuzaki; tsuzaki.koji@b4.kepco.co.jp

Academic Editor: Peter Berlit

Visual impairment can occur because of several mechanisms, including optic nerve disease and occasionally fungal sinusitis. An 87-year-old man presented with the loss of right visual acuity; he was diagnosed with optic neuritis. Steroid pulse therapy was not effective. One month later, he became unconscious because of meningitis, following which treatment with ceftriaxone and acyclovir was initiated. However, his consciousness deteriorated because of a subarachnoid hemorrhage caused by a ruptured aneurysm. Meningitis and vascular invasion caused by fungal rhinosinusitis were suspected, and the sinus mucosa was biopsied. He was pathologically diagnosed with invasive *Aspergillus* rhinosinusitis. Despite continuous liposomal amphotericin B administration, he died of cerebral infarction, following a right internal carotid artery occlusion. It is important to consider the possibility of *Aspergillus* as an etiological agent, especially when cerebrovascular events are associated with visual impairment.

1. Introduction

Unilateral visual loss is commonly caused by problems of the optic media, retina, or neural visual pathway. The optic nerve is included in the neural visual pathway. Causes of optic neuropathy include ischemia, inflammatory, or infectious process. When optic neuritis is diagnosed, it is commonly treated with steroid pulse therapy [1]. However, it should be noted that fungal rhinosinusitis (FRS), such as *Aspergillus* rhinosinusitis, infrequently causes unilateral visual loss.

The presentation of FRS could vary from being irritating to potentially fatal [2]. FRS is categorized as invasive because the fungus invades the surrounding tissues, such as bone, or maybe noninvasive [2]. Invasive FRS cases are subdivided into acute, granulomatous, and chronic [2]. In acute invasive FRS, vascular invasion rapidly progresses within 4 weeks [2]. Acute invasive FRS, though rare, has a 50–80% mortality rate [3]. An immunosuppressed status, including neutrophil dysfunction, chemotherapy, and human immunodeficiency virus infections, is the risk factor for FRS [4]. In this report, we describe a case of invasive *Aspergillus* rhinosinusitis that presented with unilateral vision loss, meningitis, subarachnoid hemorrhage, and cerebral infarction.

2. Case Presentation

An 87-year-old man presented with vision loss of the right side one and a half months before admission. He had consulted an ophthalmologist one month before admission. There was no abnormality in the fundus, and computed tomography (CT) of the head revealed no abnormal findings, except sinusitis on the right side (Figure 1(a)). On brain magnetic resonance imaging (MRI), mass lesions in the right maxillary sinus were seen with a high signal intensity on T1-weighted images and with a low signal intensity on T2-

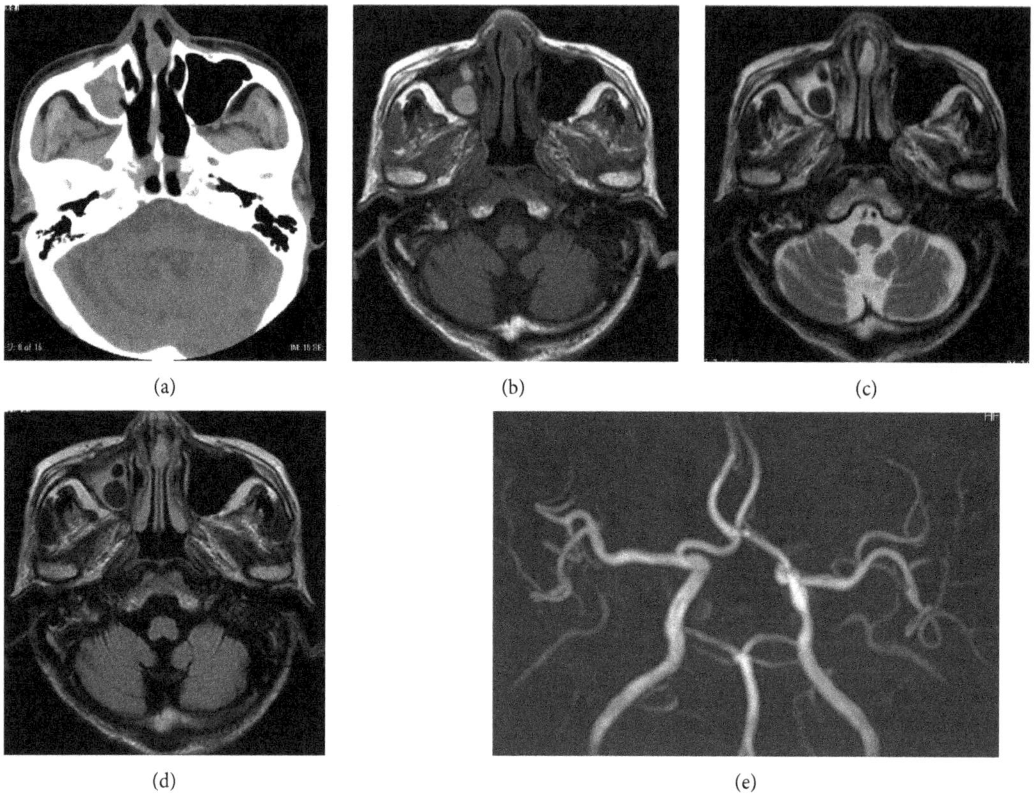

Figure 1: One month before admission: imaging included CT (a), T1-(b), and T2-weighted (c) images, fluid attenuated inversion recovery images (d), and MRA (e).

weighted and fluid-attenuated inversion recovery images (Figures 1(b)–1(d)). No aneurysm was found on magnetic resonance angiography (MRA) (Figure 1(e)). He was subsequently diagnosed with optic neuritis and treated with steroid pulse therapy. However, his visual acuity did not improve, and hearing disturbance developed in the right ear. In the evening on the day of admission, he became unresponsive, and abnormal behavior, such as wandering, was observed. He was brought to our hospital by ambulance. He had a medical history of hypertension and benign prostatic hyperplasia. He had not taken steroids or immunosuppressants.

At the time of admission, the patient's Glasgow coma scale was E4V4M6, and he could spontaneously open eyes. He was disorientated and could follow only simple instructions. Both light blink and direct light reflexes disappeared in the right eye, and a relative afferent pupillary defect was observed in the right eye. His eye position was midline. Although he could not move his eyes as instructed, he spontaneously moved them in all directions. Visual acuity could not be assessed because of disturbance of consciousness. There were no abnormalities in motor and sensory examinations. His deep tendon reflexes were normal, and signs of meningeal irritation were absent.

On laboratory examination results, his white blood cell count was mildly elevated (10700 cells/μL; normal range, 3500–9000), and C-reactive protein level was elevated (4.68 mg/dL; normal range, 0–0.3). β-D glucan level was normal (3.259 pg/mL; normal range, <11.0; colorimetric assay). Tests for the presence of autoantibodies, including antinuclear antibodies and antineutrophil cytoplasmic antibodies, were negative. Cerebrospinal fluid (CSF) examination findings showed slightly elevated cell counts (65 cells/μL; mononuclear cells, 50 cells/μL; polymorphonuclear cells, 15 cells/μL), an elevated protein level of 900.0 mg/dL, and a low glucose level of 59 mg/dL (blood glucose, 136 mg/dL). Both blood and CSF cultures were negative, and results of India ink staining of CSF samples were normal. Brain MRI showed no abnormalities in the cerebral parenchyma (Figure 2(a)). An aneurysm (3 mm diameter) was found in the siphon of the right internal carotid artery on MRA (Figure 2(b)).

Septic meningitis or herpes encephalitis was suspected, and ceftriaxone (2 g/day) and acyclovir (1500 mg/day) were administered. However, serum IgM antibodies to herpes simplex virus (HSV) were negative, and HSV DNA was undetected in the patient's CSF samples. His consciousness deteriorated to E3V1M5 on the sixth day of hospitalization. Repeated head CT revealed a subarachnoid hemorrhage, likely due to the rupture of the aneurysm in the right internal carotid artery (Figures 3(a) and 3(b)). Because treatment with antibiotic and antiviral drugs was ineffective, a fungal infection was suspected. Liposomal amphotericin B (150 mg/day) was administered. On serum examinations, *Cryptococcus neoformans* antigen was negative, *Candida* antigen level was 4 times the normal value (normal range, <2), and *Aspergillus* antigen level was 0.8 ng/mL (normal range, <0.5).

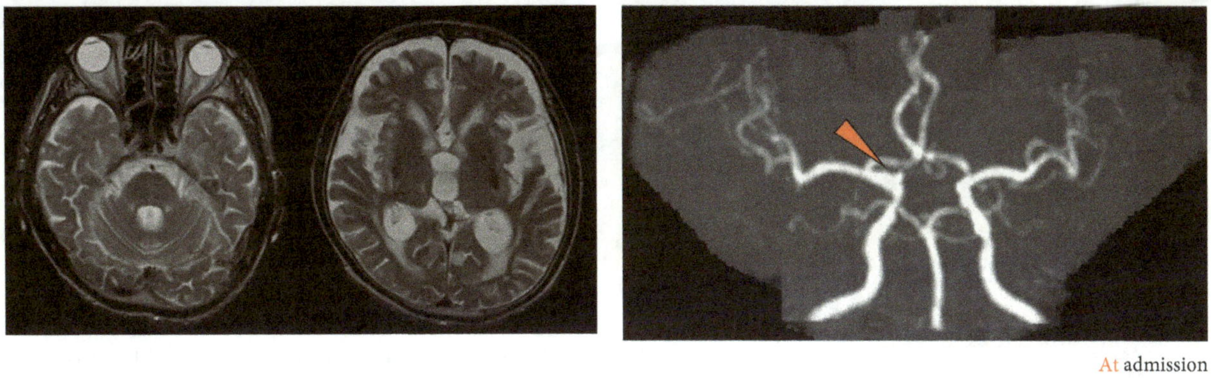

(a) (b)

FIGURE 2: On admission: brain MRI showing no abnormalities in the cerebraand parenchyma on T2-weighted images (a). MRI shows a 3 mm aneurysm in the siphon of the internal carotid (arrow head) (b).

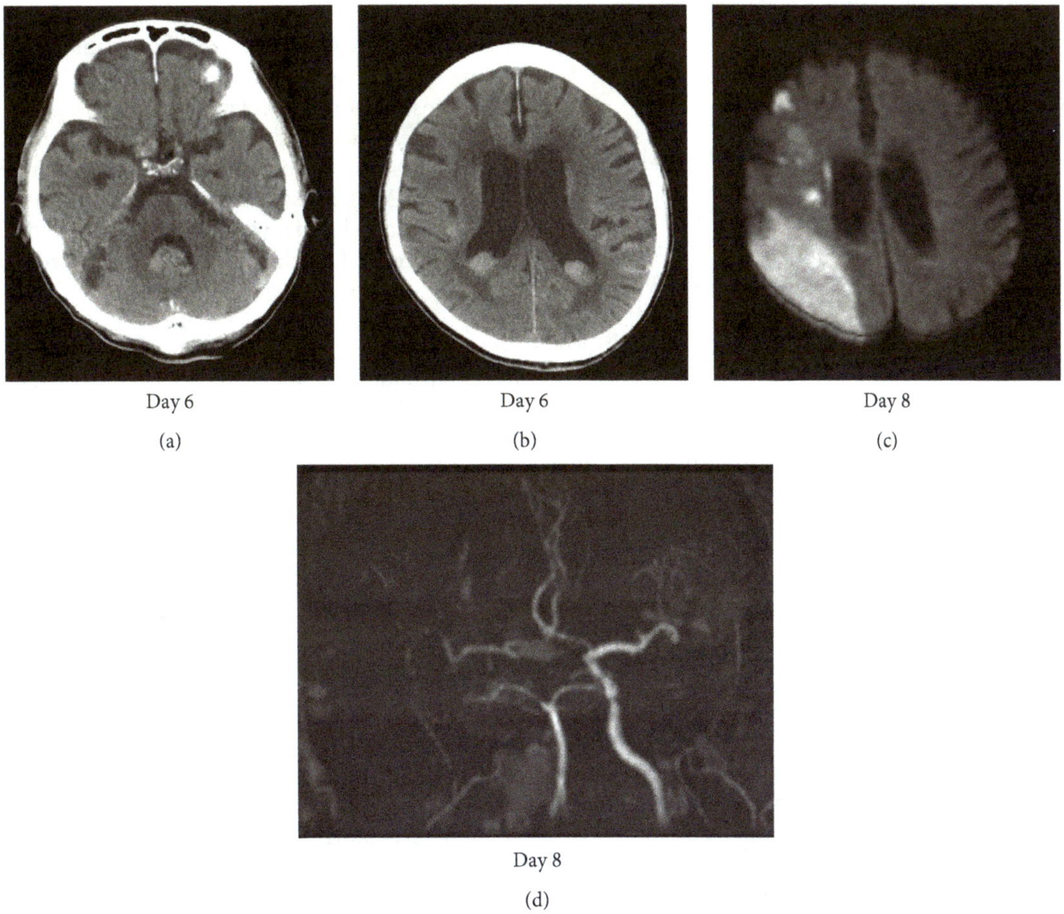

FIGURE 3: Day 6: head CT showing a subarachnoid hemorrhage (a), (b). Day 8: brain MRI showing a right middle cerebral artery infarction on DWI (c) and MRI showing right internal carotid artery occlusion (d).

Rhinoscopy revealed a fungal mass attached to the middle nasal meatus. Pathological examination of this mass showed numerous spores and mycelium with septae (Figure 4). A culture test characterized the specimen as *Aspergillus*. The patient was diagnosed with invasive *Aspergillus* rhinosinusitis. However, the patient developed left hemiplegia, and his consciousness deteriorated to E1V1M2 on the eighth day of hospitalization. Brain MRI revealed a cerebral infarction in the middle cerebral artery territory and right internal carotid artery occlusion (Figures 3(c) and 3(d)). Although treatment with liposomal amphotericin B was continued, the patient died on the sixteenth day of hospitalization.

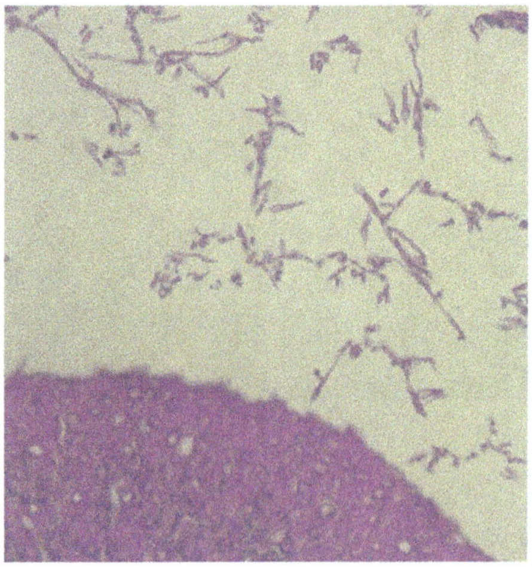

Figure 4: Sinus mucosal biopsy hematoxylin and eosin staining (magnification 400). CT: compound tomography, MRA: magnetic resonance angiography, MRI: magnetic resonance imaging, DWI: diffusion weighted imaging.

3. Discussion

The occurrence of meningitis shortly after steroid pulse therapy for visual impairment and the sequential subarachnoid hemorrhage and cerebral infarction, in this case, suggested acute invasive FRS. It is important to consider the possibility of invasive FRS in the differential diagnosis, especially when patients in an immunosuppressed state have meningitis, visual loss, and radiologically proven sinusitis.

Mucor and *Aspergillus* are the common causes of acute invasive FRS [5]. When fungal sinusitis is associated with intracranial lesions, it is necessary to consider *Aspergillus* as a causative agent. Pathological confirmation of fungal invasion is necessary to diagnose invasive FRS [5]. When invasive FRS is suspected, a rhinoscopic inspection of the sinuses and mucosal biopsy is necessary [6]. Because different antifungal drugs are used to treat *Mucor* and *Aspergillus* infections, species identification using culture of the biopsied specimen is indispensable. In the case of invasive aspergillosis, the lung is the most frequent site of infection; it rarely occurs only in the sinuses [7]. Immune suppression is a risk factor for acute invasive FRS [4]. However, in this case, the patient was not immunosuppressed. Antinori et al. found that 41 of the 93 patients with *Aspergillus* meningitis were immunosuppressed [8]. In addition, 52 patients of the 93 examined patients did not have a risk for invasive aspergillosis, and 6 of them were suspected to have direct extension of *Aspergillus* from the orbit, ear, or paranasal sinuses to the central nervous system [8]. In this case, we suspected that the Aspergillus spreads from the right maxillary sinus to the right orbital and intracranial regions.

In this case, the patient's β-D glucan level was normal. The sensitivity and specificity of the β-D glucan test for the detection of invasive fungal infection have been reported to be 63% and 96%, respectively, with a cutoff value of 7 pg/mL [9]. However, in cases of invasive fungal infection, pathological examination and culture are the standard measures for diagnosis, and β-D glucan testing has limited utility.

Typical CT findings in FRS are mucus, calcified lesions, and hematomas in the sinuses [10]. On MRI, acute invasive FRS shows high intensity on T2-weighted images, reflecting inflammatory edema and cellular infiltration. In contrast, chronic noninvasive FRS and indolent FRS show low intensity on T2-weighted images [10]. *Aspergillus* rhinosinusitis has marked low intensity on T2-weighted images because of the presence of iron and manganese [11, 12]. In this case, MRI acquired from the previous hospital showed a low-intensity mass in the right maxillary sinus on a T2-weighted image, indicative of *Aspergillus* rhinosinusitis.

In patients with acute invasive FRS due to *Aspergillus*, early recognition and therapeutic intervention are important [13]. Treatments include administration of antifungal drugs and surgical resection or debridement [13]. Amphotericin B and itraconazole have been used for FRS. Recently, voriconazole has been recommended when mucormycosis is excluded and aspergillosis is suspected [13].

Causes of visual impairment in patients with acute invasive FRS involve direct infectious infiltration into the orbit, inflammatory edema, osteomyelitis in the orbit, subperiosteal nodules and abscess, cellulitis in the orbit and face, abscess in the orbit, or thrombosis of the ocular vein [10]. In this case, the cause of visual impairment was unclear in the CT/MRI images. Since no apparent abscess, osteomyelitis, or cellulitis were observed during the clinical course, direct infiltration and inflammatory edema may have possibly caused the visual impairment.

Aspergillus is known to invade the vascular wall, causing cerebral infarction and hemorrhage [11]. *Aspergillus* invasion was likely the cause of the sudden aneurysm formation in the right internal carotid artery because prior MRI did not reveal any aneurysms. Direct extension of *Aspergillus* in the right maxillary sinus may have caused infiltration of the vessel walls, leading to the cerebral infarction and subarachnoid hemorrhage.

When sudden visual impairment occurs, and optic neuritis is suspected, steroids are often administered. However, as in the present case, sinusitis due to *Aspergillus* might have been the cause of the patient's manifestations. Therefore, it is necessary to consider all potential causes of visual impairment, especially when cerebrovascular events, such as cerebral infarction, cerebral hemorrhage, or subarachnoid hemorrhage, are involved.

Consent

Informed consent for publishing this case report was obtained from the patient's family.

Acknowledgments

The authors thank Dr. Jun Kawai from the Kansai Electric Power Hospital Department of Pathology for useful advice.

References

[1] A. T. Toosy, D. F. Mason, and D. H. Miller, "Optic neuritis," *The Lancet Neurology*, vol. 13, no. 1, pp. 83–99, 2014.

[2] A. Chakrabarti, D. W. Denning, B. J. Ferguson et al., "Fungal rhinosinusitis," *The Laryngoscope*, vol. 119, no. 9, pp. 1809–1818, 2009.

[3] J. R. Craig, "Updates in management of acute invasive fungal rhinosinusitis," *Current Opinion in Otolaryngology & Head and Neck Surgery*, vol. 27, no. 1, pp. 29–36, 2019.

[4] R. D. Deshazo, "Fungal sinusitis," *The American Journal of the Medical Sciences*, vol. 316, no. 1, pp. 39–45, 1998.

[5] C. C. Melancon and J. D. Clinger, "The use of frozen section in the early diagnosis of acute invasive fungal sinusitis," *Otolaryngology-Head and Neck Surgery*, vol. 157, no. 2, pp. 314–319, 2017.

[6] J. M. DelGaudio and L. A. Clemson, "An early detection protocol for invasive fungal sinusitis in neutropenic patients successfully reduces extent of disease at presentation and long term morbidity," *The Laryngoscope*, vol. 119, no. 1, pp. 180–183, 2009.

[7] W. J. Steinbach, K. A. Marr, E. J. Anaissie et al., "Clinical epidemiology of 960 patients with invasive aspergillosis from the PATH alliance registry," *Journal of Infection*, vol. 65, no. 5, pp. 453–464, 2012.

[8] S. Antinori, M. Corbellino, L. Meroni et al., "*Aspergillus* meningitis: a rare clinical manifestation of central nervous system aspergillosis. case report and review of 92 cases," *Journal of Infection*, vol. 66, no. 3, pp. 218–238, 2013.

[9] L. Senn, J. O. Robinson, S. Schmidt et al., "1,3-β-D-glucan antigenemia for early diagnosis of invasive fungal infections in neutropenic patients with acute leukemia," *Clinical Infectious Diseases*, vol. 46, pp. 1864–1870, 2008.

[10] M. F. Mafee, B. H. Tran, and A. R. Chapa, "Imaging of rhinosinusitis and its complications: plain film, CT, and MRI," *Clinical Reviews in Allergy & Immunology*, vol. 30, no. 3, pp. 165–186, 2006.

[11] S. S. Baeesa, R. F. Bokhari, K. B. Alghamdi et al., "Invasive aspergillus sinusitis with orbitocranial extension," *Asian J Neurosurg*, vol. 12, pp. 172–179, 2017.

[12] S. J. Zinreich, D. W. Kennedy, J. Malat et al., "Fungal sinusitis: diagnosis with CT and MR imaging," *Radiology*, vol. 169, no. 2, pp. 439–444, 1988.

[13] T. J. Walsh, E. J. Anaissie, D. W. Denning et al., "Treatment of aspergillosis: clinical practice guidelines of the infectious diseases society of America," *Clinical Infectious Diseases*, vol. 46, no. 3, pp. 327–360, 2008.

18

Extensive Longitudinal Transverse Myelitis Temporally Related to the use of AZD1222, AstraZeneca COVID-19 Vaccine: Cerebrospinal Fluid Analysis and Recent Data Review

Paulo Diniz da Gama,[1] Tiago Gomes de Alcantara,[2] Rafaela Ramos Smaniotto,[1] Penélope de Lima Petuco,[1] Wammer Alves de Almeida,[1] Rodrigo Assad Diiniz da Gama,[2] and Yara Dadalti Fragoso[3]

[1]*Faculty of Medical Sciences of Sorocaba, PUC-SP - Campus Sorocaba, São Paulo, Brazil*
[2]*The Conjunto Hospitalar de Sorocaba, Sorocaba, Brazil*
[3]*Universidade Metropolitana de Santos, Santos SP, Brazil*

Correspondence should be addressed to Paulo Diniz da Gama; inst.cerebro@gmail.com

Academic Editor: Isabella Laura Simone

While mass immunization against coronavirus disease 2019 (COVID-19) rolls out around the globe, safety concerns and adverse events that need prompt evaluation are also emerging. Neurological complications such as transverse myelitis raise concerns as cases were observed in clinical trials. Cerebrospinal fluid analysis is routine in these cases and the characteristics of the abnormalities found are of great help not only in establishing the diagnosis but also in understanding this rare condition. We present a case of extensive longitudinal transverse myelitis after vaccination with AZD1222, AstraZeneca COVID-19 vaccine, which was the first case reported in Brazil. The abnormalities found in the study of the cerebrospinal fluid in our case are reported and discussed using data from recent publications.

1. Introduction

Coronavirus disease 2019 (COVID-19), caused by severe acute respiratory syndrome coronavirus 2 (SARS-CoV-2) was declared to be a pandemic on March 11, 2020, by the World Health Organization [1]. Up to the present moment, several neurological symptoms and complications related to SARS-CoV-2 have been reported, irrespectively of disease severity [2–4]. In order to combat this pandemic disease, vaccines for COVID-19 have been developed at an exceptional rate. Therefore, due to the emergency situation of needing to hold back the pandemic, there are no medium to long-term studies on the efficacy and possible adverse events of these vaccines [5]. Here, we report a case of longitudinal extensive transverse myelitis (LETM) that appeared 18 days after the patient received the first dose of COVID-19 vaccine (AZD1222, AstraZeneca). We consider that the temporal relationship between the vaccine and the myelitis could mean a causal association. The cerebrospinal fluid (CSF) analyses were given with greater interest, with a subsequent review of our recent literature.

2. Case Report

A 47-year-old woman was admitted to our emergency unit on June 4, 2021, reporting having received the first dose of AZD1222, AstraZeneca vaccine, for COVID-19 18 days prior to her admission. Twelve hours after receiving the vaccine, she had an episode of chills, headache, retroocular pain, neck pain, tiredness, nausea, stomach pain, and shortness of breath. The symptoms diminished with symptomatic medications. After the initial improvement, the symptoms got worse again. The patient felt mild weakness in the lower limbs that evolved over 5 days until she could no longer stand up.

At the admission examination, she was conscious, with no apparent cognitive deficit, presenting motor weakness (grade 2 in the lower limbs and grade 3 in the upper limbs), hyporeflexia, bilateral Babinski's sign, mild hypoesthesia in the lower limbs without a notable sensory level, preserved coordination, and preserved function of the cranial nerves. She presented urinary retention, requiring bladder catheterization.

Routine blood tests were carried out at the time of her admission, and no hydroelectrolytic, metabolic, or systemic inflammatory changes were found. A magnetic resonance imaging (MRI) study on neuroaxis showed extensive spinal cord demyelination. This lesion, shown in Figures 1 and 2, was hyperintense in T2 sequence and extended from the C6 cervical level to the medullary cone. It was mildly tumefactive with no gadolinium enhancement. Brain MRI was unremarkable regarding any inflammatory process.

Cerebrospinal fluid (CSF) analysis showed a pleocytosis of 205 cells/mm^3 with predominance of lymphocytes (88%), and also eosinophils (7%), neutrophils (4%), and monocytes (1%). There were increased protein levels (56.7 mg/dL) and normal levels of glucose (56 mg/dL) and chlorine (125 mEq/L). Isoelectric focusing of CSF protein and serum showed identical oligoclonal IgG bands (OCB) in both (type 4 pattern), suggestive of systemic inflammation. Testing for anti-aquaporin 4 antibody and anti-MOG antibody was negative. A nasopharyngeal swab was negative for SARS-CoV-2 in RT-PCR.

The patient received methylprednisolone 1.0 g intravenously per day for five days and symptomatic medications. She showed a gradual improvement in her motor disability and was discharged for outpatient follow-up after seven days of hospitalization. Oral methylprednisolone was prescribed at a dose of 60 mg/day, which continued in use over a 45-day gradual withdrawal regimen.

On June 17, 2021, she came back to our outpatient clinic for reassessment of her condition and reported having had gradual improvement in her motor deficit. She was already walking with little disability. She was evaluated again on July 29, 2021, showing some further improvement with strength recovery in all limbs, but still showing exacerbated deep tendon reflexes with bilateral positive Babinski's sign.

3. Discussion

During the current COVID-19 pandemic, a growing number of neurological manifestations and complications have been described [2–4]. Most cases consisted of post-infectious immune-mediated myelitis, and only a few have been considered parainfectious or infectious [6,7]. Particularly regarding COVID-19 vaccines, a case of transverse myelitis was reported during a preapproval clinical trial for AZD1222, AstraZeneca vaccine [8]. National health surveillance boards have already received several spontaneous reports on myelitis following COVID-19 vaccines, but no further data on diagnostic findings are available and, generally, no distinction has been made between infectious and other etiologies [9]. Hence, the implication of these spontaneous reports remains vague and assessment of potential causality is not possible.

Pagenkopf and Sudmeyer [10] recently described a very well-documented case of a 45-year-old male with LETM after application of the AZD1222, AstraZeneca COVID-19 vaccine. This showed many similarities to our clinical case regarding the time of symptom onset, duration, degree of involvement of disabilities in the acute phase, and residual state of symptoms. We also noticed similarities regarding the MRI of the spinal cord in their study, which also showed a lesion with no gadolinium enhancement. In our case, the lesion was more extensive with a minor swelling effect. Their CSF evaluation also showed similarities regarding the increased protein levels and pleocytosis. However, possibly due to the different CSF collection periods, our patient did not present glucose consumption and had a predominance of lymphocytes in CSF, just like in the follow-up CSF of that reported case. In addition, our patient presented OCB in CSF and in serum (pattern 4), which were not visualized in the abovementioned case [10]. Notghi et al. [11] also described a case of a 58-year-old man who developed initial LEMT symptoms 7 days after receiving the AstraZeneca vaccine. The CSF analysis showed a large increase in proteins, lymphocyte pleocytosis predominantly in addition to the presence of OCB in the CSF and serum, pattern 4. In this description, the clinical history, with good evolution of their disabilities, the MRI and especially all data from the CSF study were similar to our case report. Other authors such as Yong Tan et al. [12] and Hsiao et al. [13]. also described cases of LEMT after receiving the AstraZeneca vaccine. The CSF study in these two cases also showed an inflammatory activity with the presence of increased proteins, but the first did not find the presence of OCB and the second did not provide this data. In these two cases, the images and the favorable clinical evolution were similar to our case. McLean and Trefts [14] reported a 69-year-old previously healthy female presented with LEMT, 2 days after vaccination with the Pfizer-BioNTech mRNA vaccine. This patient also revealed OCB in the CSF with matching bands in the serum (pattern 4) just like our case report, although other data from the CSF analysis were normal. MRI and the favorable clinical evolution also showed similarities. Ali Alshararni [15] also reported a case of a 38-year-old man who started his symptoms two days after also using Pfizer's vaccine. An increase in CSF proteins showing inflammatory activity was described, but there were no data provided regarding the number of cells and the study of OCB. Gao et al. [16] report a case of LETM that occurred two days after vaccination with the Moderna COVID-19 (mRNA-1273) vaccine, as well as Khan et al. [17] that report one day after the same vaccine. Both authors showed an inflammatory pattern in the CSF due to the increase in proteins, and the first found the presence of OCB in CSF and serum (pattern 4) without cell increase and the second described lymphocytic cell increase and did not find the presence of OCB (pattern 1). Tahir et al. [18] reported a case of a 44-year-old woman who presented LEMT 10 days after receiving the Johnson & Johnson COVID-19 vaccine. This patient

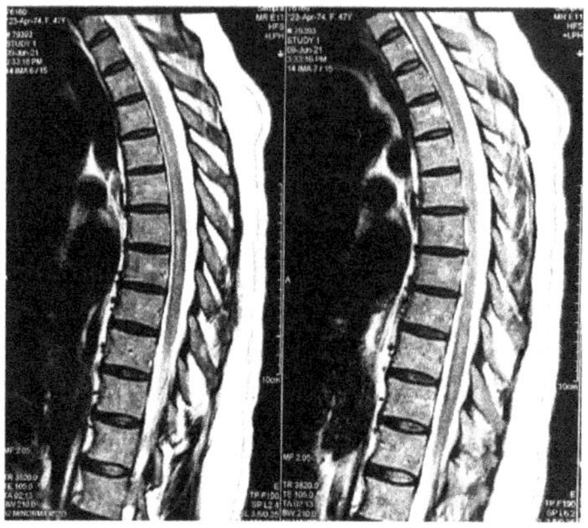

FIGURE 1: Extensive longitudinal lesion starting in C8 to the terminal cone.

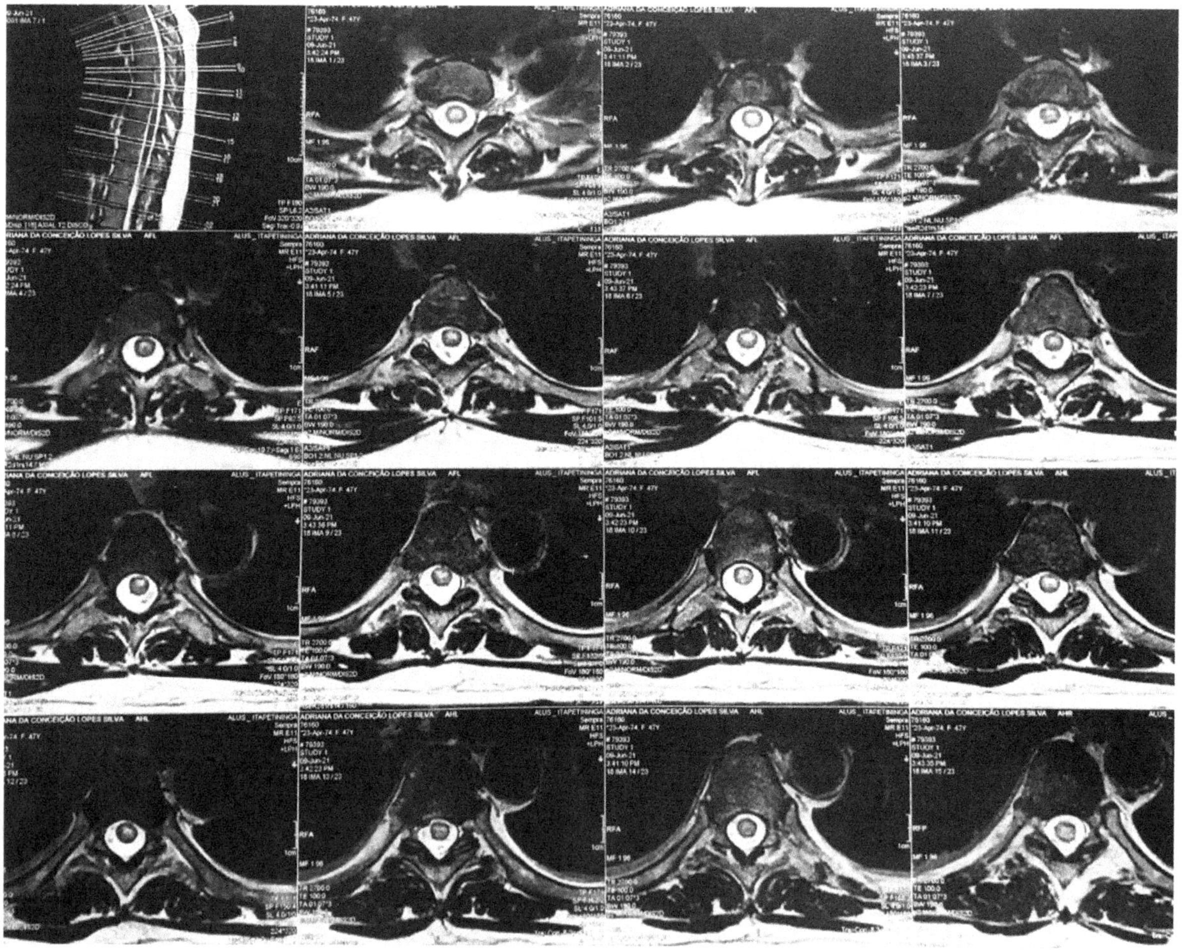

FIGURE 2: Central spinal cord lesion.

presented clinical and image manifestations with similar characteristics to our reported case, including the CSF evaluation, which showed increased protein, normal glucose, and pleocytosis with an expressive lymphocytic predominance. In this case, there was an absence of OCB in CSF and serum (pattern 1). Erdem et al. [19] reported a case of a 78-year-old woman who also presented LEMT with symptom onset 3 weeks prior to receiving the second dose of CoronaVac vaccine (Sinovac Life Sciences, China). In this case, the only data that evidenced an inflammatory activity in the CSF was an increase in protein concentration. Table 1 shows a schematic summary of all these reported cases.

Because the specific pathogenesis of postvaccinal LEMT are unknown, there is no specific test, be it lab-based or otherwise available, which is why one needs to rely on "circumstantial evidence." The diagnosis is based on typical,

Table 1: Characteristics of cerebrospinal fluid analysis in reported cases of longitudinal extensive transverse myelitis (LEMT) post COVID-19 vaccine.

Author/country	Type of vaccine	CSF protein mg/dL	CSF glucose mg/dL	CSF white blood cells x u/L	CSF OCB	Serum OCB
Our case Brazil	AstraZeneca	56.4	56 (123 serum)	205 (88% lymphocytes)	Positive	Positive
Pagenkopf and Sudmeyer [10] ermany	AstraZeneca	1400 7 days after normal	Decreased 7 days after normal	481 (67% neutrophil) 7 days after 76 (100% lymphocyte)	Negative	Negative
Notghi et al. [11] United Kingdom	AstraZeneca	168.0	76 (140 serum)	11 (100% lymphocytes)	Positive	Positive
Yong Tan et al. [12] Malaysia	AstraZeneca	54.6	31 (56 serum)	<5	Negative	Negative
Hsiao et al. [13] Taiwan	AstraZeneca	44.3	No data	11 (100% lymphocytes)	No data	No data
McLean and Trefts [14] USA	Pfizer	<40	Normal	<5	Positive	Positive
Ali Alshararni [15] Saudi Arabia	Pfizer	62.1	46 (- serum)	No data	No data	No data
Gao et al. [16] Taiwan	Moderna	57.2	71 (117 serum)	15 (73% neutrophil)	Negative	Negative
Khan et al. [17] USA	Moderna	56.0	77 (125 serum)	2	Positive	Positive
Tahir et al. [18] USA	Johnson and Johnson	43	71	227 (96% lymphocytes)	Negative	Negative
Erdem et al. [19] Turkey	CoronaVac	56.0	104 (150 serum)	2	Negative	Negative

yet not limited to, clinical findings, magnetic resonance imaging, and CSF analysis as well as other investigations.

Detection of intrathecal IgG synthesis is part of the routine CSF work-up [20]. Isoelectric focusing and subsequent immunoblotting is the gold standard to visualize clonally restricted IgG OCB in CSF [21]. Five different patterns of isoelectric focusing have been defined: pattern 1: normal; pattern 2: OCB IgG restricted to CSF; pattern 3: OCB IgG in CSF with additional identical bands in CSF and serum (combination of patterns 2 and 4); pattern 4: identical OCB in CSF and serum (a mirror effect); pattern 5: monoclonal IgG bands in CSF and serum (myeloma or monoclonal gammopathy of uncertain significance). The appearance of OCB in CSF without corresponding bands in serum constitute a local intrathecal synthesis of IgG and supports the diagnosis of a variety of inflammatory central nervous system (CNS) diseases extending from an autoimmune to infectious pathology [20, 21]. Apart from multiple sclerosis, there is a long list of diagnoses with OCB restricted to CSF reported: neuromyelitis optica spectrum disorder, MOG-IgG antibody associated syndromes, systemic lupus erythematosus, Behcet's disease, CNS vasculitis, acute and chronic infections, anti-NMDA and other autoimmune encephalitis, cerebral tumors including lymphomas, among others [20, 21]. Of most interest for neurological diagnosis are patterns 1, 2, and 3, because they reject (pattern 1) or confirm (patterns 2 and 3) the intrathecal IgG production. Furthermore, blood-derived OCB in CSF (patterns 3 and 4) can give additional information because it provides evidence of both systemic and intrathecal (pattern 3) or only systemic immune activation (pattern 4). Lastly, the "mirror-pattern" (pattern 4) is most frequently associated with various peripheral inflammatory neuropathies (e.g., Guillain-Barré) and very less frequently seen with systemic infections, systemic autoimmune diseases, or neoplastic disorders. Often this disease involving CNS synthesizes IgG intrathecally more common (pattern 3) [20, 21].

Of the 11 cases of LEMT post COVID-19 vaccine that we describe in this article, 4 of them had OCB with a distribution pattern 4 and no case was described OCB with other patterns of distribution, and this attracted a lot of attention.

The observation of the clinical characteristics of post-vaccination LEMT, with its favorable evolution, together with the peculiar data of MRI and the analysis of the CSF, which demonstrates not only an inflammatory activity in the CNS by the presence of increased proteins and pleocytosis but also by the observation of cases with this OCB "mirror-pattern" (pattern 4) which may not only be decisive for a better understanding of the pathophysiology of postvaccination LEMT but also may now better suggest the diagnosis of this rare condition.

There was no outstanding feature regarding clinical-evolutionary aspects, MRI features, or CSF presentation regarding the types of vaccine, which could lead to suggest a different inflammatory response. What we can conclude is still very initial, due to the low number of cases reported in the literature.

Nevertheless, despite the adverse effects reported by COVID-19 vaccines, which to date can be considered rare, it is essential to emphasize that the protective effects of vaccination can still greatly contribute to the health of individuals and the world.

4. Conclusion

LEMT has apparently been shown to be a temporal-related effect of COVID-19 vaccines and should be considered promptness to the onset of symptoms. The study of CSF with the presence of inflammatory activity and the demonstration of the presence of OCB equally distributed in CSF and in serum may help to consider this rare condition, until new evidence is confirmed.

Disclosure

The funder played no role in the approval and editing of this manuscript or the decision to publish it.

Acknowledgments

This study was funded by the Faculty of Medical Sciences of Sorocaba, PUC-SP, as part of Dr. Paulo Diniz da Gama's professorship.

References

[1] N. Zhu, D. Zhang, W. Wang et al., "A novel coronavirus from patients with pneumonia in China, 2019," *New England Journal of Medicine*, vol. 382, no. 8, pp. 727–733, 2020.

[2] E. Meppiel, N. Peiffer-Smadja, A. Maury et al., "Neurologic manifestations associated with COVID-19: a multicentre registry," *Clinical microbiology and infection: The Official Publication of the European Society of Clinical Microbiology and Infectious Diseases*, vol. 27, no. 3, pp. 458–466, 2021.

[3] Y. B. Ferreira, F. M. R. F. Freire, F. M. R. Freire et al., "Neurological manifestations associated with COVID- 19: a review," *Brazilian Journal of Case Reports*, vol. 1, no. 4, pp. 31–44, 2021.

[4] S. H.-Y. Chou, E. Beghi, R. Helbok et al., "Global incidence of neurological manifestations among patients hospitalized with COVID-19-A report for the GCS-NeuroCOVID consortium and the ENERGY consortium," *JAMA Network Open*, vol. 4, no. 5, Article ID e2112131, 2021.

[5] W. Health Organization, "Coronavirus disease (COVID-19): Vaccines safety," 2021, https://www.who.int/emergencies/diseases/novel-coronavirus-2019/question-and-answers-hub/q-a-detail/coronavirus-disease-(covid-19)-vaccines-safety.

[6] A. Artemiadis, A. Liampas, L. Hadjigeorgiou, and P. Zis, "Myelopathy associated with SARS-COV-2 infection. A systematic review," *A systematic review Neurological Research*, vol. 43, no. 8, pp. 633–641, 2021.

[7] G. C. Román, F. Gracia, A. Torres, A. Palacios, K. Gracia, and D. Harris, "Acute transverse myelitis (ATM):Clinical review of 43 patients with COVID-19-associated ATM and 3 post-vaccination ATM serious adverse events with the ChAdOx1 nCoV-19 vaccine (AZD1222)," *Frontiers in Immunology*, vol. 12, Article ID 653786, 2021.

[8] M. Voysey, S. A. C. Clemens, C. Costa et al., "Safety and efficacy of the ChAdOx1 nCoV-19 vaccine (AZD1222) against SARS-CoV-2: an interim analysis of four randomised controlled trials in Brazil, South Africa, and the UK," *Lancet (London, England)*, vol. 397, no. 10269, pp. 99–111, 2021.

[9] "COVID-19 Vaccine AstraZeneca Analysis Print," 2021, https://assets.publishing.service.gov.uk/government/uploads/system/uploads/attachment_data/file/1025766/COVID-19_AstraZeneca_Vaccine_Analysis_Print_DLP_06.10.2021.pdf.

[10] C. Pagenkopf and M. Südmeyer, "A case of longitudinally extensive transverse myelitis following vaccination against Covid-19," *Journal of Neuroimmunology*, vol. 358, Article ID 577606, 2021.

[11] A. A. Notghi, J. Atley, and M. Silva, "Lessons of the month 1: longitudinal extensive transverse myelitis following AstraZeneca COVID-19 vaccination," *Clinical Medicine*, vol. 21, no. 5, p. e535, 2021.

[12] W. Yong Tan, A. H. K. Yusof Khan, M. N. M. Yaakob et al., "Longitudinal extensive transverse myelitis following ChAdOx1 nCOV-19 vaccine: a case report," *BMC Neurology*, vol. 21, p. 395, 2021.

[13] Y.-T. Hsiao, M.-J. Tsai, Y.-H. Chen, and C.-F. Hsu, "Acute transverse myelitis after COVID-19 vaccination," *Medicina*, vol. 57, no. 10, p. 1010, 2021.

[14] P. McLean and L. Trefts, "Transverse myelitis 48 hours after the administration of an mRNA COVID 19 vaccine," *Neuroimmunology Reports*, vol. 1, Article ID 100019, 2021.

[15] A. Ali Alshararni, "Acute transverse myelitis associated with COVID-19 vaccine: a case report," *International Journal of Research in Pharmacy and Science*, vol. 12, no. 3, pp. 2083–2087, 2021.

[16] J.-J. Gao, H.-P. Tseng, C.-L. Lin et al., "Acute transverse myelitis following COVID-19 vaccination," *Vaccines*, vol. 9, no. 9, p. 1008, 2021.

[17] E. Khan, A. K. Shrestha, and M. A. Colantonio, "Acute transverse myelitis following SARS-CoV-2 vaccination: a case report and review of literature," *Journal of Neurology*, vol. 269, 2021.

[18] N. Tahir, G. Koorapati, S. Prasad et al., "SARS-CoV-2 vaccination-induced transverse myelitis," *Cureus*, vol. 13, no. 7, Article ID e16624, 2021.

[19] N. Ş. Erdem, D. Seden, Ö. Tuğba et al., "Acute transverse myelitis after inactivated COVID-19 vaccine," *Ideggyogyaszati Szemle*, vol. 74, no. 07-08, pp. 273–276, 2021.

[20] F. Deisenhammer, A. Bartos, R. Egg et al., "Guidelines on routine cerebrospinal fluid analysis. Report from an EFNS task force," *European Journal of Neurology*, vol. 13, no. 9, pp. 913–922, 2006.

[21] M. S. Freedman, E. J. Thompson, F. Deisenhammer et al., "Recommended standard of cerebrospinal fluid analysis in the diagnosis of multiple sclerosis," *Archives of Neurology*, vol. 62, no. 6, pp. 865–870, 2005.

19

Rescue Revascularisation in Acute Internal Carotid Artery Occlusion with a Super Extended Time Window of More than 48 hours

Katharina Berger,[1,2,3] Jennifer Sartor-Pfeiffer,[1,3,4] Annerose Mengel,[1,3,4] Ulrike Ernemann,[1,5] Ulf Ziemann,[1,3,4] Florian Hennersdorf,[1,5] and Katharina Feil[1,3,4]

[1]*Centre for Neurovascular Diseases Tübingen, ZNET: University of Tübingen, Tübingen, Germany*
[2]*Department of Neurology & Epileptology, University of Tübingen, Tübingen, Germany*
[3]*Hertie Institute for Clinical Brain Research, University Tübingen, Tübingen, Germany*
[4]*Department of Neurology & Stroke, University of Tübingen, Tübingen, Germany*
[5]*Department of Diagnostic & Interventional Neuroradiology, University of Tübingen, Tübingen, Germany*

Correspondence should be addressed to Katharina Berger; katharina.berger@med.uni-tuebingen.de

Florian Hennersdorf and Katharina Feil contributed equally to this work.

Academic Editor: Isabella Laura Simone

Background and Aim. Mechanical thrombectomy (MT) and intravenous thrombolysis are the gold standard treatment for large vessel occlusion (LVO) strokes. 10–20% of LVO patients present as "minor strokes" with a National Institutes of Health Stroke Scale (NIHSS) ≤5 points. Therefore, MT is often not primarily performed. These patients rely on collateral blood flow but are prone to clinical deterioration and unfavourable outcome. MT is performed after clinical deterioration, often in an extended time window within 24 hours. No scores identify patients at risk for clinical deterioration. *Methods.* We present the case of a 71-year-old Caucasian male "minor stroke" patient with LVO, good collateral flow via the ophthalmic artery, receiving rescue MT following clinical deterioration after >48 hours. NIHSS and modified Rankin scale (mRS) were used for follow-up and modified treatment in cerebral infarction (mTICI) score for angiographic results. *Results.* Excellent angiographic result (mTICI 3) and clinical improvement were achieved (NIHSS preintervention 18, on discharge 2 points). 90-day follow-up showed excellent outcome (mRS 1). *Conclusions.* Late intervention MT should be encouraged when clinical deficit exceeds infarct demarcation. Standardized identification based on clinical and imaging data is required to target critical patients with LVO and low NIHSS, favouring a primary intervention.

1. Introduction

Mechanical thrombectomy (MT) in combination with intravenous thrombolysis (IVT) has become the gold standard treatment for stroke patients caused by large vessel occlusion (LVO) [1]. Although LVO typically leads to severe stroke, at least 10–20% of stroke patients presenting with LVO have only mild symptoms (National Institutes of Health Stroke Scale (NIHSS) ≤5, i.e., minor stroke). These patients are at high risk of clinical neurological deterioration and poor outcome [1, 2]. Therefore, treatment guidelines in minor stroke patients remain controversial [3]. Whilst recanalization rates in LVO with recombinant tissue plasminogen activator (rtPA) alone are unsatisfactory, endovascular treatment can be associated with higher mortality rates due to the increased risk of symptomatic intracerebral hemorrhage [4]. Recent observational studies comparing immediate MT in these patients and best medical therapy followed by rescue MT in deteriorating cases have shown superior outcomes following immediate MT in minor stroke patients [2]. Current guidelines suggest MT within 6 hours, with the option for late window interventions after 6 hours [1]. Results given by the

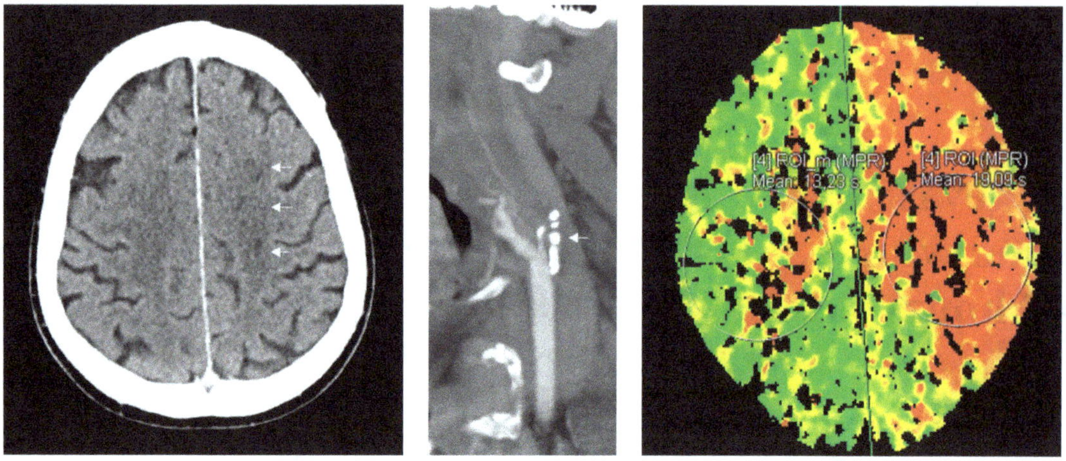

(a) (b) (c)

FIGURE 1: (a) Noncontrast CT: small border zone infarcts (white arrows) ASPECTS 10. (b) CT angiography: occlusion of the left ICA caused by a preexisting atherosclerotic stenosis (white arrow). (c) Time-to-peak map of CT perfusion: delay in maximum attenuation of 5.7 seconds.

DEFUSE3 and DAWN studies also encourage late interventions in selected patients [1, 5]. The decision for or against MT in LVO patients with minor stroke symptoms and clinical deterioration is currently based on interdisciplinary single case discussion. Predictive measures which determine the patient's risk for deterioration in case of withholding MT are not established. Here, we report on a case of a super extended time window of more than 48 hours after symptom onset until rescue MT was performed.

2. Case Report

A 71-year-old Caucasian male patient (premorbid modified Rankin scale (pmRS) 0), with a medical history of hypertension, presented with aphasia and right hemiparesis (National Institutes of Health Stroke Scale (NIHSS) 8 points) in a regional hospital; symptoms had persisted for more than six hours at time of admission. Initial cerebral computed tomography (cCT) with CT angiography (CTA) showed no infarct demarcation, but proximal LVO of the left internal carotid artery (ICA). Due to the expired time window, IVT was not performed, and the patient was transferred via "drip and ship" to the Center of Neurovascular Diseases of the University Hospital of Tuebingen (ZNET). On in-house admission, the patient presented with only a mild neurological deficit (NIHSS 3 points given for Broca's aphasia and mild right arm paresis). cCT with CTA and CT perfusion (CTP) showed a persistent occlusion of the left ICA, with beginning border zone infarct demarcation between the anterior and middle cerebral artery territories and an extensive perfusion deficit within the territory of the middle and anterior cerebral arteries with a delay in a time-to-peak of 5.7 s in comparison to the nonaffected hemisphere (Figure 1).

Due to the low NIHSS on admission, the late time window, as well as the assumed collateralization (due to only minor neurological symptoms), a decision was made in favour of a conservative treatment, and invasive blood pressure measurement was initiated for monitoring. The patient initially remained clinically stable for more than 24 hours after stroke onset. The patient received a dual antiplatelet and high-dose statin-therapy with atorvastatin. Afterwards, he began to develop fluctuating neurological symptoms dependent on variations in systolic blood pressure. In follow-up imaging, the ICA remained occluded, with a reduced blood flow in the middle cerebral artery (MCA) and a retrograde blood flow in the ophthalmic artery in duplex sonography.

Any systolic blood pressure dropping below 230 mmHg resulted in global aphasia, as well as right-sided hemiplegia (NIHSS 18 points), whereas systolic blood pressure levels above 230 mmHg resulted in immediate symptom improvement (minimal NIHSS 3 points), indicating that collateral blood flow was maintained only through high perfusion pressure. Further investigations showed that the cerebral infarct demarcation remained the same as on initial presentation with a persisting perfusion deficit indicating a small core infarct with a large volume of tissue at risk. Despite the extended time window of more than 48 hours after stroke symptom onset, an interdisciplinary decision for off-label rescue MT was made. No drugs with a potential blood pressure lowering effect were administered prior to intervention.

Angiograms of the left common carotid artery showed the occluded ICA with distal filling at the level of the skull base through multiple collaterals from the external carotid artery indicating insufficient intracranial crossflow (Figures 2(a) and 2(b)). The procedure has been performed under general anaesthesia, using an 8F balloon guide catheter (Corail Plus™, Balt). The occluded vessel was passed with a microwire, and angioplasty was performed using a percutaneous transluminal angioplasty (PTA) catheter. Thromboaspiration was performed on site of the protruded guider, enabling revascularisation of the left ICA, however, with a remaining high-grade stenosis of the revascularized vessel. The remaining stenosis was then treated by placement of a stent (Precise Pro RX™, Cardinal Health).

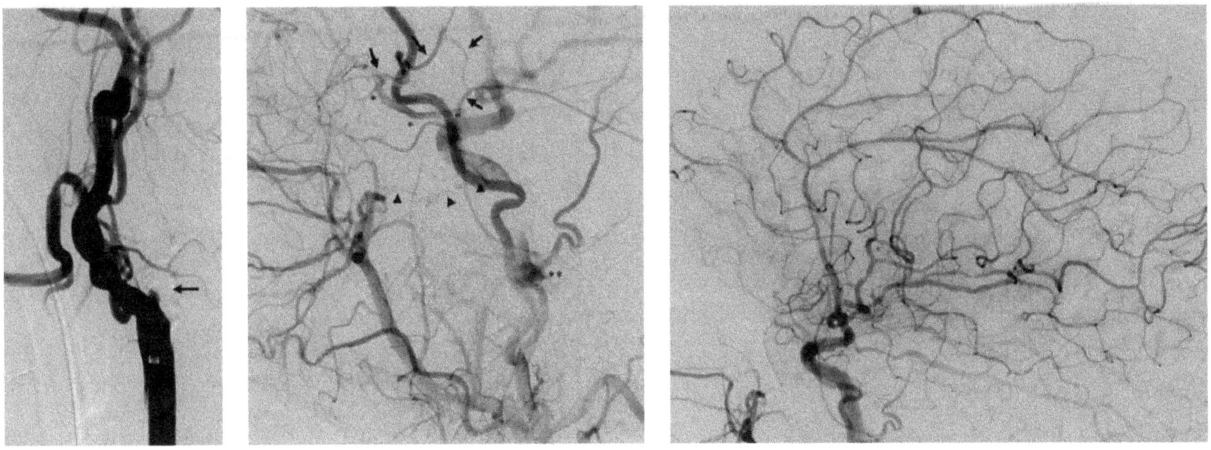

(a) (b) (c)

FIGURE 2: (a) Lateral angiogram of the common carotid artery (CCA) showing occlusion of the ICA. (b) Lateral CCA angiogram: exclusive filling of the intracranial vessels through multiple collaterals (*), retrogradely filled ophthalmic artery (OA); arrows depict a connection between the middle meningeal artery (MMA) and OA. Dural anastomoses from MMA to ICA at the level of the skull base (**); arrow heads depict a branch of the sphenopalatine artery feeding the cavernous ICA (superimposed by the superficial temporal artery). (c) Lateral angiogram after intervention: (TICI3). Vessel wall irregularities are rated as atherosclerotic.

Despite concerns about thromboembolism from the long-term persisting long-distance occlusion, the final angiograms showed no intracranial vessel occlusions (modified treatment in cerebral infarction (mTICI) score 3) (Figure 2(c)). The post-MT cCT did not show any further infarct demarcation or secondary intracranial hemorrhage.

Thereafter, the patient's clinical presentation improved significantly; blood pressure values normalized into the high-normal range. The patient was discharged to neurological rehabilitation with NIHSS 2 points (mRS 2) given for disorientation in time and space, due to a hyperactive delirium, which occurred as a complication. In the further clinical course at 90-day follow-up, the patient had an excellent clinical outcome (mRS 1).

3. Discussion

Our case presents a patient with minor stroke despite proximal LVO of the ICA turning to massive clinical deterioration after initial decision for conservative treatment. Although efficacy of MT is time-dependent [1, 2], the results of DAWN and DIFFUSE3 showed that selected patients benefit from MT in an extended time window of 6–24 hours. In our case, this window has been exceeded by far, based on a second cCT presenting still without clear infarct demarcation except for small watershed infarctions (Alberta stroke program early CT score (ASPECTS) 10) and extensive tissue at risk with only small core infarct volume on CTP. Despite concerns about thromboembolism from the long-term persisting, long-distance occlusion, the procedure was successfully performed with an excellent angiographic result (mTICI 3) and clinical outcome, and postinterventional imaging showed no increase in infarct volume.

Studies suggest that a preexisting good collateral flow is predictive for a favourable outcome after MT and can be also used as a selection criterion for patients [6]. In the present case, the clinical deficits fluctuated in association with blood pressure variation, indicating that the cerebral perfusion provided by the collateral blood flow (Figure 2(b)) was insufficient and maintained only through high perfusion pressure as any systolic blood pressure dropping below 230 mmHg resulted in a massive clinical deterioration with NIHSS increasing from 3 to 18 points. Taking the results of DEFUSE3 and DAWN into consideration, collateral blood flow has not been a selection criterion for or against MT. Contrary, criteria for intervention were LVO in the anterior circulation, small infarct volume, as well as high NIHSS. In summary, despite the late time window, our patient fulfilled the described criteria favouring MT.

Furthermore, this case once more highlights that the NIHSS cannot alone be used as a score to evaluate which primary treatment is the most appropriate regarding LVO, although to date, it is the only validated clinical score used for decision making, especially regarding rescue MT [7]. Currently, there are no clear clinical indicators, in which minor stroke patients are at high risk of clinical deterioration and accordingly would likely benefit from primary intervention. Lately, possible scores based on thrombus length and site of occlusion were discussed as easily applicable but require clinical validation [6].

4. Conclusion

Late window MT should be considered in patients with minor stroke and LVO based on standardized criteria. Especially in the context of clinical deterioration and the clinical deficit exceeding the infarct demarcation but rather matching the perfusion deficit, a reevaluation towards MT should be made. A high initial NIHSS score in the context of early improvement can imply a high likelihood of secondary deterioration as it stresses the significance of the occlusion and the clinical impact in case of collateral circulation break down. A standardized procedure based on clinical and imaging data might help to identify such critical patients for early reperfusion. Prospective studies are required for confirmation and validation.

Consent

Written informed consent was obtained from the patient's legal guardian for publication of this case report and any accompanying images.

Authors' Contributions

Florian Hennersdorf and Katharina Feil contributed equally to this study. All authors have read and approved the manuscript before submission. KB drafted and revised the manuscript for content, including medical writing, medical care, and examination of patient. JSP provided medical care of patient and revised manuscript for content. AM revised manuscript for content and provided medical care of patient. UE and UZ revised manuscript for content. FH provided medical neurointerventional care of the patient and revised manuscript for content, including medical writing. KF provided idea and drafted and revised the manuscript for content, including medical writing, medical care, and examination of patient.

Acknowledgments

The authors thank MD Roshan Rupra for copy-editing the manuscript and the patient for the participation. The authors acknowledge the support by Open Access Publishing Fund of the University of Tübingen.

References

[1] W. J. Powers, A. A. Rabinstein, T. Ackerson et al., "Guidelines for the early management of patients with acute ischemic stroke: 2019 update to the 2018 guidelines for the early management of acute ischemic stroke: a guideline for healthcare professionals from the American heart association/ American stroke association," *Stroke*, vol. 50, no. 12, p. e344, 2019.

[2] S. A. Alqahtani, A. B. Stemer, M. F. McCullough et al., "Endovascular management of stroke patients with large vessel occlusion and minor stroke symptoms," *Cureus*, vol. 9, no. 6, p. e1355, 2017.

[3] K. Feil, M. Matusevicius, M. Herzberg et al., "Minor stroke in large vessel occlusion: a matched analysis of patients from the German stroke registry-endovascular treatment (GSR-ET) and patients from the safe implementation of treatments in stroke-international stroke thrombolysis register (SITS-ISTR)," *European Journal of Neurology*, 2022.

[4] O. Volny, C. Zerna, A. Tomek et al., "Thrombectomy vs medical management in low NIHSS acute anterior circulation stroke," *Neurology*, vol. 95, no. 24, pp. e3364–e3372, 2020.

[5] M. J. Alberts, M. D. Ollenschleger, and A. Nouh, "Dawn of a new era for stroke treatment," *Circulation*, vol. 137, no. 17, pp. 1767–1769, 2018.

[6] B. Kim, C. Jung, H. S. Nam et al., "Comparison between perfusion- and collateral-based triage for endovascular thrombectomy in a late time window," *Stroke*, vol. 50, no. 12, pp. 3465–3470, 2019.

[7] P. Seners, W. Ben Hassen, B. Lapergue et al., "Prediction of early neurological deterioration in individuals with minor stroke and large vessel occlusion intended for intravenous thrombolysis alone," *JAMA Neurology*, vol. 78, no. 3, pp. 321–328, 2021.

20

Epileptic Patient with Mild Malformation of Cortical Development with Oligodendroglial Hyperplasia and Epilepsy (MOGHE): A Case Report and Review of the Literature

A. Verentzioti,[1] I. Blumcke,[2] A. Alexoudi,[1] P. Patrikelis,[1] A. Siatouni,[1] S. Korfias,[1] D. Sakas,[1] and S. Gatzonis[1]

[1]*Department of Neurosurgery, National & Kapodistrian University of Athens, Evangelismos Hospital, Athens, Greece*
[2]*Department of Neuropathology, University Hospital Erlangen, Germany*

Correspondence should be addressed to A. Verentzioti; nverentzioti@gmail.com

Academic Editor: Hidetoshi Ikeda

Introduction. There is an emerging interest in the literature about MOGHE (Mild Malformation of Cortical Development with Oligodendroglial Hyperplasia and Epilepsy). We report the case of an epileptic patient with MOGHE. *Case Report.* A 33-year-old male patient was suffering from refractory focal epilepsy since adolescence. MRI demonstrated increased T2/FLAIR signal intensity of right frontal lobe. Presurgical evaluation led to definition of epileptogenic network in a specific area of right frontal lobe. The resected specimen revealed MOGHE. *Discussion.* MOGHE appears to be a brain entity which shares some unique histopathological features. Review of the literature is in accordance with our patient's findings. The major neuropathological finding consists of areas with blurred gray-white matter boundaries due to heterotopic neurons in white matter and increased numbers of subcortical oligodendroglial cells with increased proliferation. MR abnormalities are present in T2/FLAIR sequences. It concerns patients with refractory frontal lobe epilepsy and appears to associate with unfavourable postsurgical outcome in seizure control. *Conclusion.* More cases are needed in order to establish more data about this distinct entity in frontal lobe epilepsy. This could be valuable knowledge to patients and doctors concerning expectations or management of undesirable outcome in frontal lobe epilepsy surgery.

1. Introduction

According to the updated classification for malformations of cortical development, there are three main categories of malformations which include the majority of histopathological findings and characteristics [1]. Nevertheless, a percentage of 2-26% of epilepsy surgery specimens are histopathologically classified as nonlesional [2].

There is an developing interest in the international literature on MOGHE (Mild Malformation of Cortical Development with Oligodendroglial Hyperplasia and Epilepsy). It is a new histopathological entity of brain lesions which cannot be included within the existent classification. We report the case of an epileptic patient with refractory epilepsy, who underwent surgical resection and had MOGHE.

2. Case Presentation

A 33-year-old male patient was suffering from epileptic seizures since the age of sixteen. He is right handed and his personal and familial medical history were free. At 16, he had three episodes with bilateral tonic clonic seizures at awakening. After the beginning of medication he presented only with focal hyperkinetic seizures with mild impairment of awareness without secondary generalization.

Because of drug-resistance he presented for presurgical evaluation. His seizure frequency was 4-8 seizures per month. His medication was lacosamide 600 mg/day, levetiracetam 3000 mg/day, and valproic acid 1000 mg/day.

Brain MRI revealed increased T2 and FLAIR signal intensity of right frontal lobe, due to possible gray matter

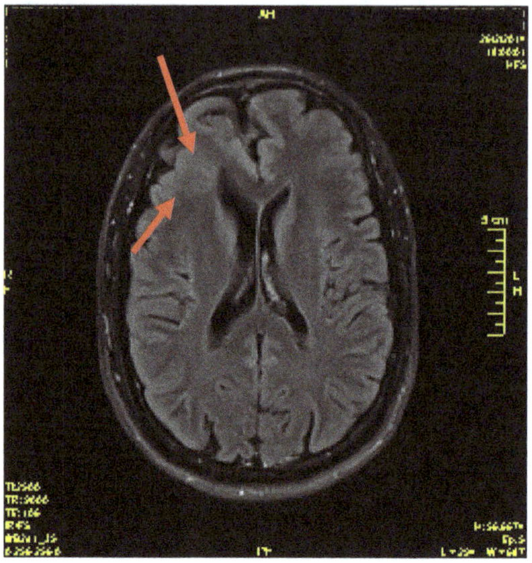

FIGURE 1: MRI-FLAIR sequence.

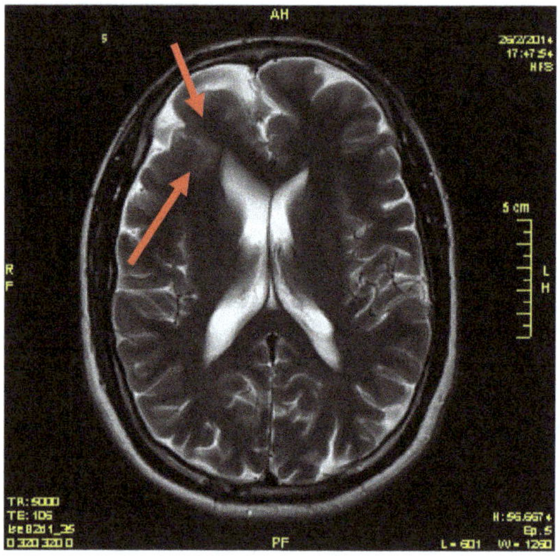

FIGURE 2: MRI-T2 sequence.

heterotopias or FCD (1.5 Tesla MR imaging study), Figures 1 and 2.

The patient underwent long term video-EEG with surface electrodes for three days, where five seizures were recorded with variable duration from 16 to 30 seconds.

Data suggested that epileptogenic network was at right frontal lobe. We proceeded thus with implantation of subdural grids and strips and depth electrodes to this specific area, in order to achieve a precise localization of caudal boundaries of epileptic network as well as to map the cortical functions, especially the kinetic area.

Second long term video-EEG and subsequent cortical stimulation led to a tailored resection of the right frontal lobe with respect to the kinetic area.

The available postoperative data concern a period of two years of seizure freedom.

The histopathological findings of the resected brain specimen revealed the emerging entity called MOGHE, Figures 3, 4, and 5.

3. Discussion

MOGHE's major neuropathological finding consists of areas with blurred gray-white matter boundaries due to heterotopic neurons in white matter and increased numbers of subcortical oligodendroglial cells [2]. Interestingly, these foci of heterotopic neurons are observed in the adjacent white matter and not in deep areas of white matter, defined as 500 μm distant from the cortical junction.

The absence of heterotopic neurons in deep white matter excludes its histopathological classification as mild malformation of cortical development (MCD) Palmini Type II [3].

Another characteristic feature is the increase of Olig2-immunoreactive oligodendroglia observed in white matter and deep cortical layers as well as increased proliferation. This increase is multifocal with patchy areas of diffuse infiltration, which differentiates it from observed perivascular clustering in specimens of temporal lobe epilepsy [4].

Furthermore, in MOGHE there is no evidence of dysmorphic neurons nor balloon cells.

There are also no signs for vertical nor a horizontal dyslamination. Consequently, it cannot be classified within the ILAE classification scheme for FCD Type I or II.

Likewise, the histopathological report for our patient's resected specimen is presented with all the above features in Figures 3, 4, and 5.

Schurr *et al.* presented a series of 1381 en bloc resected epilepsy surgery brain specimens from which 3.7% could not be histopathologically classified and were considered nonlesional [2]. In 22 of these patients (42%) the above-mentioned histopathological findings of MOGHE were present.

All patients suffered from frontal lobe epilepsy, as our patient.

Clustered oligodendroglial hyperplasia with increased proliferative activity in white matter involving the gray-white matter junction was a common finding in all specimens.

Proliferation activity of oligodendrocytes was age varied. Specifically, it was higher in young patients undergoing operations compared with older patients of their series.

Authors suggested either a maldevelopmental or secondary regenerative component in the pathogenesis of these lesions. In our specimen no signs of diffuse neuroepithelial tumor infiltration (in particular oligodendroglioma) were observed. Furthermore, IDH mutations were absent, and detection of chromosomal 1p/19q losses did not reveal any codeletion in the oligodendroglial cell component.

There is a wide histopathological spectrum of epilepsy-associated brain lesions, including malformation of cortical development (MCD) as well as focal cortical dysplasias (FCD) which are a localized forms of MCD [5].

Their classification is well established and includes FCD Type I (Ia, Ib, Ic), Type II (IIa, IIb), and Type III (IIIa, IIIb, IIIc, IIId) [6].

Palmini's classification proposed in 2004 was widely used [3] whereas in 2011 Blumcke et al. recommended a new

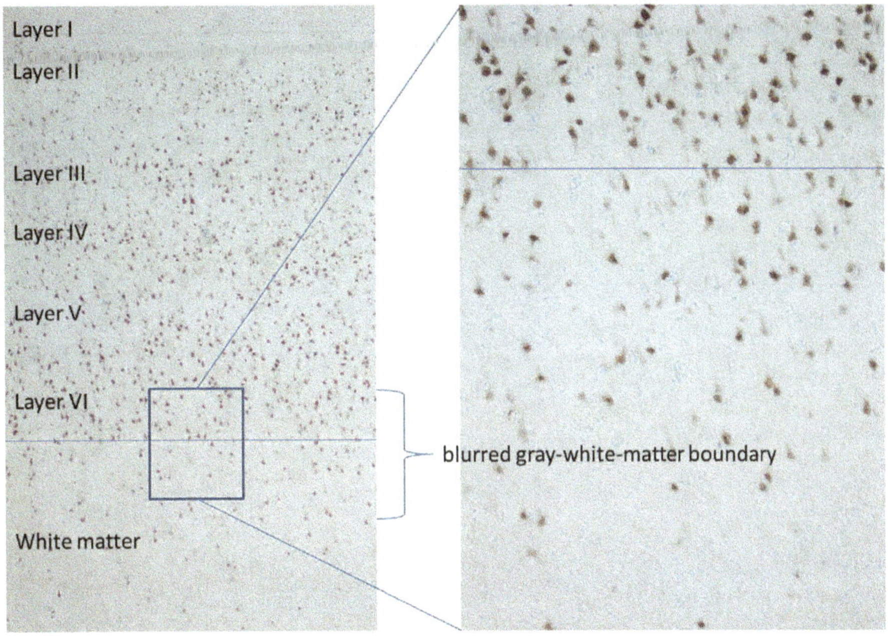

FIGURE 3: NeuN immunohistochemistry (neurons are labeled).

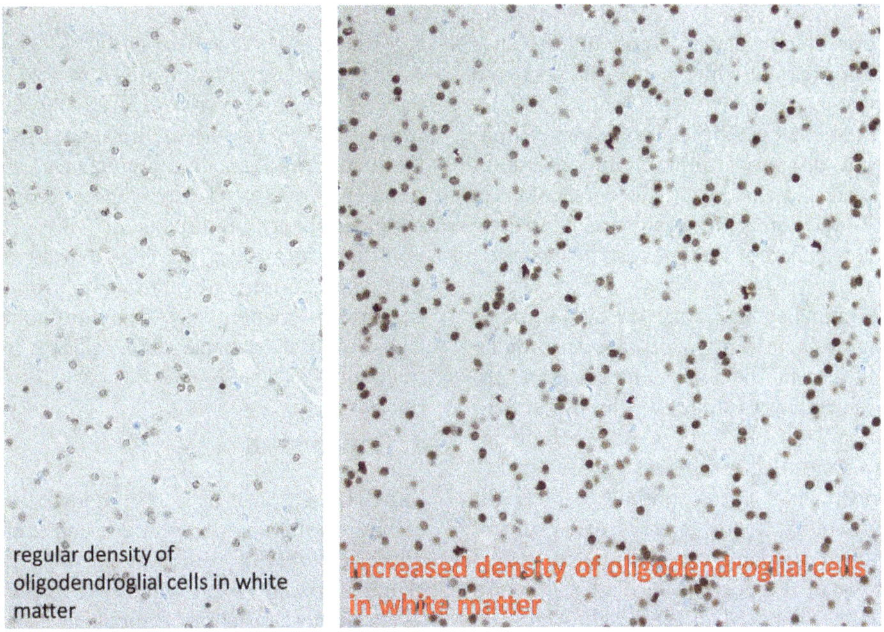

FIGURE 4: Olig2 immunohistochemistry (oligodendroglial cells are labeled).

system for classifying FCD, resulting in the first international consensus classification of FCD proposed by the International League against Epilepsy (ILAE) in 2011 [7].

Nevertheless, MOGHE cannot be classified within this sort as it presents with the above unique histopathological features.

Oligodendroglial hamartoma is another lesion that should also be under consideration. Marucci et al. [8] described a case report of this particular lesion situated in frontal lobe, associated with drug resistant epilepsy and composed exclusively of mature oligodendroglial cells. Despite the scarcity of this extratemporal location, as well as the unusual histopathological feature of exclusive mature oligodendroglial cells, their lack of proliferative activity would help the differential diagnosis.

In 2018, Till Hartlieb *et al.* presented a series of 40 preoperative MRIs of twenty-five epileptic patients with histologically confirmed MOGHE in the resected brain specimens [9]. Mean age was 9.3 years old (pediatric population) and median age at MRI imaging was 5.2 years. They resulted in 2 age-related MR subtypes.

Subtype I consists of increased T2 and fluid attenuated inversion recovery (FLAIR) signal at the corticomedullary junction and occurred at a median of 2.6 years. Subtype II

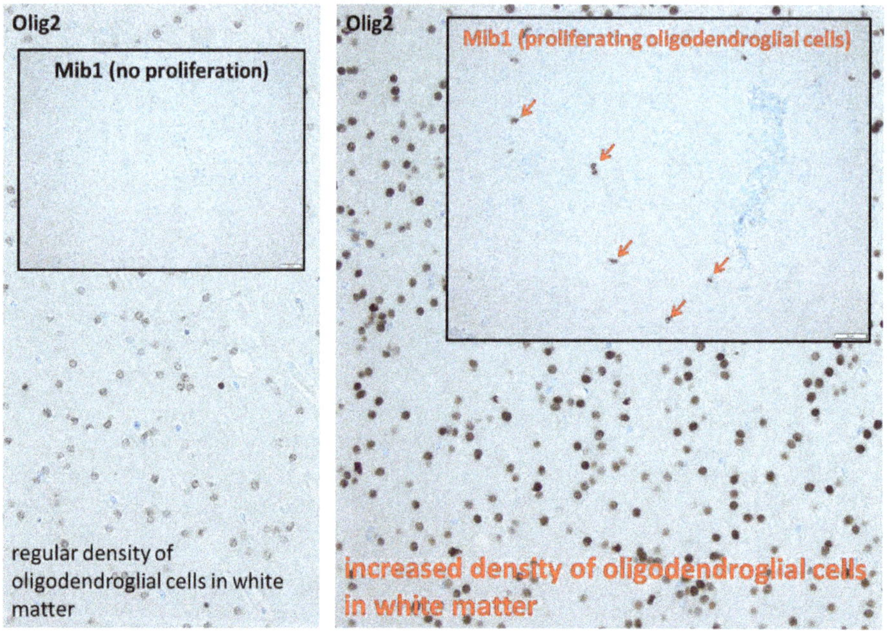

FIGURE 5: MIB1 (Ki67) immunohistochemistry (proliferating cells are labeled).

consists of reduced corticomedullary differentiation because of increased signal of the adjacent white matter and occurred at a median of 14.1 years.

The authors concluded that patchy areas of hypomyelination in histology seem to disappear during brain maturation and may therefore represent the histologic correlation of laminar T2 and FLAIR hyperintensities in subtype I. Furthermore, an age-related conversion of subtypes can be observed between 3 and 5 years.

Reviewing the literature on this field, we also found a reference of MR imaging identification of oligodendroglial hyperplasia by Hamilton *et al.* The authors presented a case of epileptic patient with refractory epilepsy who underwent a presurgical evaluation [10]. Findings of 1.5T MR imaging study revealed no abnormality, whereas subsequent 3T findings revealed abnormalities corresponding to the right frontal lobe electrophysiologic focus. Specific MR protocol for epilepsy evaluation was used and revealed subtle cortical thickening and blurring of the gray-white matter junction in the right frontal lobe compared to the residual normal cortex. Histologically, the resected specimen demonstrated oligodendroglial hyperplasia, which is characterized by the presence of increased number of normal-appearing oligodendroglial cells in the cortex and juxtacortical white matter. Oligodendroglial hyperplasia is considered to be at the mildest end of the spectrum of cortical migrational disorders [10]. It is a common characteristic with MOGHE and they share analogous MR findings.

Schurr *et al.* presented MR findings of MOGHE patients in their series, demonstrating the following features: frontal lobe localization, involvement of gray-white matter boundaries, increased signal intensity in FLAIR protocols, and presence of multifocal lesions. The authors suggested that the latter indicates a large anatomical extent of MOGHE, so this could account for surgical failure due to subtotal resections in their patient series. More specifically, postoperative seizure evaluation was available in 18 of 22 MOGHE patients. 33% were free of disabling seizures, whereas the majority (61%) of patients presented with ongoing seizures. One patient had rare disabling seizures, and two patients were reoperated due to seizure relapse. Second resection revealed histopathological remnants of MOGHE in both patients. This indicates that MOGHE could be associated with unfavourable outcome in surgery of frontal lobe in drug resistant epilepsy patients [2]. This does not apply to our patient so far, as the available data indicate two years of seizure freedom.

4. Conclusion

MOGHE seems to be an emerging histopathological entity of brain lesions which shares some unique characteristics. These features, in combination with the absence of other characteristics of well-established malformations of cortical development, raise the difficulty of classifying this entity within the existent classification scheme.

Findings of our case report are in accordance with the provided data of the reviewed literature on this field.

The potential unfavourable outcome in seizure control could unequivocally be valuable knowledge to patients along with doctors. It concerns expectations for seizure freedom as well as management of undesirable outcome.

More cases of epileptic patients are definitely needed in order to establish more data about this distinct entity in frontal lobe epilepsy.

Abbreviations

MRI: Magnetic resonance imaging
FLAIR: Fluid attenuated inversion recovery

IDH mutations: Mutations in isocitrate dehydrogenase
EEG: Electroencephalogram.

References

[1] A. J. Barkovich, R. Guerrini, R. I. Kuzniecky, G. D. Jackson, and W. B. Dobyns, "A developmental and genetic classification for malformations of cortical development: Update 2012," *Brain*, vol. 135, no. 5, pp. 1348–1369, 2012.

[2] J. Schurr, R. Coras, K. Rössler et al., "Mild malformation of cortical development with oligodendroglial hyperplasia in frontal lobe epilepsy: a new clinico-pathological entity," *Brain Pathology*, vol. 27, no. 1, pp. 26–35, 2017.

[3] M. S. Okun, M. R. DeLong, J. Hanfelt, M. Gearing, and A. Levey, "Plasma testosterone levels in Alzheimer and Parkinson diseases," *Neurology*, vol. 62, supplement 3, no. 3, pp. 411–413, 2004.

[4] H. Stefanits, T. Czech, E. Pataraia et al., "Prominent oligodendroglial response in surgical specimens of patients with temporal lobe epilepsy," *Clinical Neuropathology*, vol. 31, no. 6, pp. 409–417, 2012.

[5] Y. Bae, H. Kang, H. D. Kim, and S. H. Kim, "New classification of focal cortical dysplasia: application to practical diagnosis," *Journal of Epilepsy Research*, vol. 2, no. 2, pp. 38–42, 2012.

[6] I. M. Najm, H. B. Sarnat, and I. Blümcke, "Review: The international consensus classification of Focal Cortical Dysplasia – a critical update 2018," *Neuropathology and Applied Neurobiology*, vol. 44, no. 1, pp. 18–31, 2018.

[7] I. Blümcke, M. Thom, E. Aronica et al., "The clinicopathologic spectrum of focal cortical dysplasias: A consensus classification proposed by an ad hoc Task Force of the ILAE Diagnostic Methods Commission," *Epilepsia*, vol. 52, no. 1, pp. 158–174, 2011.

[8] G. Marucci, M. Giulioni, M. Martinoni, L. Volpi, and R. Michelucci, "Oligodendroglial hamartoma: a potential source of misdiagnosis for oligodendroglioma," *Journal of Neuro-Oncology*, vol. 101, no. 2, pp. 325–328, 2011.

[9] T. Hartlieb, P. Winkler, R. Coras et al., "Age-related MR characteristics in mild malformation of cortical development with oligodendroglial hyperplasia and epilepsy (MOGHE)," *Epilepsy & Behavior*, 2018.

[10] B. E. Hamilton and G. M. Nesbit, "MR imaging identification of oligodendroglial hyperplasia," *American Journal of Neuroradiology*, vol. 30, no. 7, pp. 1412-1413, 2009.

21

Treatment of Recurrent Painful Ophthalmoplegic Neuropathy: A Case Where Pregabalin was Successfully Employed

Laura N. Zamproni, Reinaldo T. Ribeiro, and Marina Cardeal

Instituto de Neurologia Funcional, Rua Padre Machado, 42 São Paulo, SP, Brazil

Correspondence should be addressed to Laura N. Zamproni; lnzamproni@yahoo.com.br

Academic Editor: Mehmet Turgut

Recurrent painful ophthalmoplegic neuropathy, previously known as ophthalmoplegic migraine, is a rare condition that affects children and young adults. Its cause and classification are still controversial and, consequently, there are no published treatment guidelines or consensus. Glucocorticoids seem to be beneficial for some patients, but there is no established treatment when failure of this therapy occurs. The aim of this study was to report a case where pregabalin was successfully used after failure of glucocorticoid therapy in a patient with recurrent painful ophthalmoplegic neuropathy.

1. Introduction

Recurrent painful ophthalmoplegic neuropathy (RPON), previously known as ophthalmoplegic migraine (OM), is a rare condition (estimated annual incidence of 0,7 per million) involving headache and ophthalmoplegia, which typically occurs in children and young adults [1]. Typical features include repeated attacks of paralysis of one or more ocular cranial nerves (III, IV, or VI) with ipsilateral headache that can start up to two weeks before the onset of eye muscle weakness [15]. The International Classification of Headache Disorders 3rd edition-beta version (ICHD3β) defined the following diagnostic criteria for RPON: (1) at least two attacks; (2) unilateral headache accompanied by ipsilateral paresis of one, two, or three ocular motor nerves; (3) the exclusion of orbital, parasellar, or posterior fossa lesions by an appropriate investigation; and (4) the absence of another diagnosis that could better account for the patient's condition [16].

RPON was used to be classified as a migraine variant, but the disease concept has changed due to lack of migraine symptoms in many cases and evidence supporting neuropathy [1]. Brain MRI reveals gadolinium enhancement of the affected cranial nerve in approximately 75 % of patients suggesting that the condition is a demyelinating disorder [15]. However, the cause and classification remain controversial.

This lack of information about the disease pathophysiology makes the treatment even more controversial. In fact, there are very few data or consensus about RPON treatment. The aim of this study is to report a case where pregabalin was successfully employed after glucocorticoid therapy failure in RPON.

2. Case Report

A 21-year-old female patient came to our service with a complaint of unilateral right-onset headache associated with diplopia initiated 6 months earlier. She had no personal or family remarkable antecedents. She never smoked. Six months earlier, the patient started to experience one-sided right throbbing headache. She denied nausea, vomiting, or photo- or phonophobia. Fifteen days after the pain onset, she noticed double vision and medial deviation of the right eye, which forced her to wear an eyepiece to perform her activities and drive. She went to several centers and used various medications such as paracetamol, nonsteroidal anti-inflammatory drugs (NSAIDs), opioids, and triptans without improvement. Three months earlier, she started using dexamethasone 4 mg daily with partial pain control but maintenance of diplopia.

At the examination, the patient had cushingoid face, violaceous striae, and right VI cranial nerve palsy with

TABLE 1: Results of blood and cerebrospinal fluid tests.

Hemoglobin (g/dL)	13.1
WBC (/mm^3)	12700
Platelets (/mm^3)	298000
Na (mmol/L)	141
K (mmol/L)	4,1
Coagulation tests	Normal
Creatinine (mg/dL)	0,5
CPK (U/L)	38
ESR (mm/h)	22
Bilirubin (mg/dL)	0,27
AST (U/L)	16
ALT (U/L)	18
ALP(U/L)	64
GGT (U/L)	47
TSH (um/L)	0,8
ANA	Negative
Anti-dsDNA	Negative
Anti-RNP	Negative
Anti-LA	Negative
Anti-RO	Negative
Anti-SM	Negative
ANCA	Negative
HIV	Negative
ACE (U/L)	31
VDRL test	Negative
Cerebrospinal fluid	
WBC (/mm^3)	1
Protein (mg/dL)	22
Glucose (mg/dL)	66
Bacteria	Negative

WBC: white blood cells; Na: sodium; K: potassium; ESR: erythrocyte sedimentation rate; CPK: creatine phosphokinase; AST: aspartate aminotransferase; ALT: alanine transaminase; ALP: *alkaline phosphatase; GGT:* gamma glutamyl transferase; TSH: thyroid stimulating hormone; ANA: antinuclear antibodies; Anti-dsDNA: anti-double stranded DNA antibodies; HIV: human immunodeficiency virus; ACE: angiotensin-converting enzyme; ANCA: anti-neutrophil cytoplasmic antibody; VDRL test: Venereal Disease Research Laboratory test.

no other neurological changes. Blood tests were normal (Table 1). A contrast-enhanced MRI scan of the brain did not show any remarkable features (Figure 1). A spinal tap released crystalline cerebrospinal fluid (CSF) with an opening pressure of 14 cm of water. Biochemical, microbiological, and cytological analyses of the CSF were normal (Table 1). CT scan of thorax did not show any evidence of lymphoma or sarcoidosis.

Prednisone 1mg / kg was then started. With one week of treatment, complete reversal of ocular paralysis and remission of pain were observed. However, when the corticoid was gradually withdrawn, the patient returned to pain and returned to paralysis of the VI right pair. The prednisone was increased again to 1 mg / kg this time with reversion of ocular paralysis but without pain control. Several prophylaxis attempts were made with beta-blockers, calcium channel blockers, topiramate, and tricyclics without any symptomatic control that would allow corticosteroid withdrawal.

The pregabalin 150mg daily was then introduced. With 7 days of medication onset there was already an important remission of pain. With 15 days of pregabalin initiation, the retitration of prednisone was started without any intercurrence and the patient reversed the exogenous Cushing syndrome. Pregabalin was maintained for one year and retracted. Currently, the patient has been free of pain for 2 years.

3. Discussion

According to the prevailing diagnostic criteria, our patients suffered from RPON given the presence of a documented VI nerve palsy associated with a unilateral ipsilateral headache with no remarkable alterations in laboratory or neuroimaging exams. Although the enhancement of the affected nerve occurs in 75% of patients [15], brain MRI is normal in a quarter of cases. We emphasize that our patient had been using a lower dose of corticosteroids for almost 3 months

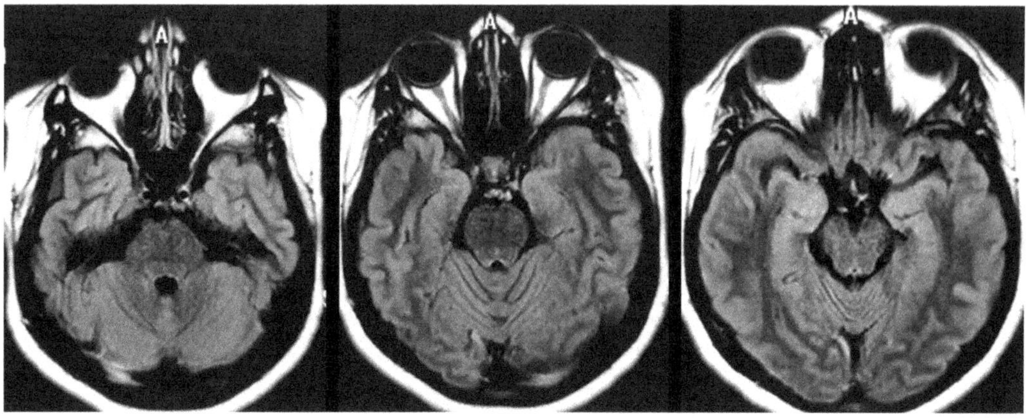

Figure 1: Axial flair brain MRI.

Table 2: Case reports.

Author	Patient age/ gender	Pain description	Nerve palsy	Treatment	Time to fully recovery
Kobayashi et al. 2017 [1]	48-year-old /female	Unilateral Throbbing Photophobia Phonophobia	Incomplete III pair	Corticosteroids	5 days Persistent Residual Mydriasis
Qureshi et al. 2017 [2]	53-year-old / female	Unilateral Throbbing Photophobia Phonophobia	Incomplete III pair	NSAIDs Serotonin receptor agonist Calcium channel blocker	NR
Huang et al. 2017 [3]	26-year-old / female	Unilateral	Incomplete III pair	Corticosteroids Topiramate	6 weeks
Tripathi et al. 2017 [4]	36-year old / female	Unilateral Throbbing Photophobia	VI pair	Gabapentin Topiramate	2 months
Okura et al. 2017 [5]	12-year-old / male	Unilateral	Incomplete III pair	Corticosteroids	8 weeks
Takizawa et al. 2016 [6]	42-year-old / female	Unilateral Throbbing	Incomplete III pair	NR	NR
Ghosh 2015 [7]	5-year-old / male	Unilateral	Incomplete III pair	Corticosteroids Immunoglobulin	3 weeks
Ramakrishnan et al. 2015 [8]	30-year-old / female	Unilateral Photophobia Phonophobia	Incomplete III pair	Valproate Corticosteroids	1 month
Wang et al. 2014 [9]	63-year-old / male	Unilateral Pressure-like Phonophobia	Incomplete III pair	Valproate Flunarizine	NR
Shetty et al. 2013 [10]	26-year-old / female	Unilateral Throbbing	Incomplete III pair	NSAIDs Propranolol	2 weeks

NR: not reported; NSAIDs: nonsteroidal anti-inflammatory drugs.

before admission, which may have reduced the sensitivity of the exam (Figure 1). Our patient responded partially to corticosteroids and absolutely to pregabalin but not to other treatment.

Since RPON is a very rare condition, it is difficult to conduct studies. There are no published treatment trials or guidelines for RPON and all evidence of effective treatments came from observational studies. Glucocorticoids seem to be beneficial for some patients. Prompt administration of steroids at the clinical onset may minimize permanent ophthalmoparesis or pupillary disfunction [17]. In a retrospective review of 80 patients, steroids were used to treat at least 31% of patients and there was a perceived benefit from corticosteroid treatment in 54 %. Only 12 % had no improvement or clinical worsening [15].

For those patients that do not respond to corticosteroids, treatment evidence is even smaller. The efficacy of drugs for migraine such as acetaminophen, NSAIDs, ergotamine, and

Table 3: Mechanisms of action of drugs used in headache.

Drug	Mechanism of action
Corticosteroids	inhibit the synthesis of inflammatory proteins, induce the expression of anti-inflammatory proteins and inhibit cyclooxygenase-2 [11]
Indomethacin	inhibition of cyclooxygenase 1 and cyclooxygenase 2 and phospholipase A2 [12]
Valproate	increases gamma-aminobutyric acid (GABA) levels in synaptosomes and in the brain, reduces the central trigeminal nerve activation (by increasing GABA levels), was shown to reduce experimental neurogenic inflammation in the peripheral trigeminal vascular system [13]
Topiramate	modifies the excitability of nerves by blocking voltage-sensitive sodium channels and L-type voltage-activated calcium channels, inhibits carbonic anhydrase activity, inhibits the excitatory glutamate pathway while enhancing the inhibitory effect of GABA [13]
Pregabalin	binds to alpha 2-delta subunits of the voltage-gated calcium cannels in the nervous system, reducing the influx of calcium in the presynaptic ending, and, consequently, reduces the release of excitatory neurotransmitters including glutamate, noradrenaline, dopamine, and serotonin in the synaptic cleft [14]

triptans is unknown [1]. Pareja et al. described two cases of PRON responsive to indomethacin [18]. Also, cyproheptadine hydrochloride has been reported to prevent recurrent attacks of RPON by targeting the vascular edema around the oculomotor nerve [1].

Some authors recommend standard migraine prophylactic therapy for patients with recurrent attacks. We searched PubMed for case reports published between 2103 and 2017 using the search terms "ophthalmoplegic migraine" and "recurrent painful ophthalmoplegic neuropathy". We found 10 case reports that are displayed at Table 2. After steroids, valproate and topiramate were the most prescribed medication. Both valproate and topiramate increase gamma-aminobutyric acid (GABA) levels in the brain and are first-line agents in migraine prevention (Table 3) [13].

In more refractory cases, injection of botulinum toxin or strabismus surgery may be considered for patients with persistent sequelae, to correct eye misalignment [15].

As far as we know, pregabalin has not been reported for RPON treatment. Pregabalin is a structural analogue of GABA. Pregabalin binds to alpha 2-delta subunits of the voltage-gated calcium cannels in the nervous system, reducing the influx of calcium in the presynaptic ending, and, consequently, reduces the release of excitatory neurotransmitters including glutamate, noradrenaline, dopamine, and serotonin in the synaptic cleft [14]. Pregabalin has been used to treat neuropathic pain. The response to pregabalin and the lack of efficacy of classic drugs used in migraine, such as NSAIDs and first-line prophylactic migraine drugs (topiramate and valproate) in this case, reinforce the neuropathic etiology of the disease and not a variant of migraine as it was formerly classified.

Consent

Informed consent has been obtained from the patient for this report.

Disclosure

No funding sources are involved in this paper.

References

[1] Y. Kobayashi, Y. Kondo, K. Uchibori, and J. Tsuyuzaki, "Recurrent painful ophthalmoplegic neuropathy with residual mydriasis in an adult: Should it be classified as ophthalmoplegic migraine?" *Internal Medicine*, vol. 56, no. 20, pp. 2769–2772, 2017.

[2] I. A. Qureshi, G. J. Rodriguez, S. Cruz-Flores, and A. Maud, "Persistent focal enhancement of the cisternal segment of oculomotor nerve in ophthalmoplegic migraine," *Neurology: Clinical Practice*, vol. 7, no. 5, pp. 381–383, 2017.

[3] C. Huang, M. Amasanti, B. Lovell, and T. Young, "Recurrent painful ophthalmoplegic neuropathy," *Practical Neurology*, vol. 17, no. 4, pp. 318–320, 2017.

[4] R. Tripathi, A. Tselis, and E. Bernitsas, "Bilateral cisternal abducens nerve involvement with ophthalmoplegic migraine," *Cephalalgia*, vol. 37, no. 12, pp. 1211-1212, 2017.

[5] Y. Okura, A. Wakayama, C. Yoshizawa, I. Kobayashi, and Y. Takahashi, "Recurrent painful ophthalmoplegic neuropathy in a 12-year-old boy," *Pediatrics International*, vol. 59, no. 11, pp. 1208–1210, 2017.

[6] T. Takizawa, M. Shibata, H. Fujiwara, T. Shimizu, S. Momoshima, and N. Suzuki, "Adult-onset recurrent painful ophthalmoplegic neuropathy displaying atypical oculomotor nerve gadolinium-enhancement pattern in the orbit and cavernous sinus," *Cephalalgia*, vol. 36, no. 2, pp. 199-200, 2016.

[7] P. S. Ghosh, "Recurrent right-sided ptosis in a child," *JAMA Pediatrics*, vol. 169, no. 7, pp. 693-694, 2015.

[8] S. Ramakrishnan, P. Kallollimath, G. B. Kulkarni, and V. Mustare, "Transient oculomotor synkinesis in a case of ophthalmoplegic migraine," *Neurology India*, vol. 63, no. 5, pp. 778–780, 2015.

[9] Y. Wang, X.-H. Wang, M.-M. Tian et al., "Ophthalmoplegia starting with a headache circumscribed in a line-shaped area: a subtype of ophthalmoplegic migraine?" *The Journal of Headache and Pain*, vol. 15, no. 1, pp. 1–4, 2014.

[10] A. Shetty, S. Khardenavis, and A. Deshpande, "Ophthalmoplegic migraine with isolated third cranial nerve palsy in a known case of juvenile myoclonic epilepsy," *BMJ Case Reports*, 2013.

[11] M. Ciriaco, P. Ventrice, G. Russo et al., "Corticosteroid-related central nervous system side effects," *Journal of Pharmacology and Pharmacotherapeutics*, vol. 4, no. 5, pp. 94–98, 2013.

[12] O. Summ and S. Evers, "Mechanism of action of indomethacin in indomethacin-responsive headaches," *Current Pain and Headache Reports*, vol. 17, no. 4, article 327, 2013.

[13] R. Shahien and K. Beiruti, "Preventive agents for migraine: Focus on the antiepileptic drugs," *Journal of Central Nervous System Disease*, vol. 4, pp. 37–49, 2012.

[14] S. M. Cain, B. Bohnet, J. LeDue et al., "In vivo imaging reveals that pregabalin inhibits cortical spreading depression and propagation to subcortical brain structures," *Proceedings of the National Acadamy of Sciences of the United States of America*, vol. 114, no. 9, pp. 2401–2406, 2017.

[15] A. A. Gelfand, J. M. Gelfand, P. Prabakhar, and P. J. Goadsby, "Ophthalmoplegic "migraine" or recurrent ophthalmoplegic cranial neuropathy: New cases and a systematic review," *Journal of Child Neurology*, vol. 27, no. 6, pp. 759–766, 2012.

[16] Headache Classification Committee of the International Headache Society (IHS), "The international classification of headache disorders, 3rd edition (beta version)," *Cephalalgia*, vol. 33, no. 9, pp. 629–808, 2013.

[17] B. D. Arasho, "Ophthalmoplegic migraine in a 15-year-old Ethiopian: Case report and literature review," *The Journal of Headache and Pain*, vol. 10, no. 1, pp. 45–49, 2009.

[18] J. A. Pareja, J. Churruca, B. De La Casa Fages, C. L. De Silanes, C. Sánchez, and F. J. Barriga, "Ophthalmoplegic migraine. Two patients with an absolute response to indomethacin," *Cephalalgia*, vol. 30, no. 6, pp. 757–760, 2010.

22

The Spectrum of Acute Disseminated Encephalomyelitis and Mild Encephalopathy with Reversible Splenial Lesion

Michel Sáenz-Farret, Mariana Aurora Cansino-Torres, Valeria Sandoval-Rodríguez, Rigoberto Navarro-Ibarra, and Carlos Zúñiga-Ramírez

Movement Disorders and Neurodegenerative Diseases Unit, Hospital Civil de Guadalajara "Fray Antonio Alcalde", Guadalajara, Mexico

Correspondence should be addressed to Carlos Zúñiga-Ramírez; c.zuniga.ramirez@gmail.com

Academic Editor: Ritsuo Hashimoto

Background. Acute disseminated encephalomyelitis and mild encephalopathy with reversible splenial lesion are autoimmune demyelinating disorders of central nervous system. Diagnosis remains clinical, aided by neuroimaging confirmation and excluding other causes. In the absence of a biological marker, the diagnosis of these entities based on clinical and imaging criteria could overlap. *Methods.* We describe a 22-year-old woman developing mild neurological signs after an upper tract infection, a brain magnetic resonance image revealed confluent, symmetrical white matter lesions with corpus callosum involvement; after extensive ancillary testing that ruled out secondary causes we concluded that this subject had a post infectious encephalitis sharing clinical and imaging criteria for acute disseminated encephalomyelitis. However, mild encephalopathy with reversible splenial lesion could be an alternate diagnosis for this subject. Treatment with methylprednisolone completely solved both the clinical and image abnormalities without relapsing for more than 3 years of follow-up. *Conclusion.* Both acute disseminated encephalomyelitis and mild encephalopathy with reversible splenial lesion share clinical and radiological features. A biological marker is needed to differentiate among these entities, since overlap is seen according to current criteria.

1. Introduction

Acute disseminated encephalomyelitis (ADEM) is a multifocal inflammatory demyelinating disease of the central nervous system (CNS) which occurs most commonly in children after a bacterial, viral process or vaccination. It is thought that an immune response against these infectious agents cross-react with self-myelin peptides, hence leading to an autoimmune response [1].

In most cases the disease has a monophasic course, although it can also present as a relapsing illness. ADEM usually begins from 2 days to 4 weeks after infection or vaccination. The typical course begins with a sudden onset of encephalopathy and several focal neurological deficits such as weakness of extremities, ataxia, cranial nerve palsies, seizures, myelitis and optic neuritis among others. Subjects also develop systemic symptoms such as headache, fever and vomiting [2].

Magnetic resonance imaging (MRI) of the brain and spine is the most useful ancillary test for acute demyelination [3]. The newest proposed criteria for ADEM diagnosis based on MRI include: 1. Diffuse, poorly demarcated, large (>1–2 cm) lesions involving predominantly the cerebral white matter, 2. White matter T1 hypointense lesions are rare, and 3. Deep gray matter lesions (e.g. thalamus or basal ganglia) can be present. Furthermore, the MRI during the acute phase should be abnormal and new lesions should not be present three months or more after the disease onset [4].

An important differential diagnosis of ADEM is mild encephalopathy with reversible splenial lesion (MERS), this entity is a clinico-radiological syndrome characterized by a transient mild encephalopathy and a reversible lesion in the splenium of the corpus callosum on MRI. This syndrome has almost universally been described in children from Japan and East Asia [5]. The aim of this article is to present a case of an adult fulfilling both clinical criteria for ADEM and MERS type 2. Based on these findings, both entities could be, at least, part of the spectrum of one disease. A biological marker capable to distinguish ADEM from MERS is needed.

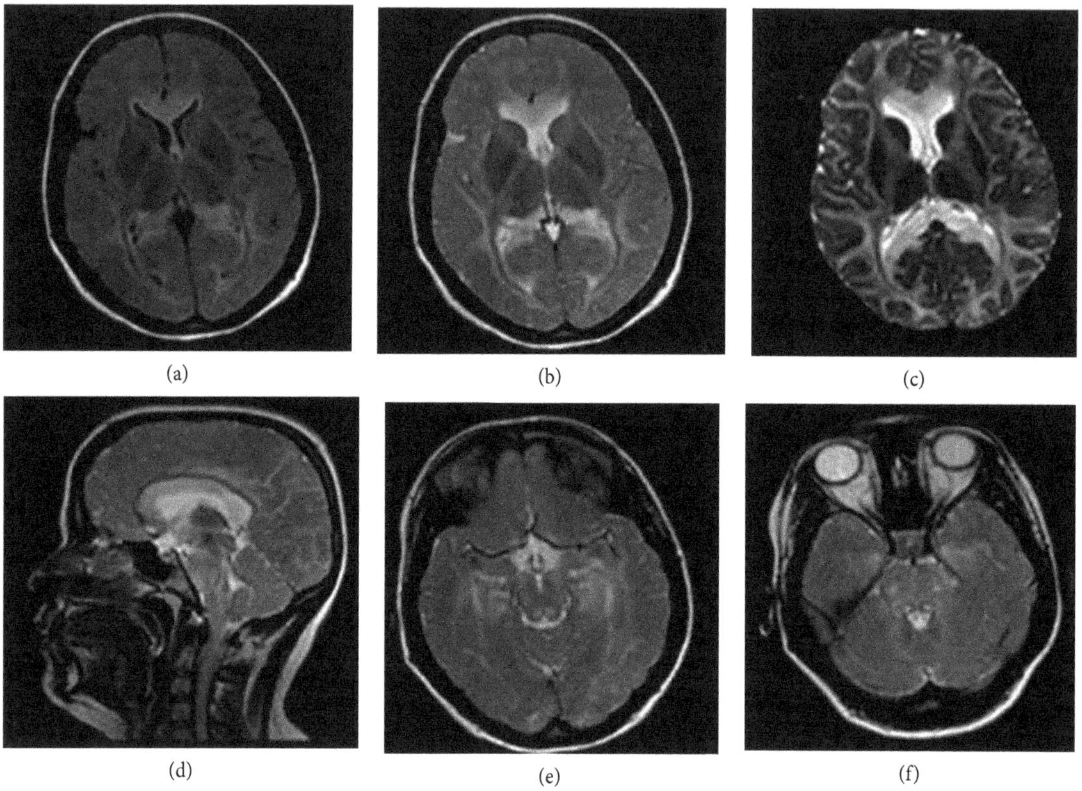

Figure 1: (a) Axial FLAIR showed hyperintense signal in supratentorial white matter. (b) Axial T2 showed hyperintense signal in supratentorial white matter. (c) Axial Diffusion showed restricted diffusion at the entire corpus callosum and at the white matter. (d) Sagittal T2 showed hyperintense signal in supratentorial white matter and also in the brainstem. (e) Axial T2 showed hyperintense signal at the mesencephalon. (f) Axial T2 showed hyperintense signal at the pons.

2. Case Presentation

A 22-year-old woman was admitted into the hospital for a 2-week course of diplopia, frontal headache and retro-ocular pain following an unspecified self-limited upper respiratory tract infection 15 day prior to the appearance of these neurological symptoms. Neurologic exam showed conjugated primary-gaze diplopia and generalized hyperreflexia. Fundoscopy showed optic nerve pallor bilaterally. Brain MRI was performed which showed extensive T2 and FLAIR white matter hyperintense lesions as well as in brainstem and splenium of corpus callosum (Figure 1). Laboratory tests including blood count, glucose, urea, creatinine, electrolytes and HIV ELISA were unremarkable. Cerebrospinal fluid was completely normal, oligoclonal bands were absent and Polymerase Chain Reaction (PCR) for Herpes Virus Simplex Type I (HSV-I) and other common viruses was performed, resulting negative as well. Somatosensory Evoked Potentials depicted only a delay at P37 wave bilaterally. Symptoms completely solved after 5 days of intravenous methylprednisolone 1 g daily. Six-weeks after treatment, a brain MRI was repeated, showing complete resolution of previous findings (Figure 2). Complete remission was achieved clinically and radiologically, remaining asymptomatic for more than three years of follow-up.

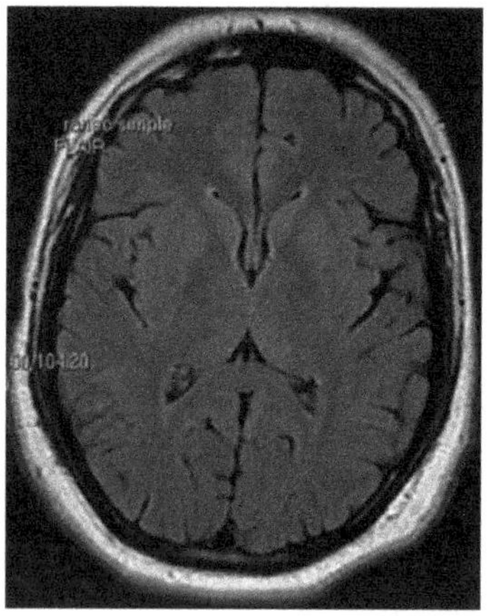

Figure 2: Axial FLAIR showed absence of abnormalities at follow up.

3. Discussion

ADEM in adults is a rare manifestation of post infectious disease [6], however it can also arise spontaneously or after vaccination [7]. Nevertheless, among these subjects, an infectious background should raise suspicion of an autoimmune demyelinating disease.

The diagnosis of ADEM remains clinical, aided by neuroimaging confirmation and the exclusion of other causes [8]. Clinical features are varied and depend mainly on the affected CNS area. In the largest prospective study of ADEM in adults, the most frequent signs of involvement were at the brainstem, mainly ocular motor deficit followed by dysarthria. It is important to note that in contrast to children, the prevalence of fever, loss of consciousness, and Meningism was low [9] as seen in our case. Brain and spine MRI is the most useful paraclinical tool to aid in the diagnosis of ADEM, distinguishing it from other inflammatory and noninflammatory neurological diseases [10].

Five patterns of cerebral involvement have been proposed to classify the MRI findings in ADEM among children and adolescents: 1. ADEM with small lesions (less than 5 mm); 2. ADEM with large, confluent, or tumefactive lesions; 3. ADEM with additional symmetrical bithalamic involvement; 4. Acute hemorrhagic encephalomyelitis (AHEM); and 5. ADEM with pseudo-leukodystrophic pattern, with a diffuse, bilateral, symmetrical, and usually non-enhanced white matter involvement [2].

The diffuse, symmetrical, and usually non-enhancing white matter involvement can be rarely found in subjects with ADEM, with all the reported cases seen during infancy and adolescence. Clinically, most of them were associated with seizures, fever and aggressive neurologic involvement. Although these findings in neuroimaging are not the most typical pattern of ADEM, the exclusion of other entities such as a history of previous infection or vaccination points toward a diagnosis of ADEM. Also, the response to methylprednisolone supports the diagnosis in a retrospective manner [11–13].

Since ADEM is a diagnosis of exclusion [7], other diseases were considered prior to diagnosing this entity in our patient. In adults, the differential diagnosis of confluent, symmetrical white matter lesions and corpus callosum involvement is broader including inflammatory conditions, infections, vascular disorders, neoplasia, and toxic causes [14]. CNS lymphoma is an entity that must be considered among subjects with large and atypical white matter lesions. Steroids can vanish white matter abnormalities in these cases, but recurrence is always seen [15]. Our case remained free from lesions after more than 3 years of follow up, making CNS lymphoma diagnosis unlikely.

Clinical clues in the present case favoring a diagnosis of ADEM are: prior upper tract infection, unremarkable laboratory studies, confluent symmetrical white matter lesions, the complete response to methylprednisolone and the monophasic course, remaining symptomatically free for more than 3 years of follow up. Nevertheless, atypical MRI findings such as corpus callosum involvement, a confluent, symmetrical white matter lesions and subtle neurological involvement makes also MERS type 2 a feasible diagnosis.

MERS is a clinical and radiological syndrome characterized by transient lesions at the splenium and associated frontal white matter [16]. The diagnostic criteria for MERS includes: onset with neuropsychiatric symptoms within one week after the onset of fever; complete recovery without sequelae within 10 days after the onset of neuropsychiatric symptoms; high-signal-intensity lesion in the splenium of corpus callosum, in the acute stage; lesion may involve the entire corpus callosum and the cerebral white matter in a symmetric fashion; lesion disappears within 1 week, with neither residual signal changes nor atrophy [17]. Additionally, parietal or frontoparietal lesions have also been reported in MERS [18] but not confluent, symmetrical white matter lesions pattern which has been described in ADEM.

Currently, availability of biomarkers have been made possible not only with the diagnosis of complex entities but also understanding of their pathophysiological processes. In the case of demyelinating diseases, the presence of antibodies against myelin oligodendrocyte glycoprotein (anti-MOG) have been associated with acute disseminated encephalomyelitis, recurrent and bilateral optic neuritis and transverse myelitis in both children and adults; however, they have not been tested in the differential diagnosis of ADEM and MERS (in case they are different and not just part of a spectrum of the same disease). Additionally, the sensitivity of this antibody for a diagnosis of ADEM is as low as of 40% [19]. We did not test either anti-MOG nor aquaporine-4 antibodies in this subject since cost and availability of both tests were limiting issues, and treatment was installed immediately after admission into the hospital. Follow up showed complete resolution of both clinical and radiological features and no recurrence was seen after more than 3 years, testing both antibodies was not justified at this point of time.

A recent article that summarizes the evidence of rotavirus associated MERS found a total of 13 reported cases of MERS and showed that 10 were from Japan, one from Korea, one from China and one from Poland; the median age at presentation was 2 years (range 1–6 years) and in all cases, MERS was preceded by symptoms of gastroenteritis, such as vomiting, diarrhea and fever; Seizures (9/13; 69%) and disturbance of consciousness (8/13; 62%) were the most common neurological signs. Twelve patients (92%) had an isolated lesion in the splenium of the corpus callosum, and one patient (8%) had lesions in the splenium and genu of the corpus callosum [17]. Another study reported five cases of older age (2–26 years), all of them had sudden onset of fever and one also experienced recurrent vomiting and watery diarrhea; with respect to nervous system involvement, seizures, headache and meningeal signs were also reported. Neuroimaging showed abnormal signals restricted to the splenium of the corpus callosum (SCC) in all patients [16].

As our subject of study did not have all the clinical features (fever, gastrointestinal symptoms, seizures or meningeal signs) or the demographic characteristics of the reported cases of MERS (Asian ethnicity), it does not seem to fulfill all the criteria for that entity, besides that, our case has also imaging features not previously described for MERS such as infratentorial hyperintense images and confluent, symmetrical white matter lesions in MRI; it is important to note that the involvement of corpus callosum and restricted diffusion has also been described in the acute phase of ADEM [10] and the proposed imaging distinction between them is that in ADEM the lesions seen in the corpus callosum usually are asymmetric and contrast-enhancing [20].

Taking together the demographic, clinical and imaging features seen in our subject makes the diagnosis of ADEM and MERS overlap, a well-known condition in the scenario of post infectious encephalitis [20], in fact, the clinical and imaging spectrum of these entities is so broad that they may converge and may be seen as a single entity with a broad spectrum of manifestations (Table 1).

In this respect, and possibly related with the same spectrum of disease, tumefactive lesions (demyelinating lesions of greater than 2 cm) involving the corpus callosum can also occur in ADEM but are most closely related with MS where they often

Table 1: Diagnostic criteria for ADEM, MERS type 1 and MERS type 2.

<table>
<tr><th></th><th>ADEM (Krupp 2013) [4]</th><th>MERS type 1</th><th>MERS type 2 (Notebaert 2013) [20]</th></tr>
<tr><td>Clinical manifestations</td><td>(i) A first polyfocal, clinical CNS event with presumed inflammatory demyelinating cause
(ii) Encephalopathy that cannot be explained by fever
(iii) No new clinical and MRI findings emerge three months or more after the onset</td><td colspan="2">(i) Clinical onset associated with neuropsychiatric symptoms within 1 week after fever onset
(ii) Encephalitis or encephalopathy: speech difficulties, drowsiness, decreased consciousness, delirium, seizures, irritability, agitation, and disorientation
(iii) Complete recovery without sequelae, mostly within 10 days after the onset of neuropsychiatric symptoms</td></tr>
<tr><td>Brain MRI</td><td>(i) Diffuse, poorly demarcated, large (>1–2 cm) lesions involving predominantly the cerebral white matter
(ii) T1 hypointense lesions in the white matter are rare
(iii) Deep grey matter lesions (e.g. thalamus or basal ganglia) can be present
(iv) Gadolinium enhancement of one or more lesions occurs in 14–30% of cases
(v) In addition to findings on brain MRI, patients with ADEM can have extensive lesions on spinal MRI</td><td>(i) High-signal-intensity lesions on T2-weighted images, isointense to hypointense lesions on T1-weighted imaged and a homogenously reduced diffusion
(ii) Lesions are seen in the midline of the splenium of the corpus callosum without contrast-enhancement
(iii) Complete resolution of the splenial lesion on repeat imaging within 1 week, with no residual signal changes or atrophy</td><td>(i) High-signal-intensity lesions on T2-weighted images, isointense to hypointense lesions on T1-weighted imaged and a homogenously reduced diffusion
(ii) Lesions affect in a variable degree the corpus callosum (from its anterior aspect to its totality) and in a bilateral and symmetrical fashion the center semiovale without contrast-enhancement
(iii) Complete resolution of the splenial lesion on repeat imaging within 1 week, with no residual signal changes or atrophy</td></tr>
</table>

ADEM = Acute disseminated encephalomyelitis, MERS = Mild encephalopathy with reversible splenial lesion, CNS = Central Nervous system, MRI = Magnetic resonance imaging.

occur at the time of first presentation, either isolated or in association with other typical MS demyelinating lesions. In the largest published series of tumefactive demyelinating lesions among 168 patients, 10 patients (7%) exhibited a so-called "butterfly" appearance with symmetrical involvement of the corpus callosum and both cerebral hemispheres [21, 22].

"Transient splenial lesions" of the corpus callosum have been used to describe more restricted lesions among MERS cases, however, this term has also been employed to describe not only CNS inflammatory diseases such as Kawasaki disease, systemic lupus erythematosus and CNS infections, but also, non-inflammatory entities such as seizures (including status epilepticus), anticonvulsant use, hypoglycemia and other metabolic disturbances [21, 23].

Regarding pharmacological management, most of the published evidence for ADEM suggests high-dose corticosteroids as the first-line of treatment. Either methylprednisolone (20–30 mg/kg/day to a maximum dose of 1 g/day), or dexamethasone (1 mg/kg/day), followed by oral prednisone tapering for 4–6 weeks are the suggested schemas [24]. In the case of MERS the available literature suggest only the use of supportive measures such as hydration and antibiotics [17]. In our case, 5 days of methylprednisolone were enough to solve both clinical and radiological abnormalities. Besides this, there was no need to reinforce treatment with any other intervention, since the clinical picture completely solved after intravenous methylprednisolone was used, and clinical relapses have been negative for more than 3 years of follow-up.

The prognosis in ADEM is more severe in adults with respect to hospitalization, intensive-care unit admission, recovery and mortality [25]. The benign course and excellent response to treatment found in our patient, seems similar to children where the extent and site of lesions on initial MRI scans are not predictive of clinical outcome [26]. In general, patients with MERS type 2 lesions have also a good prognosis [20].

4. Conclusion

The present case showing confluent, symmetrical white matter lesions and corpus callosum involvement after an infectious disease shares clinical and radiological features of acute disseminated encephalomyelitis and mild encephalopathy with reversible splenial lesion. If MERS and ADEM are not part of the same spectrum, it is necessary to develop a biological marker that clearly distinguishes between these two entities, however due to the overlap they may be part of the same spectrum of disease.

References

[1] A. Javed and O. Khan, "Acute disseminated encephalomyelitis," *Handbook of Clinical Neurology*, vol. 123, pp. 705–717, 2014.

[2] S. N. Tenembaum, "Acute disseminated encephalomyelitis," *Handbook of Clinical Neurology*, vol. 112, pp. 1253–1262, 2013.

[3] S. Tenembaum, T. Chitnis, J. Ness, and J. S. Hahn, "Acute disseminated encephalomyelitis," *Neurology*, vol. 68, no. 16, Suppl 2, pp. S23–S36, 2007.

[4] L. B. Krupp, M. Tardieu, M. P. Amato et al., "International Pediatric Multiple Sclerosis Study Group criteria for pediatric multiple sclerosis and immune-mediated central nervous system demyelinating disorders: revisions to the 2007 definitions," *Multiple Sclerosis Journal*, vol. 19, no. 10, pp. 1261–1267, 2013.

[5] A. Ka, P. Britton, C. Troedson et al., "Mild encephalopathy with reversible splenial lesion: an important differential of encephalitis," *European Journal of Paediatric Neurology*, vol. 19, no. 3, pp. 377–382, 2015.

[6] C. E. Otten and C. J. Creutzfeldt, "Fulminant acute disseminated encephalomyelitis presenting in an adult," *JAMA Neurology*, vol. 71, no. 5, p. 648, 2014.

[7] E. Marchioni, E. Tavazzi, L. Minoli et al., "Acute disseminated encephalomyelitis," *Neurological Sciences*, vol. 29, Suppl 2, pp. 286–288, 2008.

[8] D. L. Koelman and F. J. Mateen, "Acute disseminated encephalomyelitis: current controversies in diagnosis and outcome," *Journal of Neurology*, vol. 262, no. 9, pp. 2013–2024, 2015.

[9] S. Schwarz, A. Mohr, M. Knauth, B. Wildemann, and B. Storch-Hagenlocher, "Acute disseminated encephalomyelitis: a follow-up study of 40 adult patients," *Neurology*, vol. 56, no. 10, pp. 1313–1318, 2001.

[10] S. E. Marin and D. J. Callen, "The magnetic resonance imaging appearance of monophasic acute disseminated encephalomyelitis: an update post application of the 2007 consensus criteria," *Neuroimaging Clinics of North America*, vol. 23, no. 2, pp. 245–266, 2013.

[11] A. Kaya, M. Acikgoz, L. Ustyol et al., "A case of acute disseminated encephalomyelitis mimicking leukodystrophy," *The Kurume Medical Journal*, vol. 57, no. 3, pp. 85–89, 2010.

[12] S. Pradhan and R. Tandon, "Acute disseminated encephalomyelitis mimicking leukodystrophys," *Pediatric Neurology*, vol. 51, no. 5, p. 749, 2014.

[13] A. Al-Futaisi, F. Al-Azri, A. A. Abdelmogheth, F. Al-Murshedi, and R. Koul, "Severe acute disseminated encephalomyelitis mimicking leukodystrophy in a child," *Sultan Qaboos University Medical Journal*, vol. 14, no. 3, pp. e409–11, 2014.

[14] D. L. Renaud, "Clinical approach to leukoencephalopathies," *Seminars in Neurology*, vol. 32, no. 1, pp. 29–33, 2012.

[15] Y. Okita, Y. Narita, Y. Miyakita et al., "Long-term follow-up of vanishing tumors in the brain: How should a lesion mimicking primary CNS lymphoma be managed?" *Clinical Neurology and Neurosurgery*, vol. 114, no. 9, pp. 1217–1221, 2012.

[16] J. J. Pan, Y. Y. Zhao, C. Lu, Y. H. Hu, and Y. Yang, "Mild encephalitis/encephalopathy with a reversible splenial lesion: five cases and a literature revisew," *Neurological Sciences*, vol. 36, no. 11, pp. 2043–2051, 2015.

[17] K. Karampatsas, C. Spyridou, I. R. Morrison, C. Y. Tong, and A. J. Prendergast, "Rotavirus-associated mild encephalopathy with a reversible splenial lesion (MERS)-case report and review of the literature," *BMC Infectious Diseases*, vol. 15, no. 1, p. 446, 2015.

[18] J. Takanashi, A. J. Barkovich, T. Shiihara et al., "Widening spectrum of a reversible splenial lesion with transiently reduced diffusion," *American Journal of Neuroradiology*, vol. 27, no. 4, pp. 836–838, 2006.

[19] S. Ramanathan, R. C. Dale, and F. Brilot, "Anti-MOG antibody: the history, clinical phenotype, and pathogenicity of a serum biomarker for demyelination demyelination," *Autoimmunity Reviews*, vol. 15, no. 4, pp. 307s–324, 2016.

[20] A. Notebaert, J. Willems, L. Coucke, R. Van Coster, and H. Verhelst, "Expanding the spectrum of MERS type 2 lesions, a particular form of encephalitis," *Pediatric Neurology*, vol. 48, no. 2, pp. 135–138, 2013.

[21] N. Garg, S. W. Reddel, D. H. Miller et al., "The corpus callosum in the diagnosis of multiple sclerosis and other CNS demyelinating and inflammatory diseases," *Journal of Neurology, Neurosurgery & Psychiatry*, vol. 86, no. 12, pp. 1374–1382, 2015.

[22] C. F. Lucchinetti, R. H. Gavrilova, I. Metz et al., "Clinical and radiographic spectrum of pathologically confirmed tumefactive multiple sclerosis," *Brain*, vol. 131, no. 7, pp. 1759–1775, 2008.

[23] H. Tada, J. Takanashi, A. J. Barkovich et al., "Clinically mild encephalitis/encephalopathy with a reversible splenial lesion," *Neurology*, vol. 63, no. 10, pp. 1854–1858, 2004.

[24] I. Steiner and P. G. Kennedy, "Acute disseminated encephalomyelitis: current knowledge and open questions questions," *Journal of NeuroVirology*, vol. 21, no. 5, pp. 473–479, 2015.

[25] I. A. Ketelslegers, I. E. Visser, R. F. Neuteboom, M. Boon, C. E. Catsman-Berrevoets, and R. Q. Hintzen, "Disease coursse and outcome of acute disseminated encephalomyelitis is more severe in adults than in children," *Multiple Sclerosis Journal*, vol. 17, no. 4, pp. 441–448, 2011.

[26] P. L. Khong, H. K. Ho, P. W. Cheng, V. C. Wong, W. Goh, and F. L. Chan, "Childhood acute disseminated encephalomyelitis: the role of brain and spinal cord MRI," *Pediatric Radiology*, vol. 32, no. 1, pp. 59–66, 2002.

23

A Case of Reverse Takotsubo Cardiomyopathy Incited by a Spinal Subdural Hematoma

Kyle Sanchez,[1] Steven Glener,[1] Nathan E. Esplin,[2] Okorie N. Okorie,[3] and Amay Parikh[3]

[1] *University of Central Florida College of Medicine, 6850 Lake Nona Boulevard, Orlando, FL 32827, USA*
[2] *Department of Neurosurgery, Allegheny General Hospital, 320 E North Ave., Pittsburgh, PA 15212, USA*
[3] *Florida Hospital, 601 E Rollins Street, Orlando, FL 32803, USA*

Correspondence should be addressed to Kyle Sanchez; kylesanchez@knights.ucf.edu

Academic Editor: Shahid Nimjee

Takotsubo cardiomyopathy is a rare syndrome of transient, reversible left ventricular systolic dysfunction. It mimics myocardial infarction clinically and includes elevated cardiac enzymes, but echocardiography reveals apical ballooning and basal hyperkinesis. Infrequently, midventricular or even reverse Takotsubo patterns have been described, involving ballooning of the basal heart without the characteristic 'Takotsubo' appearance. There are cases in the literature that support a connection between reverse Takotsubo cardiomyopathy (r-TTC) and neurological insults as inciting factors. We report a case of r-TTC in an otherwise healthy 23-year-old man presenting with back pain, urinary retention, bradycardia, and hypertension. Troponin levels and brain natriuretic peptide (BNP) were elevated, and echocardiogram revealed an ejection fraction (EF) of less than 20%. In addition, MRI demonstrated a spinal subdural hematoma from T1-S1 with no cord compression. Repeated echocardiogram demonstrated an EF of 20-25% with a reverse Takotsubo pattern of cardiomyopathy. With supportive care, his clinical picture improved with normalization of cardiac enzyme and BNP values. This case represents a r-TTC presenting as heart failure in a young, apparently healthy male likely incited by a spinal subdural hematoma. To our knowledge, it is the first of its kind reported.

1. Introduction

Takotsubo Cardiomyopathy (TTC), also called stress-induced cardiomyopathy or broken heart syndrome, is a rare syndrome of transient and reversible left ventricular systolic dysfunction in the absence of coronary stenosis. TTC is characterized by ballooning of the left ventricular apex that is provoked by an emotionally or physically stressful experience [1], although the mechanism is still debated. The clinical presentation of TTC mimics acute coronary syndrome, as it presents with symptoms ranging from isolated chest pain to severe dyspnea and cardiogenic shock, often accompanied by elevation of troponin level and T-wave and ST-segment abnormalities on echocardiogram (ECG) [2]. Classically, echocardiogram shows apical ballooning and basal hyperkinesis, resembling a 'crab pot' or 'octopus trap' that, from the Japanese word for such, gives this disorder its name.

The four known patterns of left ventricular involvement in TTC include classical type, reverse type, midventricular type, and localized type [2]. In the classical pattern of TTC, the most common type, the base of the ventricle contracts normally or is hyperkinetic while the rest of the ventricle is dyskinetic or akinetic [3], causing the classical ballooning of the left ventricular apex. Reverse, or inverted type, Takotsubo cardiomyopathy (r-TTC) is a rare variant characterized by hypokinesis of the base with relative sparing of the midventricle and apex [1], causing ballooning to occur at the base of the heart.

In comparison to other patterns of TCC, r-TCC usually presents in a younger patient population with higher troponin levels, lower ejection fraction, and a paradoxically faster recovery [4]. The higher troponin levels are believed to be the result of a larger region of myocardial involvement in r-TTC in comparison to the apex alone [2]. On the contrary, natriuretic peptides are often more elevated in apical and midventricular patterns of TCC and account for the higher prevalence of severe symptoms and higher NYHA functional class [2] seen in comparison to r-TTC. The higher prevalence

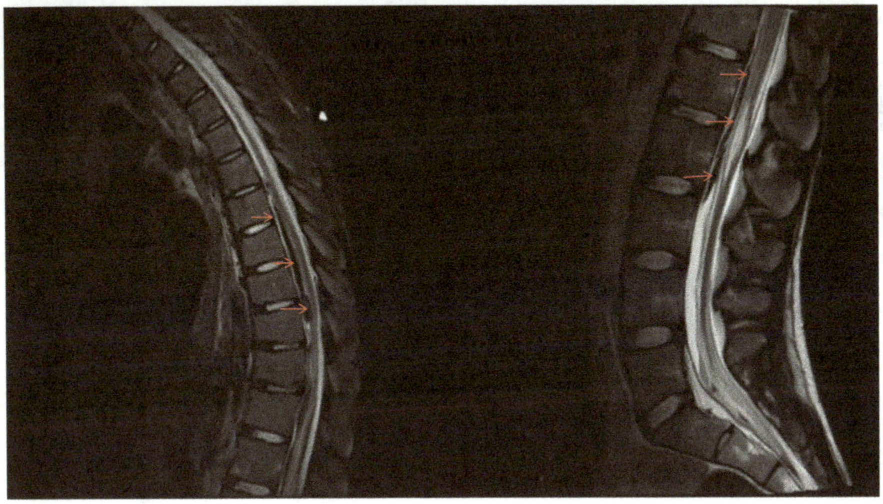

FIGURE 1: MRI showing thoracic (*left*) and lumbar (*right*) subdural hematomas (arrows).

of symptoms despite less damage to cardiomyocytes may be explained by the frequent coexistence of mitral regurgitation caused by apical ballooning [2]. Predictors of mortality from r-TTC include decreased left ventricular ejection fraction, development of atrial fibrillation, and neurologic disease."

The precise etiology of TCC/r-TCC is unknown, but evidence indicates that both patterns are associated with strong surges of adrenergic outflow that occur following intense emotional or physical stress [5–9], where high circulating levels of epinephrine may cause coronary spasm, endothelial dysfunction, and indirect myocardial damage [2]. A few case studies have suggested a potential connection between r-TTC and neurological insults as inciting factors. Reported neurological stressors which have induced r-TCC include cerebellar hemorrhage [2], medulla oblongata hemorrhage [5], subarachnoid hemorrhage [10], inadvertent intrathecal injection [11], and multiple sclerosis [12]. Additionally, the presence of neurologic disease may be a good predictor of mortality in patients with r-TTC [13]. To the best of our knowledge, this is the first report of a case of r-TTC presenting after a spinal subdural hematoma.

2. Case Presentation

A 23-year-old man presented to an outside Emergency Department (ED) with difficulty in voiding both bowel and bladder, and significant mid-back pain with associated weakness, numbness, and tingling in bilateral lower extremities. He reported a two-week history of headache, nonproductive cough, nasal congestion, nausea, and vomiting but denied flank pain and dysuria. On physical exam, he was significantly hypertensive (225/119 mmHg) and bradycardic (57 bpm), with paraspinal muscle tenderness, but there was no vertebral point tenderness. He was also found to have hypoactive deep tendon reflexes at the patella and Achilles tendons.

He had visited the ED twice in the two days prior to this admission for constant, "achy" back pain in the lumbar region, exacerbated by movement, which he attributed to lifting boxes at work. During these hospital visits, the patient denied bowel and bladder dysfunction, saddle anesthesia, fever, and chills. On both occasions, he was discharged home with the diagnosis of acute lumbar paraspinal muscle strain.

On this third visit, now with urinary retention, he was admitted to the outside facility. The patient was catheterized, yielding 1400 mL of urine, which tested positive for THC and oxycodone and revealed trace amounts of ketones. Initial laboratory evaluation was significant for leukocytosis (14,580 cells/μL, neutrophil 81.6%) and elevated N-terminal BNP at 734 pg/mL (0 – 125 pg/mL).

Computed tomography (CT) of the head showed no evidence of significant intracranial pathology. CT of the abdomen and pelvis showed no acute findings with no evidence of intra-abdominal trauma. Computed tomography angiogram (CTA) of the chest revealed symmetric infiltrates and interlobular septal thickenings of the lungs, presumed to be pulmonary edema, although diffuse multifocal pneumonia and pneumocystis pneumonia were considered. It also revealed dilation of left ventricle and left atrium, pneumomediastinum, and fluid in the esophagus. MRI of the lumbar spine revealed abnormally decreased T2 signal and mildly increased T1 signal involving the ventral central canal spanning from T5 to L2-L3, which likely reflected a subdural hematoma (Figure 1). It also demonstrated a likely superimposed subdural hygroma with fluid signal present that was most prominent beginning at the L2-L3 level and progressing caudally to the L5-S1 level within the ventral thecal sac. There was associated dorsal displacement of the nerve roots of the cauda equina and crowding of the nerve roots. These findings resulted in diffuse narrowing of the lumbar thecal sac most severely between T7-T8 and the mid-T10 vertebral body, where the subdural hematoma was largest. Narrowing of the thecal sac was most severe at the T9-T10 level where there was moderate to severe narrowing of the thecal sac present with deformation of the anterior surface of the cord that was worse on the left. Small active Schmorl's nodes were demonstrated along the inferior endplate of L1. There was

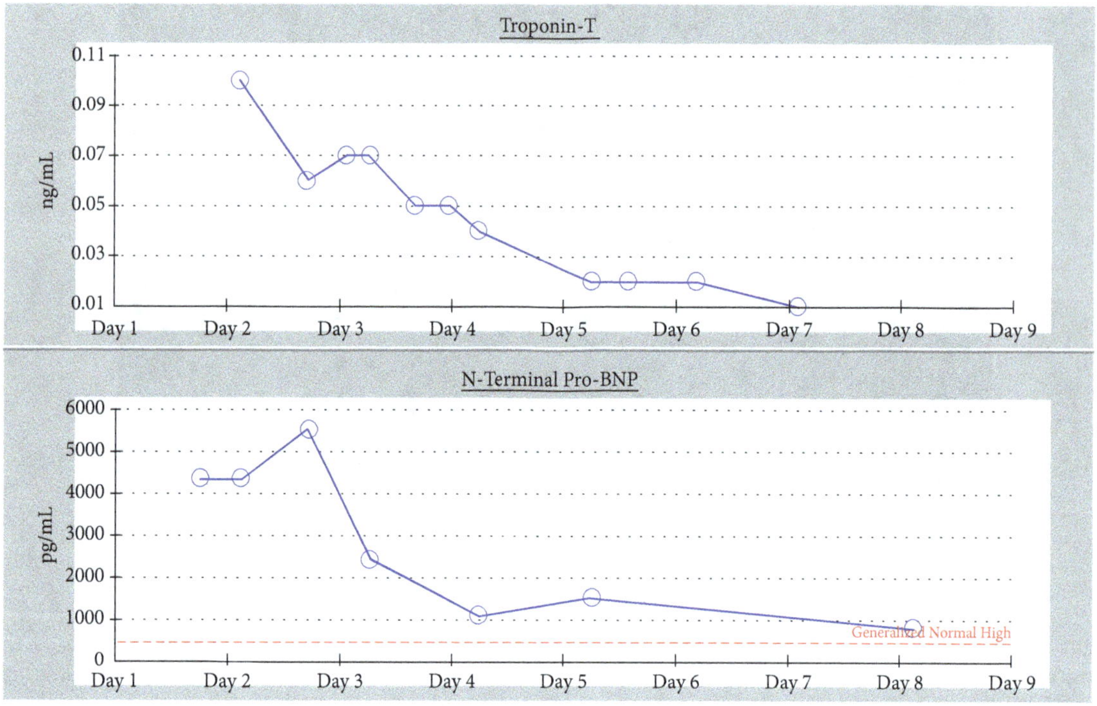

FIGURE 2: Troponin-T and N-Terminal Pro-BNP levels over the course of hospital stay.

also an abnormal signal within the subarachnoid spaces of the lower lumbar spine that was most prominent at the L5-S1 level. The decreased T2 signal and increased T1 signal present at this level likely reflected a subarachnoid hemorrhage. There was no enhancement on the study to suggest infection and no fracture or subluxation. After experiencing a hypoxic event with O2 saturation dropping to 70%, he was then transferred to our tertiary care center.

On admission, physical exam revealed full strength in upper and lower extremities with normal light touch sensation. However, he reported quadricep and calf numbness, despite the normal light touch sensation. Laboratory evaluation was significant for leukocytosis (20,970 cells/μL) (neutrophil 77.1%), elevated N-terminal BNP level (4,325 pg/mL), and troponin T level elevation at 0.6 ng/mL (0 - 0.14 ng/mL).

Repeated noncontrast MRI of the thoracic spine ordered by neurosurgery showed acute subdural hematoma involving the thoracic spine and the ventral central canal that was worse on the left, spanning from the T5 level caudally to involve the lumbar spine. Despite prior suspicion of increased T2 signal involving the ventral cord spanning the T7-T8 level to mid-T10 vertebral body, evaluation for cord signal abnormality was deemed severely limited secondary to motion artifact. There were small areas of acute subdural hemorrhage within the dorsal aspect of the thecal sac most prominent at the T4-T5 level with suspicion for a small amount of dorsal subdural hygroma involving the thoracic spine (Figure 1). No fracture or subluxation was seen. It also demonstrated airspace consolidation involving the bilateral lung bases and the dependent portion of the right upper lobe of the lung. These findings were believed to have reflected severe pulmonary edema. CT of the head without contrast was negative for large territorial acute infarction, acute intracranial hemorrhage, and mass effect. CT angiogram of the head showed no evidence of significant intracranial arterial pathology. Repeated MRI of the lumbar spine showed loss of T2 prolongation in the ventral subdural region from the level of L1-L3, which was originally felt to represent a flow-related artifact. Upon further review, this may have represented a true fluid collection. From the level of L3-L5, there may have been a possible subdural hygroma (Figure 1). However, the etiology of subdural hematoma was unclear; infectious or traumatic etiologies were suspected.

ECG showed sinus bradycardia with possible left atrial enlargement and left ventricular hypertrophy. Echocardiogram revealed an ejection fraction of 20-25%. The etiology of cardiomyopathy was also unclear, but viral infection was suspected.

Antibody testing was conducted for HIV, *Toxoplasma* spp., and EBV; PCR testing was conducted for HHV-6 and Parvovirus B19; serological testing was conducted for Coxsackieviruses A and B; and blood cultures were taken, all of which were negative. During his stay, the patient's N-terminal BNP level steadily declined after peaking at 5,516 pg/mL, as did his troponin T levels (Figure 2). A repeated echocardiogram on hospital day six revealed an ejection fraction of 45-50%, with normal left ventricular size, mild right ventricular dilation, mild mitral regurgitation, trace tricuspid regurgitation, and normal systolic function. An additional echocardiogram the following day showed an ejection fraction of 55-60% with mild mitral regurgitation, trace

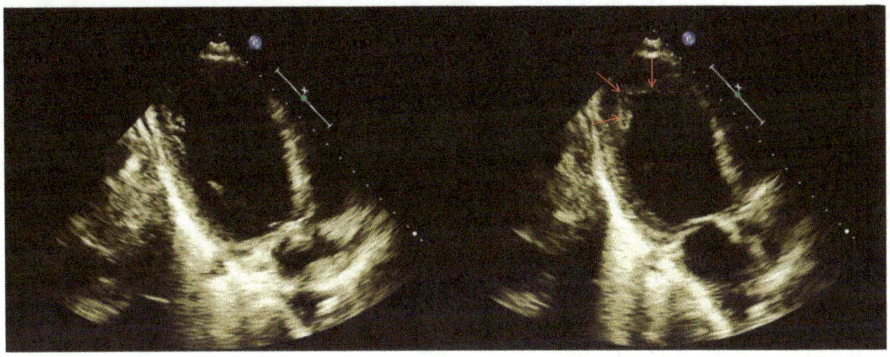

FIGURE 3: TTE apical two-chamber view of left ventricle in End Diastole (*left*) and End Systole (*right*), demonstrating poor ventricular compression and low EF. r-TTC pattern is indicated by contraction of ventricular apex (arrows) and hypokinesis of base during systole.

tricuspid regurgitation, and greater than 50% respiratory change in the inferior vena cava dimension from normally sized chambers.

The patient was diagnosed with a case of likely reverse Takotsubo cardiomyopathy potentially secondary to subdural hematoma of the thoracic and lumbar spine.

3. Discussion

We believe this to be a case of r-TTC presenting as heart failure in a young, apparently healthy man likely incited by a spinal subdural hematoma.

TTC is a rare syndrome of transient, reversible left ventricular dysfunction that is provoked by physical or emotional stressors [1]. Of the four types of TTC, the hallmark of r-TTC is the presence of an inverted Takotsubo pattern with hypokinesis of the left ventricular base and sparing of the apex, causing ballooning of the base rather than apex, which was observed on the patient's echocardiogram (Figure 3). All patterns of TTC typically mimic acute coronary syndrome and related cardiovascular complications [1], but r-TTC is associated with higher troponin levels and lower EF [2]. In this patient, we believe that r-TTC explains the heart failure with reduced EF. The transient nature of the patient's condition, as evidenced by the resolution of symptoms and normalization of Troponin-T levels, N-terminal BNP levels, and EF, is consistent with the spontaneous resolution of all cases of TTC, especially those of r-TTC [2]. In addition, the patient's young age is typical of r-TTC [2, 14].

While all patterns of Takotsubo cardiomyopathy are typically preceded by emotional or physical stressors [1], the patient's history did not indicate that he experienced any intense stressor before his condition developed. We recognize that this is atypical, even for r-TTC. However, there have been multiple cases that suggest a potential connection between r-TTC and neurological insults as inciting factors [4–12]. The patient initially presented with back pain, which was likely the result of his underlying subdural hematoma. Etiology of the subdural hematoma was unclear, and infectious or injury-induced causes were suspected. However, infectious workup was negative, and patient denied any overt injury aside from his back pain. Regardless of the etiology of his subdural hematoma, we believe that it then incited a r-TTC presenting as heart failure with reduced EF.

To our knowledge, this is the first case reported of a spinal subdural hematoma inciting r-TTC. It demonstrates the critical nature of this rare presentation of poorly understood pathology and drives home the need to keep it on the differential in a case of cardiomyopathy or heart failure.

Disclosure

An earlier version of this manuscript was presented as a poster in the 2018 Neurocritical Care Society Annual Meeting.

References

[1] D. Belliveau and S. De, "Reverse takotsubo cardiomyopathy following exogenous epinephrine administration in the early postpartum period," *Journal of Echocardiography*, vol. 33, no. 7, pp. 1089–1091, 2016.

[2] S. Piérard, M. Vinetti, and P. Hantson, "Inverted (reverse) takotsubo cardiomyopathy following cerebellar hemorrhage," *Case Reports in Cardiology*, vol. 2014, Article ID 781926, 4 pages, 2014.

[3] K. A. Bybee, T. Kara, A. Prasad et al., "Systematic review: transient left ventricular apical ballooning: a syndrome that mimics ST-segment elevation myocardial infarction," *Annals of Internal Medicine*, vol. 141, no. 11, pp. 858–865, 2004.

[4] T. Tagami, A. Mertens, D. Rothschild, and P. Chowdhury, "A case of reverse takotsubo cardiomyopathy caused by an eating disorder," *Journal of Cardiology Cases*, vol. 15, no. 3, pp. 77–79, 2017.

[5] K. T. Gobeske, M. E. Sarano, J. E. Fugate, and E. F. Wijdicks, "Medulla oblongata hemorrhage and reverse takotsubo cardiomyopathy," *Neurocritical Care*, vol. 29, no. 3, pp. 508–511, 2018.

[6] F. Pelliccia, J. C. Kaski, F. Crea, and P. G. Camici, "Pathophysiology of takotsubo syndrome," *Circulation*, vol. 135, no. 24, pp. 2426–2441, 2017.

[7] O. Chehab, A. Ioannou, A. Sawhney, A. Rice, and S. Dubrey, "Reverse takotsubo cardiomyopathy and cardiogenic shock associated with methamphetamine consumption," *The Journal of Emergency Medicine*, vol. 53, no. 5, pp. e81–e83, 2017.

[8] B. Flam, M. Broomé, B. Frenckner, R. Bränström, and M. Bell, "Pheochromocytoma-induced inverted takotsubo-like cardiomyopathy leading to cardiogenic shock successfully treated with extracorporeal membrane oxygenation," *Journal of Intensive Care Medicine*, vol. 30, no. 6, pp. 365–372, 2015.

[9] T. Kudaiberdiev, I. Akhmedova, G. Imanalieva et al., "Surgical treatment of left ventricular wall rupture, regarded as a consequence of Takotsubo cardiomyopathy," *SAGE Open Medical Case Reports*, vol. 5, Article ID 2050313x16689210, 2017.

[10] T. Kumai, J. Inamasu, E. Watanabe, K. Sugimoto, and Y. Hirose, "Differences between Takotsubo cardiomyopathy and reverse Takotsubo cardiomyopathy associated with subarachnoid hemorrhage," *IJC Heart and Vasculature*, vol. 11, pp. 99–103, 2016.

[11] C. Lee, J. Son, and U. Kim, "Reverse takotsubo cardiomyopathy following inadvertent intrathecal injection during percutaneous epidural neuroplasty," *Heart, Lung and Circulation*, vol. 25, no. 9, pp. e148–e151, 2015.

[12] F. London, N. Gonzalez Rodriguez de Azero, M. Philippart, J. Higny, and N. Mulquin, "Reverse takotsubo cardiomyopathy triggered by a multiple sclerosis relapse," *Acta Neurologica Belgica*, vol. 119, no. 2, pp. 295–297, 2019.

[13] H. H. Awad, A. R. McNeal, and H. Goyal, "Reverse takotsubo cardiomyopathy: a comprehensive review," *Annals of Translational Medicine*, vol. 6, no. 23, pp. 460-460, 2018.

[14] D. Rosu, S. Askandar, and R. N. Khouzam, "Why is reverse takotsubo 'reverse'?" *Southern Medical Journal*, vol. 110, no. 5, pp. 381–385, 2017.

24

MELAS Missed for Years: Stroke-Like Lesions are No Indication for Brain Biopsy

J. Finsterer

Krankenanstalt Rudolfstiftung, Messerli Institute, Vienna, Austria

Correspondence should be addressed to J. Finsterer; fipaps@yahoo.de

Academic Editor: Peter Berlit

A 56-year-old female with a history of chronic alcoholism until age 38 y with a relapse between ages 45 and 46 y developed seizures, psychosis, and hemianopia to the left at age 46 y. Imaging revealed a right parieto-occipital lesion with intralesional bleeding. Five months after the first lesion she developed a second left parieto-occipital lesion, resulting in cortical blindness. Extensive workup, including brain biopsy, was noninformative. Retrospectively, the occipital abnormalities were identified as stroke-like lesions (SLLs). Further manifestations of the mitochondrial disorder (MID) were tremor, cerebral atrophy, bilateral basal ganglia, calcification, glaucoma, hypoacusis, short stature, hyperostosis frontalis, hyperthyroidism, sick-sinus syndrome and AV-block-1, and myopathy. According to the Walker criteria, a possible MID was diagnosed. In conclusion, adult-onset MID may be missed for years, SLLs may be easily misinterpreted entailing brain biopsy, and psychosis may contribute to a reduced impact for proper workup of a MID.

1. Introduction

Despite recent advances in the management of mitochondrial disorders (MIDs), diagnosing and treating MIDs remains challenging [1]. This is not only due to unawareness of the condition in adults but frequently also due to misinterpretation of diagnostic tests and ignorance. Therapy is challenging as well, as no causal treatment is currently available for most of the conditions [2], but progress has been achieved in preventing transmission of MIDs via the maternal line (maternal spindle transfer and pronuclear transfer) [3]. Here, we present a patient with a late-onset, multisystem MID, which remained undiagnosed for 10 y.

2. Case Report

The patient is a 56-year-old Caucasian female, with height 168 cm and weight 57 kg, who was referred for replacing carbamazepine (CBZ) by another antiepileptic drug (AED), which does not cause hyponatremia or thrombocytopenia. She had a long-term medical history suggestive of a slowly progressive multisystem disease (Table 1), including fracture of the petrosal bone after a collapse of unknown cause at age 16 y, right bimalleolar fracture at age 23 y, chronic alcoholism until age 38 y with a relapse between ages 45 and 46 y, and icterus and hepatopathy at age 39 y. At age 43 y she received bilateral breast implants. At age 46 y, she developed epilepsy initially with a series of partial complex and generalized seizures, being attributed to chronic alcoholism, but the latter occurred during abstinence. Additionally, she experienced a first psychotic episode with optic hallucinations and developed hemianopia to the left. Workup with imaging initially revealed a right occipital lesion hyperintens on diffusion-weighted imaging (DWI), apparent diffusion coefficient (ADC), and T2-weighted images with bleeding in the center of the lesion in the absence of arterial hypertension or coagulopathy and a small lesion on the left precentral gyrus. Five months later, a left occipital lesion (hyperintense on DWI, ADC, and T2-weighted images) not confined to a vascular territory developed (Figure 1). Workup by means of imaging, functional studies, cerebrospinal fluid (CSF) investigations, blood tests, electroencephalography (EEG), and

Table 1: Disease trajectory of the presented patient.

Onset, age	Manifestation	Therapy
16 y	Collapse with TBI (petrous bone fracture)	Conservative
23 y	Right bimalleolar fracture	Np
Until 38 y	Chronic alcoholism	Withdrawal
39 y	Icterus, hepatopathy	None
43 y	Small breasts	Breast silicon implants
45–46 y	Relapse of alcoholism	Successful withdrawal
46 y	Epilepsy with focal and generalized seizures	Levetiracetam
46 y	1 SLL with intralesional bleeding (right occipital) hemianopia and neglect to the left, psychosis	Neuroleptics
46 y	Hepatopathy, steatosis hepatis	None
Until age 46 y	Smoking	Withdrawal
46 y	Acne rosacea	Topic ointments
46 y	Arachnoidal cyst (left temporo-basal)	None
46 y	Folic acid deficiency	Folic acid
46 y	Hyperlipidemia	Diet
46 y	2 SLE (left occipital (epilepsy, psychosis, cortical blindness, and optic hallucinations))	Brain biopsy via drill-hole quetiapin
47 y	Arterial hypertension	Bisoprolol
47 y	AV-block-1	None
47 y	Hyponatremia after adding OXC	OXC replaced with CBZ
Since age 47 y	Thrombocytopenia after adding CBZ	CBZ withdrawal
47 y	Myoclonic seizure	Levetiracetam
49 y	Glaucoma	Latanoprost
Until 49 y	Recurrent syncopes due to sinus arrests	Pacemaker
49 y	Hyperthyroidism	None
53 y	Capsular fibrosis	Replacement of breast implants
53 y	Ischemic strokes (PCAS territory, PCAS stenosis)	Antithrombotics
56 y	Barrett esophagus	Esomeprazole
56 y	Hyperostosis frontalis	None
56 y	Generalized brain atrophy	None
Since years	Carpopedal spasms	Magnesium
Since years	Hypoacusis	None

PCAS: left posterior cerebral artery syndrome, PRES: posterior reversible encephalopathy syndrome, SLE: stroke-like episode, AEDs: antiepileptic drugs, SSS: sick-sinus syndrome, TBI: traumatic brain injury, CBZ: carbamazepine, and np: not provided.

brain biopsy via a left occipital drill-hole, for primary cerebral neoplasm, metastasis, extrapontine myelinolysis, hepatic encephalopathy, Macchia-Fava disease, neuro-Whipple disease, the Heidenhain type of Creutzfeldt-Jakob disease, cerebral vasculitis, including neuro-Behcet, Wernicke-encephalopathy, and dementia, was negative. Thus, the occipital lesions were interpreted as posterior reversible encephalopathy syndrome (PRES). The lesions were followed up during the succeeding years, evolving into gliosis, cysts, and siderosis and retrospectively interpreted as stroke-like lesions (SLLs). Cortical blindness, psychosis, and epilepsy persisted.

At age 47 y, transient arterial hypertension without requiring long-term medication and hyponatremia, first recognized after adding oxcarbazepine (OXC), became apparent. OXC was replaced with CBZ. An AV-block-1 was recorded. At age 49 y, a pacemaker was implanted because of recurrent syncopes due to sinus arrest. Additionally, bilateral glaucoma was diagnosed. At age 53 y, ischemic stroke in the left posterior cerebral artery territory occurred. She reported muscle cramps of the small foot muscles (carpopedal spasms) and hypoacusis since years (Table 1). The patient had various AEDs since onset of epilepsy, including levetiracetam (LEV), OXC, LTG, lacosamide (LAC), and CBZ, but adherence to these drugs was poor. The family history was positive for breast cancer in her mother. Since age 53 y, the index patient was supported by a legal representative.

Clinical neurologic exam at age 56 y revealed short stature, hypoacusis, bilateral ptosis, marked bilateral visual impairment , left-sided intention tremor, wasting of the distal lower limb muscles, and reduced Achilles tendon reflexes bilaterally. Creatine kinase (CK) and resting serum lactate were normal. There was mild hyponatremia and thrombocytopenia being attributed to CBZ and mild hepatopathy. Though the CBZ serum level was within the normal range, CBZ was replaced by LEV (1500 mg/d). ECG showed an AV-block-I. Gastroscopy revealed a Barrett esophagus, and why esomeprazole was given. EEG showed occasional spikes in the right temporal projection. Cerebral computed tomography (CT) showed generalized atrophy and the known left temporal and bilateral occipito-temporal defects. The mitochondrial multiorgan disorder syndrome (MIMODS) score was 46 (number of organs affected: 6, number of organ manifestations: 15: PubMed hits: 25) (Table 2) [4]. Possible MID was diagnosed [4]. The patient refused to undergo further diagnostic workup for MID and announced not to take the AEDs prescribed.

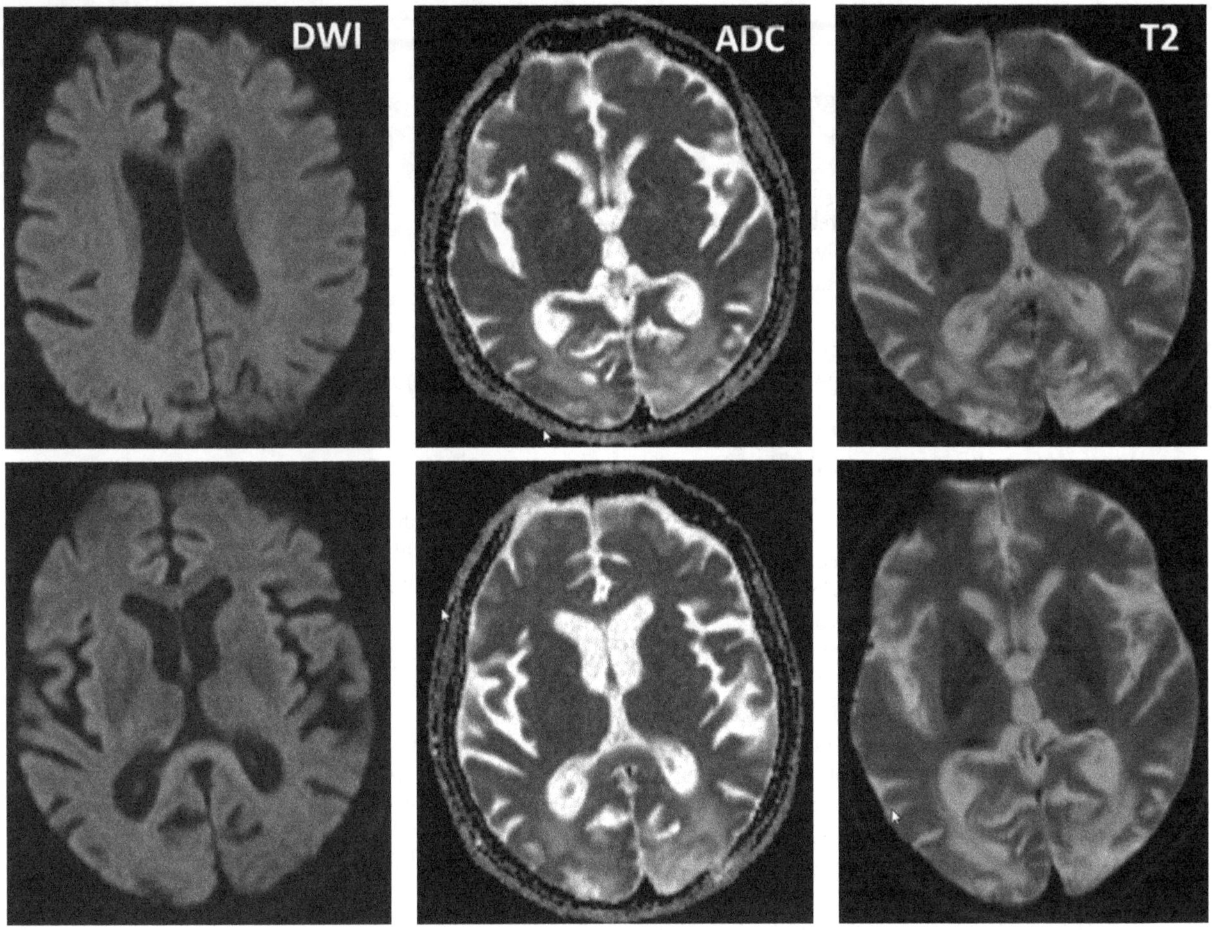

(a) (b) (c)

FIGURE 1: Cerebral MRI, 2 months after onset of psychosis, epilepsy, and visual impairment showing a slightly hyperintense right occipital lesion and a slightly hypointense similar lesion in the left occipital area, which were both hyperintense on ADC and hyperintense on T2-weighted images. Within the right occipital lesion, cortical and subcortical bleeding was identified. The occipital lesions were retrospectively interpreted as consecutive, subacute SLLs.

TABLE 2: MIMODS score calculated as the sum of three items.

(1) Number of affected organs (range: 0–14) (muscle, CNS, endocrine organs, heart, intestines, nerves, ears, eyes, bone marrow, kidneys, skin, bones, lungs, and arteries)
(2) Number of manifestations per organ
Muscle (ophthalmoplegia (3), ptosis (3), easy fatigability (exercise intolerance) (3), limb weakness (2), hyper-CK-emia (2), wasting (1), respiratory insufficiency (1), myoglobinuria (1), cramping (1), myalgia (1), abnormal lactate stress test (1), double vision (diplopia) (1), muscle stiffness (1), fasciculations (1), muscle rupture (1))
CNS (epilepsy (3), atrophy (3), ataxia (3), Parkinson (3), dementia (3), stroke-like episodes (2), migraine (2), dystonia (1), tremor (1), leukoencephalopathy (white matter lesions) (1), spasticity (1), dysarthria (1), psychosis (1), confusion (1), mild cognitive impairment (1), basal ganglia calcification (1), dilative arteriopathy (1), delayed visually evoked potentials (1), myelopathy (1))
Heart (hypertrophic, dilated, restrictive CMP (3), heart failure (2), systolic dysfunction (2), arrhythmias (1), arterial hypertension (1), noncompaction (1), pulmonary hypertension (1), aortic root ectasia (1), coronary heart disease (1), congenital heart disease (1))
Intestines (hepatopathy (3), vomiting (1), diarrhea(1), pancreatitis (1), steatosis hepatis (1), nonspecific colitis (1), diverticulosis (1), sialadenitis (1))
Nerves (neuropathy (3), neuronopathy (1))
Eyes (optic atrophy (3), retinopathy (3), cataract (1), glaucoma (1))
Ears (hypoacusis (3), tinnitus (1))
Kidneys (renal insufficiency (2), renal failure (2), tubular acidosis (1), Fanconi syndrome (1), cysts (1), nephrolithiasis (1))
Arteries (dissection (1), spontaneous rupture (1), aneurysm (1), ectasia (1), dilative arteriopathy (1), atherosclerosis (1))
Bone marrow (anemia (2), leukopenia (1), thrombopenia (1))
Bones (skeletal deformities (1), polyarthralgia (1), arthrosis (1))
Dermis (psoriasis (1), lipomatosis (1), vitiligo (1), edema (1), hypertrichosis (1), baldness, alopecia (1), madarosis (1), skin rashes (1), seborrheic eczema (1)*)
(3) Frequency of citations in PubMed (>100 citations: 3 points, 50–100 citations: 2 points, <50 citations; 1 point); *appropriate scores are provided in parenthesis above

A score >11 suggests definite MID; *the PubMed value is provided in parenthesis after each manifestation.

3. Discussion

The presented patient is interesting for slowly progressive multimorbidity with onset at age 46 y, suggesting a MID and matching with the diagnostic criteria for possible MID [5, 6]. Arguments for the diagnosis of MID are seizures, tremor, psychosis, cerebral atrophy, bilateral basal ganglia calcification, and the bilateral SLLs, suggesting cerebral involvement, glaucoma suggesting ophthalmologic involvement, hypoacusis suggesting involvement of the ears, short stature, hyperostosis frontalis, and hyperthyroidism suggesting endocrine involvement, sick-sinus syndrome and AV-block-1 suggesting cardiac involvement, and bilateral ptosis, distal lower limb wasting, and carpopedal spasms, suggesting myopathy. A further argument for MID is the MIMODS score of 46. MIMODS scores >10 have been shown to be indicative for a MID [4]. A late-onset MID is likely also in the light of an increasing number of mtDNA mutations with advanced age [7].

According to a recent consensus statement, a SLE can be diagnosed solely upon clinical presentation, cerebral MRI, and EEG [personal communication]. No advance genetic confirmation is required. The reason why the SLE had been misinterpreted and the SLL missed on MRI remains elusive. Most likely, a SLL was not considered as a differential and only those mentioned above were excluded. Arguments for a SLE are the MRI findings, the clinical presentation, the disease trajectory, and the multisystem nature of the condition. An argument against the right occipital SLL could be the bleeding since SLLs usually do not go along with intracerebral bleeding, but it is conceivable that in the course of laminar cortical necrosis, bleeding and consecutive siderosis developed. A further argument for a SLL is the dynamics of the lesions ending up as atrophy, gliosis, cysts, and siderosis. Arguments against PRES in the presented patient are that the occipital lesions did not resolve (PRES last maximally for three months), that arterial hypertension was well controlled even without antihypertensive drugs, that epilepsy and psychosis are only rare manifestations of PRES [8, 9], and that cortical blindness did not resolve. An argument against a reversible cerebral vasoconstriction syndrome is that the lesion lasted >3 months.

To which degree the right occipital stroke at age 53 y further deteriorated visual acuity remains speculative as the patient could not specify if visual acuity further deteriorated after this cerebrovascular event. Whether the 10 y history of psychosis contributed to the delayed suspicion and diagnosis of a MID remains speculative, but it is conceivable that psychiatric disease may generally prevent from a thorough workup for neurological disease as in nonpsychiatric patients with similar complaints [10]. Limitations of the study were that first-degree relatives were not systematically investigated and that muscle biopsy and genetic workup were refused by the patient and her legal representative.

4. Conclusions

This case shows that late-onset MIDs may be missed for years, that SLLs may be easily misinterpreted even entailing brain biopsy, and that the history of psychosis may contribute to a reduced impact for a proper workup of an underlying MID.

References

[1] M. Paiva Coelho, E. Martins, and L. Vilarinho, "Diagnosis, management, and follow-up of mitochondrial disorders in childhood: a personalized medicine in the new era of genome sequence," *European Journal of Pediatrics*, vol. 178, no. 1, pp. 21–32, 2019.

[2] J. Finsterer and P. S. Bindu, "Therapeutic strategies for mitochondrial disorders," *Pediatric Neurology*, vol. 52, no. 3, pp. 302–313, 2015.

[3] M. Tachibana, T. Kuno, and N. Yaegashi, "Mitochondrial replacement therapy and assisted reproductive technology: a paradigm shift toward treatment of genetic diseases in gametes or in early embryos," *Reproductive Medicine and Biology*, vol. 17, no. 4, pp. 421–433, 2018.

[4] J. Finsterer and S. Zarrouk-Mahjoub, "Mitochondrial multiorgan disorder syndrome score generated from definite mitochondrial disorders," *Neuropsychiatric Disease and Treatment*, vol. 13, pp. 2569–2579, 2017.

[5] U. A. Walker, S. Collins, and E. Byrne, "Respiratory chain encephalomyopathies: a diagnostic classification," *European Neurology*, vol. 36, no. 5, pp. 260–267, 1996.

[6] J. Finsterer and S. Z. Mahjoub, "Presentation of adult mitochondrial epilepsy," *Seizure*, vol. 22, no. 2, pp. 119–123, 2013.

[7] H. Li, J. Slone, L. Fei, and T. Huang, "Mitochondrial DNA variants and common diseases: a mathematical model for the diversity of age-related mtDNA mutations," *Cells*, vol. 8, no. 6, p. 608, 2019.

[8] L. Bastide, B. Legros, N. Rampal, E. J. Gilmore, L. J. Hirsch, and N. Gaspard, "Clinical correlates of periodic discharges and nonconvulsive seizures in posterior reversible encephalopathy syndrome (PRES)," *Neurocritical Care*, vol. 29, no. 3, pp. 481–490, 2018.

[9] G. S. Díaz-Ramírez, C. A. Salgado-Cifuentes, G. Zúñiga-Escobar, and C. D. Morales-Plaza, "Síndrome de leucoencefalopatía posterior reversible asociado a psicosis: una presentación inusual," *Neurología*, vol. 34, no. 8, pp. 549–551, 2019.

[10] W. M. M. Albers, D. P. K. Roeg, Y. Nijssen, J. van Weeghel, and I. M. B. Bongers, "Profiling of victimization, perpetration, and participation: a latent class analysis among people with severe mental illness," *PLoS One*, vol. 13, no. 11, Article ID e0208457, 2018.

25

The Successful use of Infliximab in a Relapsing Case of Susac's Syndrome

Suran L. Fernando,[1,2,3] **Therese Boyle**,[1] **Annika Smith**,[2] **and John D.E. Parratt**[3,4]

[1]*Immunology Laboratory, New South Wales Health Pathology, Royal North Hospital, Sydney, Australia*
[2]*Department of Clinical Immunology and Allergy, Royal North Hospital, Sydney, Australia*
[3]*Sydney Medical School, University of Sydney, Sydney, Australia*
[4]*Department of Neurology, Royal North Hospital, Sydney, Australia*

Correspondence should be addressed to Suran L. Fernando; suran.fernando@health.nsw.gov.au

Academic Editor: Peter Berlit

Susac's syndrome is a rare and debilitating disease characterized by the triad of encephalopathy, branch retinal artery occlusions, and sensorineural hearing loss. All manifestations may not be clinically apparent at presentation resulting in delayed diagnosis. Early recognition of the syndrome may prevent disease sequelae such as permanent cognitive, visual, and hearing loss. We present such a case of Susac's syndrome that was also refractory to conventionally prescribed combination of immunosuppressive treatments including high-dose potent corticosteroids, intravenous cyclophosphamide, methotrexate, plasma exchange, rituximab, and mycophenolate. His disease was stabilized with infliximab in combination with a tapering course of low-dose prednisone. After 2 years of remission with TNF treatment, consideration is being given to ceasing therapy. He has the sequelae of bilateral sensorineural hearing loss but no visual impairment or cognitive deficits on follow-up with neuropsychometric testing. This is the first case report to our knowledge of the successful use of infliximab for a patient with Susac's syndrome that was necessary following treatment with cyclophosphamide and then rituximab.

1. Introduction

Susac's syndrome is a rare and potentially debilitating disease affecting small cerebral and retinal arteries and the cochlea, resulting in the triad of encephalopathy, branch retinal artery occlusions, and sensorineural hearing loss [1]. The pathogenesis of the disease is not fully understood but is likely to be a cytotoxic CD8+ cell-mediated endotheliopathy with consequent microinfarctions [2]. A potent immunosuppressive therapy is often required to reduce disease sequelae. We describe the effect of infliximab upon acute and chronic disease activity in this case of Susac's syndrome that was refractory to other immunosuppressive and immunomodulatory agents.

2. Case Presentation

A 30-year-old previously well man presented with a four-week history of progressive right-sided hearing loss, wide-based gait, and cognitive disturbance characterized by short-term memory loss, impaired attention span, and verbal fluency. The patient had neither a personal nor family history of pertinent medical problems, and he did not smoke, drink excessive alcohol, or take illicit drugs.

On examination, he had cerebellar signs characterized by dysdiadochokinesis and ataxia of gait.

MRI of the brain at presentation demonstrated multiple hyperintense lesions in the corpus callosum, periventricular white matter, cerebellar hemispheres, and leptomeninges (Figure 1).

MRI of the spine was normal. The CSF showed a small pleocytosis with normal cytology and an elevated protein 3.06 g/L. There was an absence of oligoclonal bands in both CSF and serum. CSF microbiologic investigations revealed a Gram-negative stain, syphilis serology, and cryptococcal antigen. PCR analysis of the CSF did not detect EBV, CMV, HSV, VZV, enterovirus, *M. tuberculosis*, or fungal pathogens. Widespread triphasic waves consistent with

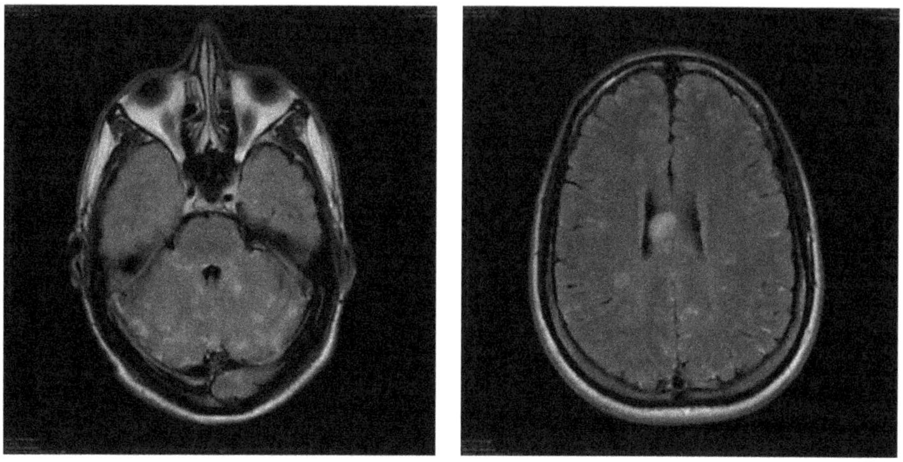

(a) (b)

Figure 1: MRI brain (T2 axial section). Extensive postcontrast T2 FLAIR enhancement of periventricular and cerebellar diseases with patchy leptomeningeal enhancement accentuated by the FLAIR technique. (a) Large T2 FLAIR signal in the body of corpus (snowball lesions) and throughout the periventricular white matter. (b) Regions of T2 FLAIR signal correlated with DWI (b1000) diffusion restriction.

encephalopathy but with no focal or generalised epileptic activity were demonstrable on an electroencephalogram (EEG). CT of the chest, abdomen, and pelvis did not reveal any lesions.

The full blood count, electrolytes, creatinine, and liver function tests were normal. The ANA, ANCA, anticardiolipin antibodies, and lupus anticoagulant were negative. Evaluation for autoimmune and paraneoplastic encephalitis with serum and CSF antibodies to NMDAR (*N*-methyl-D-aspartate receptor), AMPAR (α-amino-3-hydroxy-5-methyl-4-isoxazolepropionic acid receptor), LGI1 (leucine-rich glioma-inactivated 1), Caspr 2 (contactin-associated protein-like 2), GABA (gamma-aminobutyric acid) B receptor, and IgLON5 were negative, and ANNA-(anti-neuronal nuclear antibody-)1, ANNA-2, PCA (Purkinje cell antibody), PCA 2, Ma 1, Ma 2, CV2/CRMP5 (collapsin response mediator protein 5), Tr, and SOX antibodies were also not detected. Antiaquaporin-4 antibodies and anti-heat shock 70 antibodies were negative.

The differential diagnosis included acute disseminated encephalomyelitis, aquaporin-4 negative neuromyelitis optica [3], neurosarcoidosis, and primary angiitis of the CNS.

Despite treatment with intravenous methylprednisolone 1 g daily for 3 days followed by a tapering course commenced at 1 mg/kg daily, he suffered progressive bilateral hearing loss over the following four weeks and impaired vision from the right eye. Audiometry demonstrated low-frequency sensorineural hearing loss bilaterally. Neuropsychometric assessment revealed severe global cognitive impairment including difficulties with verbal fluency, as well as deficits in short-term memory and executive function.

A biopsy of the cerebellum and meninges was performed due to disease progression and lack of response to the high-dose corticosteroid therapy. The histopathology showed mild, nonspecific perivascular inflammation and a diffuse pial infiltrate dominated by CD8 T lymphocytes and macrophages with microinfarctions in the territory of the small pial arteries. There was no evidence of vasculitis or malignancy. Culture and PCR analysis of the specimen excluded mycobacterial or fungal infection.

The patient developed painless scotomata, and a branch retinal artery occlusion (BRAO) of the right temporal retina was identified on fundal photography and retinal fluorescein angiography (Figure 2). Subsequently, Susac's syndrome was diagnosed based on the triad of encephalopathy, right BRAO, and bilateral sensorineural hearing loss.

Methylprednisolone 1 g daily for 3 days was subsequently readministered followed by oral prednisolone 1 mg/kg daily concurrently with intravenous cyclophosphamide 1 g (15 mg/kg) monthly for 6 months and intravenous immunoglobulin (IVIg) 2 g/kg loading and 0.4 g/kg per month for 6 months. Adjunctive treatments included cotrimoxazole prophylaxis against *Pneumocystis jiroveci*, risedronate for osteoprotection, and aspirin to aid vessel patency.

Clinical remission was achieved by 6 weeks, but there was no improvement in the sensorineural deafness on the right side. Maintenance of remission was attempted with methotrexate 20 mg (0.3 mg/kg) weekly following cyclophosphamide.

Another clinical relapse, however, occurred 3 months after the maintenance therapy with methotrexate was started, characterized by recurrent bilateral hearing loss, bilateral BRAOs, and new T2 hyperintensities shown by MRI of the brain. Further remission was achieved with methylprednisolone 1 g daily for 3 days, and plasma exchange was administered daily for four consecutive days. In addition, rituximab 375 mg/m^2 weekly for four weeks was used as an induction agent, and methotrexate was replaced with mycophenolate mofetil (MMF) 1.5 g BD. Prior to rituximab, enumeration of lymphocyte subsets on peripheral blood revealed 302×10^6 CD19+ cells/L with CD19 suppression ($<25 \times 10^6$ cells/L) maintained for 18 months following therapy. Oral prednisolone was slowly tapered to a maintenance dose of 12.5 mg (0.18 mg/kg) daily.

Despite this treatment, the patient relapsed again two months later, i.e., 11 months following initial treatment,

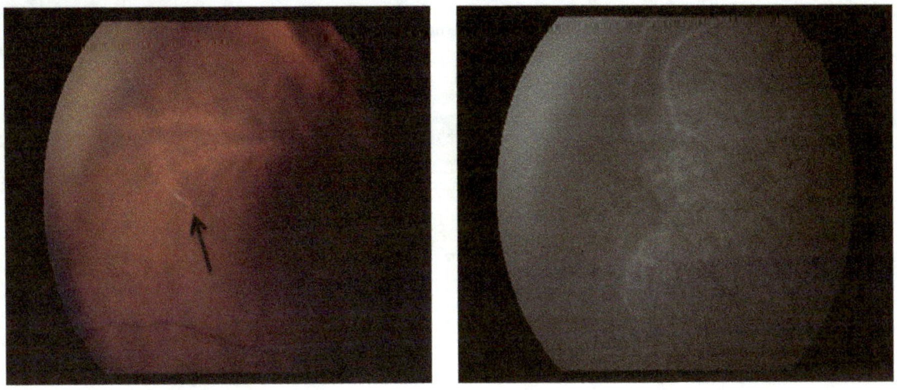

(a) (b)

FIGURE 2: Fundal photography (right eye) showing a ghost vessel, likely secondary to previous branch retinal artery occlusion (arrow) (a). Late-phase fundal angiography with no perfusion noted in the corresponding territory (b).

suffering a generalised tonic-clonic convulsion, encephalopathy, recurrent bilateral hearing loss, fresh BRAOs, and new MRI lesions. His neurological status improved after methylprednisolone 1 g daily was administered for 3 days. His dose of oral prednisolone was increased to 1 mg/kg daily, IVIg 2 g/kg monthly was recommenced, and MMF continued at a dose of 1.5 g BD. MRI brain with MR venogram demonstrated right transverse venous sinus thrombosis. A procoagulant screen was positive for the lupus anticoagulant. Review of a previous MR venogram 3 months prior showed that the thrombus had been present for some time and was not changing in morphology or size. For these reasons, aspirin rather than warfarin was continued as an anticoagulant.

A further clinical relapse occurred 3 months later, i.e., 14 months (Figure 3) after initial treatment was commenced, characterized by sudden painless partial visual loss in the right eye with new BRAO encroaching on the central retina, persisting hearing loss, and MRI changes demonstrating diffuse cerebellar, leptomeningeal, and parenchymal enhancement. Infliximab 5 mg/kg was started using a loading regimen at 0, 2, and 6 weeks for induction and then 8 weekly treatments for maintenance. Over the following 4 weeks, there was both clinical and radiological remission of disease. His dose of prednisone was tapered completely from 12.5 mg daily over 4 months. The thrombus resolved, and the patient returned to work. Two years after remaining on the maintenance infliximab therapy, the patient has been free of relapses, the visual acuity is normal, and there are no cognitive deficits on follow-up neuropsychological testing. He continues to be troubled by partial bilateral deafness, for which cochlear implantation has proven helpful. Consideration is being given to stepping down immunosuppression to MMF.

3. Discussion

Susac's syndrome is a very rare condition consisting of the clinical triad of encephalopathy, BRAO, and sensorineural deafness with an annual incidence of 0.024/100,000 (95% CI 0.010–0.047) [4]. It has a female preponderance with the peak age at onset occurring in the third and fourth decades of life [2]. A substantial proportion of patients including our patient did not present with the classical triad of manifestations, and therefore, diagnosis is often delayed, during which time disability may accrue [4]. The European Susac Consortium (EuSaC) proposed criteria for a definitive diagnosis characterized by the presence of the clinical triad, which was present in 56% of 192 patients, and probable Susac comprising 2 of the 3 clinical features in the remainder of the cohort [5]. This will allow for heightened suspicion for diagnosing, monitoring, and investigating undeclared or clinically subtle or silent manifestations enabling effective therapies to be implemented without delay.

The aetiology and pathogenesis of Susac's syndrome are unclear. The disease is proposed to be an autoimmune endotheliopathy characterized by cerebral microinfarction, hyalinised vessel walls due to collagen deposition, CD8+ lymphocytic inflammation, and perivascular lymphocytic cuffing in the leptomeninges, with enlarged and reactive endothelial cells leading to near occlusion of the vessel [6, 7]. The microvascular changes are indistinguishable from dermatomyositis [8]. Changes of vasculitis have been recently described in an autopsy case [9]. Antiendothelial cell antibodies have been identified, but whether they are pathogenic or epiphenomenon requires clarification [10, 11]. Recently, Gross et al. used immune profiling and phenotyping of blood and CSF samples with histopathologic studies of neural tissue from Susac's patients and patients with demyelinating diseases to reveal distinct mechanisms in these two neuroinflammatory conditions. Mouse models were also used to determine the effects of an antigen-specific cytotoxic CD8+ T cell (CTL) inflammatory effect against the CNS endothelium. They demonstrated that cytotoxic CD8+ T (CTL) cells mediated the vascular CNS injury, and they identified CTL-mediated endotheliopathy as a major pathogenic process in the disease [2]. Amelioration of disease was achieved in the mouse model by blocking adhesion and trafficking of CTLs using an anti-$\alpha4$ integrin monoclonal antibody [2].

Coagulation abnormalities might modify or play a role in the pathogenesis of the disease. Although a procoagulant

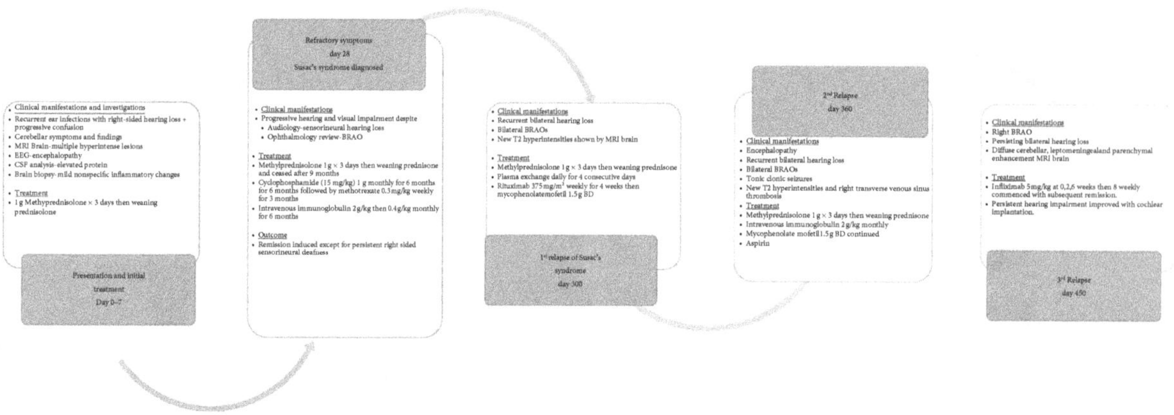

Figure 3: Timeline of case presentation with relapses and treatment moldalities.

state is not consistently reported, protein S deficiency and factor V Leiden mutations have been described in case reports [12, 13]. Anticardiolipin antibodies and lupus anticoagulant have also been found in patients with Susac's syndrome [14, 15], but it is uncertain whether these are pathogenic. This is the first case of cerebral vein thrombosis described in Susac's syndrome suggesting that macrovascular as well as microvascular thrombosis can occur.

The optimal treatment for Susac's syndrome is not established, particularly in refractory or relapsing disease, due to the rarity of this condition. Therapeutic recommendations were initially largely based on anecdotal reports, case series, and pathological similarities with dermatomyositis [16]. In an early case series and review of the literature, most patients respond to oral prednisone (91% of 22 patients), IV methylprednisolone (87% of 8 patients), or IV cyclophosphamide (92% of 11 patient) although one patient who received cyclophosphamide developed hemorrhagic cystitis [17]. Hence, initial recommendations were for IV or the oral corticosteroid therapy and IV cyclophosphamide for refractory cases. IVIg was then introduced in the treatment regimen (usually 2 g/kg initially with the option of further doses at 0.4 g/kg monthly for a total of 6 months) in combination with either corticosteroids and/or adjuvant immunosuppression, e.g., azathioprine, mycophenolate, or cyclophosphamide [18–20]. Plasma exchange may be useful as an alternative to IVIg in combination with the adjunctive therapy, as was shown in eight patients who received between 3 and 10 exchanges, with six patients showing improvement and two demonstrating stabilization [21].

The biologic therapy was initially used in patients with Susac's disease refractory to conventional immunosuppression and immunomodulation in the mid-2000s due to its early success in patients with recalcitrant dermatomyositis [16] and especially in patients with sight-threatening BRAO [18]. Rituximab is frequently an effective therapy in immune-mediated diseases by removing the precursors of autoantibody-producing plasma cells and inhibiting autoantigen presentation to CD4 T-cells, perhaps in this case by abrogating the pathogenic effect of antiendothelial cell antibodies [2]. However, our patient relapsed following the rituximab therapy. The lack of efficacy of rituximab in our patient suggests that the pathogenesis of Susac's syndrome may not be mediated by autoantibodies alone. The successful induction of remission with cyclophosphamide suggests that potent inhibition of cell-mediated inflammation is required in severe and recalcitrant cases such as our patient.

Infliximab is a chimeric monoclonal antibody that binds to human tumor necrosis factor (TNF), thereby rapidly blocking with theendogenous TNF activity. TNF induces the production of proinflammatory cytokines (interleukins) by macrophages and endothelial cells, enhances leukocyte migration to sites of inflammation, activates neutrophils and eosinophils at inflammatory sites, and enhances production of acute phase reactants. Hence, the anti-TNF therapy has the advantage of disabling a final common pathway of inflammation irrespective of the initiating process. The effect of infliximab is relatively rapid as TNF is a preformed cytokine contained in the cytoplasm [22]. Furthermore, infliximab has been shown in diseases such as inflammatory bowel disease to induce apoptosis of T lymphocytes and enhance T regulatory cell function [23].

Infliximab was first successfully utilised in Susac's syndrome in 2011, in which a single dose was administered in a patient who was not responding to prednisone. The patient's symptoms of headache and ataxia improved within 24 hours [24]. However, follow-up treatment consisted of IVIG 2 g/kg administered 24 hours following clinical improvement, as well the commencement of cyclophosphamide 1 g monthly for 5 months. A multicentre retrospective case series demonstrated durable disease remission of ocular disease in 5 cases of Susac's syndrome with the TNF inhibitor therapy refractory to, on average, 3.2 immunosuppressive agents including prednisone, IVIg, mycophenolate, cyclophosphamide, azathioprine, methotrexate, and cyclosporine but not rituximab [25]. Three patients were treated with infliximab and two with adalimumab for a mean period of 2.86 years resulting in a reduction in the number of ocular relapses from 5.54 to <0.35 per year of follow-up during therapy. Studies in the prebiologic era revealed that immunosuppression had a minimal effect on the development of sensorineural deafness [26]. Further studies are required to determine whether biologic therapies given earlier for refractory disease improve auditory outcomes in Susac's patients. The finding of blocking T cell adhesion by anti-$\alpha4$ integrin-intervention through the use of natalizumab in 4 patients in the study by Gross et al. for patients with progressive relapsing disease was encouraging despite the relapse in 2 patients once the therapy was ceased [2].

This is the first case to our knowledge of the successful use of infliximab for a patient with Susac's syndrome that was necessary following treatment with cyclophosphamide and then rituximab. It must be stated, however, that in a case series comprising three patients with Susac's syndrome successfully treated with infliximab, one was previously treated with rituximab. However, none of these patients had the cyclophosphamide therapy, and the precise time course between the administration of rituximab and infliximab was not presented in detail in this report [7]. It is also unknown as to when to cease the infliximab therapy. The natural history of Susac's syndrome is still unclear, but the disease seems to follow 3 different patterns: monocyclic (remission within 1-2 years without recurrence), polycyclic (recurrences over a period of greater than 2 years alternating with periods of remission), or chronic (prolonged, continuous course for more than 2 years) [27].

In conclusion, prompt and aggressive treatment of Susac's syndrome is recommended to improve prognosis [21]. The anti-TNF therapy may be an effective induction and maintenance therapy in refractory cases of Susac's syndrome. Further studies including elucidation of the pathogenesis are required to determine whether it should be incorporated earlier into therapeutic strategies in order to improve long-term outcomes. Consideration should also be given to its addition as a therapeutic option for refractory disease in the treatment algorithm and guidelines in Susac's syndrome [28].

Consent

The patient provided written consent for publication.

Authors' Contributions

SLF, JDP, AS, and TB developed the concept. All four authors edited and approved the final manuscript.

References

[1] J. O. Susac, "Susac's syndrome: the triad of microangiopathy of the brain and retina with hearing loss in young women," *Neurology*, vol. 44, no. 4, p. 591, 1994.

[2] C. C. Gross, C. Meyer, U. Bhatia et al., "CD8$^+$ T cell-mediated endotheliopathy is a targetable mechanism of neuro-inflammation in Susac syndrome," *Nature Communications*, vol. 10, no. 1, p. 5779, 2019.

[3] R. Marignier, R. Bernard-Valnet, P. Giraudon et al., "Aquaporin-4 antibody-negative neuromyelitis optica: distinct assay sensitivity-dependent entity," *Neurology*, vol. 80, no. 24, pp. 2194–2200, 2013.

[4] T. Seifert-Held, B. J. Langner-Wegscheider, M. Komposch et al., "Susac's syndrome: clinical course and epidemiology in a central European population," *International Journal of Neuroscience*, vol. 127, no. 9, pp. 776–780, 2017.

[5] I. Kleffner, J. Dörr, M. Ringelstein et al., "Diagnostic criteria for Susac syndrome," *Journal of Neurology, Neurosurgery & Psychiatry*, vol. 87, no. 12, pp. 1287–1295, 2016.

[6] J. Dorr, H. Radbruch, M. Bock et al., "Encephalopathy, visual disturbance, and hearing loss recognizing the symptoms of Susac syndrome," *Nature Reviews Neurology*, vol. 5, no. 12, pp. 683–688, 2009.

[7] T. A. Hardy, B. O'Brien, N. Gerbis et al., "Brain histopathology in three cases of Susac's syndrome: implications for lesion pathogenesis and treatment," *Journal of Neurology, Neurosurgery & Psychiatry*, vol. 86, no. 5, pp. 582–584, 2015.

[8] A. N. Crowson and C. M. Magro, "The role of microvascular injury in the pathogenesis of cutaneous lesions of dermatomyositis," *Human Pathology*, vol. 27, no. 1, pp. 15–19, 1996.

[9] D. P. Agamanolis, C. Klonk, K. Bigley, and R. M. Rennebohm, "Neuropathological findings in Susac syndrome: an autopsy report," *Journal of Neuropathology & Experimental Neurology*, vol. 78, no. 6, pp. 515–519, 2019.

[10] J. O. Susac, R. A. Egan, R. M. Rennebohm, and M. Lubow, "Susac's syndrome: 1975–2005 microangiopathy/autoimmune endotheliopathy," *Journal of the Neurological Sciences*, vol. 257, no. 1-2, pp. 270–272, 2007.

[11] C. M. Magro, J. C. Poe, M. Lubow, and J. O. Susac, "An organ-specific autoimmune endotheliopathy syndrome associated with antiendothelial cell antibodies," *American Journal of Clinical Pathology*, vol. 136, no. 6, pp. 903–912, 2011.

[12] V. P. J. Saw, P. A. Canty, C. M. Green et al., "Susac syndrome: microangiopathy of the retina, cochlea, and brain," *Clinical and Experimental Ophthalmology*, vol. 28, no. 5, pp. 373–381, 2000.

[13] R. A. Barker, J. R. Anderson, P. Meyer, D. J. Dick, and N. J. Scolding, "Microangiopathy of the brain and retina with hearing loss in a 50-year-old woman: extending the spectrum of Susac's syndrome," *Journal of Neurology, Neurosurgery & Psychiatry*, vol. 66, no. 5, pp. 641-643, 1999.

[14] M. W. Nicolle and R. S. McLachlan, "Microangiopathy with retinopathy, encephalopathy, and deafness (RED-M) and systemic features," *Seminars in Arthritis and Rheumatism*, vol. 21, no. 3, pp. 123–128, 1991.

[15] S. Bucciarelli, R. Cervera, M. Martinez, X. Latorre, and J. Font, "Susac's syndrome or catastrophic antiphospholipid syndrome?" *Lupus*, vol. 13, no. 8, pp. 607-608, 2004.

[16] R. M. Rennebohm, R. A. Egan, and J. O. Susac, "Treatment of susac's syndrome," *Current Treatment Options in Neurology*, vol. 10, no. 1, pp. 67–74, 2008.

[17] H. S. O'Halloran, P. A. Pearson, W. B. Lee, J. O. Susac, and J. R. Berger, "Microangiopathy of the brain, retina, and cochlea (Susac syndrome). A report of five cases and a review of the literature," *Ophthalmology*, vol. 105, no. 6, pp. 1038–1044, 1998.

[18] R. Rennebohm, J. O. Susac, R. A. Egan, and R. B. Daroff, "Susac's syndrome—update," *Journal of the Neurological Sciences*, vol. 299, no. 1-2, pp. 86-91, 2010.

[19] R. M. Rennebohm and J. O. Susac, "Treatment of Susac's syndrome," *Journal of the Neurological Sciences*, vol. 257, no. 1-2, pp. 215–220, 2007.
[20] E. Capiluppi, L. Romano, S. V. Luccarelli, A. Macerollo, and G. Cislaghi, "Aggressive immunosuppression in Susac's syndrome: 10 years of follow-up," *Neurological Sciences*, vol. 39, no. 10, pp. 1807–1809, 2018.
[21] F. J. Mateen, A. Y. Zubkov, R. Muralidharan et al., "Susac syndrome: clinical characteristics and treatment in 29 new cases," *European Journal of Neurology*, vol. 19, no. 6, pp. 800–811, 2012.
[22] C. F. Ware, "Protein therapeutics targeted at the TNF superfamily," *Advances in Pharmacology*, vol. 66, pp. 51–80, 2013.
[23] J. M. H. V. D. Brande, H. Braat, G. R. V. D. Brink et al., "Infliximab but not etanercept induces apoptosis in lamina propria T-lymphocytes from patients with Crohn's disease," *Gastroenterology*, vol. 124, no. 7, pp. 1774–1785, 2003.
[24] T. A. Hardy, R. J. Garsia, G. M. Halmagyi et al., "Tumour necrosis factor (TNF) inhibitor therapy in Susac's syndrome," *Journal of the Neurological Sciences*, vol. 302, no. 1-2, pp. 126–128, 2011.
[25] T. Buelens, J. O.-V. Norel, J. H. D. Boer et al., "Evaluation of tumor necrosis factor inhibitor therapy in Susac syndrome," *Retina*, vol. 40, no. 3, pp. 581–590, 2020.
[26] F. Aubart-Cohen, I. Klein, J.-F. Alexandra et al., "Long-term outcome in Susac syndrome," *Medicine*, vol. 86, no. 2, pp. 93–102, 2007.
[27] A. Saux, G. Niango, M. Charif et al., "Susac's syndrome, a rare, potentially severe or lethal neurological disease," *Journal of the Neurological Sciences*, vol. 297, no. 1-2, pp. 71–73, 2010.
[28] R. A. Egan, "Diagnostic criteria and treatment algorithm for Susac syndrome," *Journal of Neuro-Ophthalmology*, vol. 39, no. 1, pp. 60–67, 2019.

26

Utility of Botulinum Injections in Stiff-Person Syndrome

L. M. Conners, A. Betcher, A. Shahinian, and P. Janda

Department of Neurology, Valley Hospital Medical Center, Las Vegas, NV, USA

Correspondence should be addressed to Lisa Conners; lisa.conners.neuro@gmail.com

Academic Editor: Peter Berlit

Stiff-person syndrome (SPS) is an uncommon neurological disorder characterized by significant rigidity and muscle spasms primarily affecting the truncal and proximal musculature. Furthermore, a wide-based gait with functional impairment is generally seen. High-dose benzodiazepines or baclofen are widely considered the optimal initial therapy; however, major adverse effects often preclude adequate dosing. Refractory cases may be treated with intravenous immunoglobulins (IVIG), plasma exchange, or B-cell depletion with rituximab, although these are also associated with major, sometimes fatal, adverse reactions. Several reports have validated the safety and utility of botulinum injections in this setting, yet botulinum remains markedly underutilized in this cohort. Below, a case report and review of the literature show botulinum can decrease pain and stiffness, improve gait and balance, and decrease dependence on powerful systemic treatments in this group.

1. Introduction

The first reports of stiff-person syndrome (formerly stiff-man syndrome) were published by Moersch and Woltman in 1956, and described "tin soldiers" that were "board-like" and "stiff" [1]. This stiffness results from dysfunction of CNS inhibitory pathways involving glutamic acid decarboxylase (GAD) and gamma amino butyric acid (GABA) in these patients. GAD is an enzyme responsible for the conversion of L-glutaminc acid to GABA and is critical in maintaining inhibitory pathways [2]. Sixty to eighty percent of those with SPS have elevated titers of antibodies against GAD-65 in their serum [3].

Epidemiologic data are somewhat limited due to underdiagnosis of the disease, but the current estimated prevalence of SPS is approximately one per million. Patients typically present between the ages of twenty and fifty. As with many autoimmune phenomena, there is a female predominance, 2 : 1. There are associations with other autoimmune processes, particularly type 1 diabetes mellitus [4].

Many describe stiff-person syndrome as a spectrum, with more than eighty percent of patients falling into the category of classic SPS [5]. Variants of SPS described in the literature include partial stiff-person syndrome, paraneoplastic stiff-person syndrome, and progressive encephalomyelitis with rigidity and myoclonus (PERM). Partial SPS, also known as stiff-limb syndrome, is the most common variant and affects ten to fifteen percent of patients on the SPS spectrum. While classic SPS is characterized by truncal and proximal spasms and rigidity, stiff-limb syndrome is typically associated with focal rigidity of a lower limb, sparing the trunk muscles. These patients typically lack auto-antibodies to GAD and respond less adequately to benzodiazepines and baclofen [6]. Functionally, they suffer significant gait disturbances due to considerable rigidity of the lower limb, and many are unable to ambulate altogether [3, 6]. Alternatively, patients with the paraneoplastic variant of SPS share clinical features of the classic stiff-person syndrome and may present with a known diagnosis of neoplasm or concomitant features of malignancy, such as unintentional weight loss. They are typically GAD seronegative. Accordingly, this diagnosis should always be considered in those with strong features of classic stiff-person syndrome who lack auto-antibodies to GAD in the serum. Paraneoplastic SPS has been associated with breast cancer, lung cancer, and Hodgkin's lymphoma, and is estimated to affect one to two percent of patients with SPS overall [3]. Finally, less than one-tenth of one percent of patients will be diagnosed with progressive encephalomyelitis with rigidity and myoclonus, which includes transient oculomotor disturbances not seen in classic SPS or other variants. Features of classic stiff-person syndrome with brainstem dysfunction, myoclonus, sensory deficits, sphincter, or autonomic dysfunction, seizures, or cognitive deficits may suggest a diagnosis of progressive encephalomyelitis with rigidity and myoclonus [3, 5]. It typically takes a relentless course, often leading to death within a few months [6].

There are no formally accepted diagnostic criteria for stiff-person syndrome, and establishing the diagnosis requires a high level of suspicion on the part of the examiner. Stiffness in the axial or limb muscles resulting in an impaired gait, in combination with episodic spasms (often provoked by sudden movement, noise or emotional upset) are generally required to make the diagnosis. Improvement with GABA-enhancing medications such as diazepam and continuous motor unit activity on EMG are expected as well. Symptoms should not be better explained by another condition. The presence of anti-GAD antibodies is not required but supports the diagnosis when present [3].

Current therapies aim to mitigate painful spasms and improve mobility. Initial therapy typically consists of diazepam, or clonazepam when diazepam is poorly tolerated. Very high dosages are usually required to adequately control symptoms, with up to thirty milligrams four times a day being a typical dose of diazepam for these patients. Benzodiazepines, however, are oftentimes limited by major adverse effects including somnolence, fatigue, mood changes, or respiratory depression. If benzodiazepines fail to adequately control symptoms or are poorly tolerated, baclofen is usually used. When baclofen is used in combination with benzodiazepines, sedation may be significant and limit adequate dosing. Benzodiazepines and baclofen improve symptoms by augmenting the inadequate GABA-ergic inhibitory pathways in these patients [3]. For those with refractory symptoms or who are intolerant of the above therapies, IVIG has been shown to improve mobility and unassisted ambulation [7]. B-cell depletion with rituximab has also been used in this cohort. Notably, IVIG and rituximab should be reserved for refractory cases given the potential for serious adverse effects. Other, therapies may include botulinum, plasma exchange, intravenous methocarbamol, sodium valproate, gabapentin, vigabatrin, and propofol [4, 8–12].

SPS is a progressive disease. Initiation of therapy is recommended as soon as a diagnosis is made as the natural course of the disease involves progressive gait dysfunction and limitations in functioning. Combination therapies are usually recommended to maximize functional status [3].

2. Discussion

Our discussion begins with a case report describing the use of botulinum injections in a patient with classic stiff-person syndrome and concludes with a review of the literature on this topic. A 38-year-old female with anxiety, depression, and Grave's disease presented with several months of diffuse muscle pain and spasms. She had previously been diagnosed with hyperthyroid myopathy as well as rhabdomyolysis. Repeat CK level in the clinic was normal, as was MRI of the brain and cervical spine, EMG/nerve conduction study, aldolase, autoimmune panel, and muscle biopsy. Notably, anti-GAD antibodies were negative in the serum at that time. One year later, she returned with a progressive worsening of her symptoms, including impaired ambulation, difficulties with activities of daily living, and hospitalizations to manage pain. Repeat serum anti-GAD-65 antibodies were 69 IU/mL (normal <5 IU/mL). EMG revealed continuous motor activity in several muscles of the neck and thoracic paraspinal muscles, where she reported significant pain and tightness. Her symptoms were not sufficiently controlled on a combination of diazepam 7.5 mg three times a day, baclofen 30 mg three times a day, Percocet 10–325 mg four times per day, tizanidine 4 mg three times a day, IVIG 400 mg/kg every 4 weeks, and physical therapy. Her initial Botox treatment consisted of 25 units Botox in the right as well as left trapezius, and 25 units in the right and left sternocleidomastoid muscle. Three months later she had a second treatment in which those dosages were exactly doubled (50 units in the right and left trapezius and 50 units in the left and right sternocleidomastoid muscles). Again, three months afterwards she received 50 units in the right and left trapezius and sternocleidomastoid muscles as well as 20 units in the right as well as left thoracic paraspinals as she noted pain and spasms in that region. 6 months later she received 40 units in the right and left trapezius, 40 units in the right and left levator scapulae, and 30 units in the right and left semispinalis capitis muscles. The Botox dosages were adjusted each treatment to target the most painful regions at that time. After the addition of Botox injections, the patient reported an improvement in pain, decreased muscle spasms, an improvement in her quality of life, although she was not able to decrease her home medications. She denied adverse effects from the Botox treatments.

In 2003, Szczepańska-Szerej et al. reported a marked functional improvement and a decreased dependence on systemic drugs for up to four months in a 41-year-old woman with SPS following botulinum injections [13]. Similarly, Shah and Bunzol described a 53-year-old-male with stiff-person syndrome with a poor response to IVIG, corticosteroids, diazepam, baclofen, gabapentin, warm baths, heating pads, transcutaneous electrical nerve stimulation, and chiropractic manipulation. Following botulinum injections to the biceps femoris, adductor magnus, and rectus femoris, the patient reported considerable pain relief, improved range of motion, and decreased stiffness. He also noted an improvement in balance and gait with fewer falls and the ability to walk longer distances [14]. Likewise, in 1993, Davis and Jabbari reported remarkable relief from pain and stiffness and a substantial improvement in ambulation in a 36-year-old male with stiff-person syndrome after botulinum injections into the lumbar paraspinal muscles. The patient suffered from an awkward and antalgic gait and was unable to stand from the sitting position without assistance due to marked stiffness and pain. EMG noted continuous activity in the lumbar paraspinals, which were injected with a total of 560 units of botulinum toxin after diazepam and baclofen provided only minimal relief. The injections were done over three sessions spanning three weeks and were divided over five sites from L1–L5. One week after the final set of injections, the patient noted almost complete relief from exertional pain and resolution of painful spasms. The injections also lead to a significant functional improvement and reduced need for systemic drugs [2].

Botulinum injections have also been shown to improve rigidity, pain, and gait in stiff-limb syndrome. In 2012, Anagnostou and Zambelis recounted a 40-year-old female with several years of progressive stiffness of the left leg. Modified Ashworth scale score of the extremity was four, signifying that the affected extremity was rigid in flexion or extension, and EMG showed continuous motor unit potentials in the left vastus medialis. Following a poor response to pharmacotherapy, several dosages of Botox were tried over time without significant subjective improvement. Ultimately, a dose of 900 units (vastus lateralis 350 units, vastus medialis 350 units, and rectus femoris 200 units) produced a marked improvement in her symptoms. She reported a dramatic improvement in rigidity and gait as well as decreased pain for two and a half months following the injections. Modified Ashworth scale score following the injections was one, denoting a slight increase in muscle tone, and repeat EMG was within normal limits. She denied adverse effects other than a slight weakness of leg extension, which she noticed only when attempting to jump. Three months following the injections, her symptoms had returned. She repeated the injections at the dose of 900 units and again reported a dramatic improvement in her symptoms [15].

3. Conclusion

SPS is a progressive neurological condition that often leads to refractory rigidity, painful spasms, and gait difficulties. The use of botulinum toxin in this cohort has been shown to improve function, gait, and quality of life, decrease pain and spasms, and decrease the need for systemic drugs; however, its use continues to remain markedly underutilized in this group.

References

[1] F. P. Moersch and H. W. Woltman, "Progressive fluctuating muscular rigidity and spasm (stiff-man syndrome); report of a case and some observations in 13 other cases," *Proceedings of the Staff Meetings of the Mayo Clinic*, vol. 31, no. 15, pp. 421–427, 1956.

[2] D. Davis and B. Jabbari, "Significant improvement of stiff-person syndrome after paraspinal injection of botulinum toxin A," *Movement Disorders*, vol. 8, no. 3, pp. 371–373, 1993.

[3] S. M. Helfgott, "Stiff-person syndrome," *UpToDate*, 2018, https://www.uptodate.com/contents/stiff-personsyndrome?search=stiff%20person%20syndrome&source=search_result&selectedTitle=1~15&usage_type=default&display_rank=1.

[4] G. Ciccotto, M. Blaya, and R. Kelley, "Stiff person syndrome," *Neurologic Clinics*, vol. 31, no. 1, pp. 319–328, 2013.

[5] H. Sarva, A. Deik, A. Ullah, and W. L. Severt, "Clinical spectrum of stiff person syndrome: a review of recent reports," *Tremor and Other Hyperkinetic Movements (New York, N.Y.)*, vol. 6, no. 340 , 2016.

[6] P. J. Shaw, "Stiff-man syndrome and its variants," *Lancet*, vol. 353, no. 9147, pp. 86–87, 1999.

[7] M. C. Dalakas, M. Fujii, M. Li, B. Lutfi, J. Kyhos, and B. McElroy, "High-dose intravenous immune globulin for stiff-person syndrome," *New England Journal of Medicine*, vol. 345, no. 26, pp. 1870–1876, 2001.

[8] J. M. Voci, M. Al-Hakim, Y. Dokko, and M. B. Katirji, "Intravenous methocarbamol in the treatment of stiff-man syndrome," *Muscle & Nerve*, vol. 16, no. 4, pp. 434–435, 1993.

[9] R. Liguori, C. Cordivari, E. Lugaresi, and P. Montagna, "Botulinum toxin A improves muscle spasms and rigidity in stiff-person syndrome," *Movement Disorders*, vol. 12, no. 6, pp. 1060–1063, 1997.

[10] R. Spehlmann, K. Norcross, S. C. Rasmus, and N. L. Schlageter, "Improvement of stiff-man syndrome with sodium valproate," *Neurology*, vol. 31, no. 9, pp. 1162–1162, 1981.

[11] M. C. Prevett, P. Brown, and J. S. Duncan, "Improvement of stiff-man syndrome with vigabatrin," *Neurology*, vol. 48, no. 4, pp. 1133–1134, 1997.

[12] E. Hattan, M. R. Angle, and C. Chalk, "Unexpected benefit of propofol in stiff-person syndrome," *Neurology*, vol. 70, no. 18, pp. 1641–1642, 2008.

[13] A. Szczepańska-Szerej, M. Kulka, J. Wojczal, and Z. Stelmasiak, "Botulinum toxin A in the treatment of stiff man syndrome," *Neurologia i Neurochirurgia Polska*, vol. 37, supplement 5, pp. 175–181, 2003.

[14] C. D. Shah and D. Bunzol, "A novel approach to the treatment of stiff-person-syndrome with botulinum toxin: a case report," *Practice Management & Leadership*, vol. 8, no. 9S, p. S244, 2016.

[15] E. Anagnostou and T. Zambelis, "Botulinum toxin in anti-GAD positive stiff-limb syndrome," *Muscle & Nerve*, vol. 46, no. 3, pp. 457–458, 2012.

27

A Case of Carbon Monoxide-Induced Delayed Neurological Sequelae Successfully Treated with Hyperbaric Oxygen Therapy, N-Acetylcysteine, and Glucocorticoids: Clinical and Neuroimaging Follow-Up

Vincenzo Spina[1], **Francesco Tomaiuolo**[2], **Lorenzo Celli**[3], **Luca Bonfiglio**[1], **Luca Cecchetti**[4], and **Maria Chiara Carboncini**[1]

[1] *Department of Translational Research and New Technologies in Medicine and Surgery, University of Pisa, Pisa, Italy*
[2] *Auxilium Vitae, Volterra (Pisa), Italy*
[3] *Neurology Department, ASLAL, San Giacomo Hospital, Novi Ligure (Alessandria), Italy*
[4] *Molecular Mind Lab, IMT School for Advanced Studies Lucca, Lucca, Italy*

Correspondence should be addressed to Vincenzo Spina; vincenzospina90@yahoo.it

Academic Editor: Jacqueline A. Pettersen

Carbon monoxide (CO) poisoning is a leading cause of intentional and unintentional poisoning worldwide, associated with mortality and severe morbidity. Some survivors of CO poisoning develop, after a lucid interval, a potentially permanent encephalopathy in the form of cognitive impairment and movement disorders, such as Parkinsonism. One of the most frequent neuroimaging findings is a cerebral white matter damage, but so far its precise cause and specific therapy are still debated. We here report the case of a 33-year-old woman with severe carbon monoxide poisoning who, after a period of lucid interval, presented symptoms of declining motor and cognitive functions. She was treated with 40 sessions of Hyperbaric Oxygen Therapy (HBOT). The therapeutic use of oxygen at supraphysiological pressures might either increase systemic oxidative stress or cause an overproduction of oxygen free radicals as drawbacks. Concurrent use of antioxidants and anti-inflammatory drugs may prevent the side effects of oxygen therapy at supraphysiological pressure due to oxidative stress. For this reason, the patient was also treated with high-dose N-Acetylcysteine and glucocorticoids. Here, we describe the longitudinal monitoring of patient's cognitive abilities and leukoencephalopathy associated with her positive clinical outcome.

1. Introduction

At present, carbon monoxide (CO) poisoning remains a leading cause of unintentional poisoning worldwide [1]. In Italy, the estimated incidence is about 6.000 cases per year, resulting in more than 350 deaths per year [2]. The clinical symptoms range from headache and confusion to coma and death, with mortality rates reaching up to 3%.

CO is a nonirritant gas generated during the incomplete combustion of carbon-based compounds. Upon exposure, CO binds to hemoglobin with an affinity known to be 200-300 times greater than oxygen, generating carboxyhemoglobin (HbCO). It decreases both the oxygen-carrying and oxygen-delivery capacity of blood, inducing tissue hypoxia (HbCO theory) [3]. While the hypoxemic hypoxia suggested by the HbCO theory is undoubtedly a key component of CO poisoning mechanisms, it is not enough to account for some of the neuropathological manifestations of CO poisoning. In recent years, researchers have demonstrated CO interaction with soluble guanylate cyclase, ion channels, nitric oxide, nitric oxide synthase, mitochondria, cytochromes, NAPDH oxidase, and xanthine oxidase. Direct effects of CO poisoning on separate organ systems are well explained by these extra-hemoglobin effects, with the most important being the effects upon nitric oxide and on reactive oxygen species (ROS). In addition, a direct effect on cardiac ion channels has been established [4].

A significant number of patients who survive CO poisoning suffer from delayed neurological sequelae (DNS) that typically develop between 27 and 270 days after injury. The DNS reported incidence varies widely from 3 to 40%, because of the lack of established diagnostic criteria. In the classic biphasic presentation, patients recovering from acute CO poisoning manifest a relapse of neurological deficits after a lucid period, including seizures, consciousness disturbances, psychiatric disturbances, movement disorders, and urinary incontinence [5].

The pathophysiology of DNS is not completely understood, though some authors suggested that the typical white matter involvement in CO poisoning reflects a transient intramyelinic edema or inflammation, due to brain lipid peroxidation [6, 7]. Biochemical and immunological studies found that myelin basic protein (MBP) undergoes antigenic alterations after CO-exposure, which suggest that delayed CO-mediated neuropathology is linked to an adaptive immunological response to chemically modified MBP [8]. In the setting of acute CO poisoning, the standard of care is high-flow oxygen, preferentially hyperbaric therapy, and general supportive care [9]. As compared to Normobaric Oxygen Therapy (NBOT), Hyperbaric Oxygen Therapy (HBOT) provides increased dissolved-oxygen content in blood and accelerated elimination of CO. Nonetheless, existing randomized trials do not establish whether the administration of HBOT to patients with CO poisoning reduces the incidence of adverse neurologic outcomes [10].

Currently, in the subacute phase of CO poisoning and/or DNS, there is no standard treatment and clinical case reports do not agree about treatment strategies (e.g., the choice between NBOT and HBOT, the number of sessions) [11–15].

Here, we describe the case of a 33-year-old woman who suffered from CO acute intoxication and was diagnosed with DNS after a period of full recovery (i.e., lucid period). Hyperbaric Oxygen Therapy associated with administration of ROS scavenger was tentatively performed and the positive clinical evolution of the patient was monitored through extensive cognitive testing and radiological assessment.

2. Case Presentation

A previously healthy 33-year-old woman was found unconscious at her house. She was exposed to CO from a faulty heater and the exposure time was unknown. She was last heard by her relatives 10 hours earlier, when she referred experiencing nausea, vomiting, and headache.

She was admitted to intensive care unit (ICU) with a Glasgow Coma Scale score of 9/15 (E4-M3-V2). Arterial blood gas sample analysis revealed metabolic acidosis and her HbCO level was 20.4 percent. Serum biochemistry disclosed elevated serum creatinine (1.33 mg/dL) and HS-Troponin T (188 ng/L). Due to her severe neurological symptoms, she was intubated and sedated with propofol. No evidence for alterations of brain tissue was found from either computed tomography (CT) or magnetic resonance imaging (MRI) at this point. HBOT (Drass Galeazzi Underwater Technology, Livorno, Italy) was performed immediately and 24 hours after admission (80 minutes' exposure at 2.5 atmospheres absolute, ATA). After 9 days, the patient showed some spontaneous movement. She gradually regained consciousness and both cardiac and kidney functions improved.

On the 15th day after her ICU admission, she started following commands and was subsequently weaned from the ventilator. She was discharged from the ICU and directed to the rehabilitation unit on the 18th day after admission. At first, the patient showed good adherence to rehabilitation program.

Disability Rating Scale (DRS) [16] measured at this time revealed a score of 8/30, corresponding to moderately severe disability.

However, approximately 40 days after the exposure to CO, she was confused and suffered from slowing of psychomotor functions, impaired short-term memory, and reduced sustained attention. She was no more able to maintain the upright position. The symptoms gradually worsened in few days and she was transferred to our hospital. The patient was hypomimic and presented stereotyped movements, especially with her hands, when she was admitted to the facility. She was not oriented in time and space, had reduced ability to sustain attention, and had optic apraxia as well. Her speech was restricted to short phrases in response to specific requests and she had anterograde memory deficits. She demonstrated very poor awareness of her cognitive deficits. The overall raw score to the Mini-Mental State Examination (MMSE) [17] was 6/30. DRS at this time reached the score of 16/30, corresponding to severe disability.

Motor system examination revealed rigid tetraparesis. There was significant truncal and nuchal extensor hypertonia. She had urinary and bowel incontinence. Examination of the other systems was normal.

Brain MRI performed on day 45 after exposition showed confluent bilateral and symmetric white matter hyperintense areas on T2 and Fluid Attenuated Inversion Recovery (FLAIR) sequences (Figure 2). The hematologic, biochemical, and serological studies as well as HbCO levels were unremarkable. Electroencephalogram showed diffuse slow brain activity. Based on the clinical history and laboratory/imaging findings, the diagnosis of DNS was assumed.

Inpatient rehabilitation program consisted of 2 up to 3 hours of physical and speech therapy per weekday. Therapeutic rehabilitation techniques focused on obtaining a good trunk control in sitting position, readjustment to upright position, muscle strengthening for upper and lower limbs, initiation of gait training, and improvement of orientation and attention.

Rehabilitative treatment was performed concurrently with HBOT and ROS scavenger administration.

HBOT consisted of 40 sessions (two 35 minutes' oxygen breathing cycles with air breathing interval for 5 minutes at 2.5 ATA) with the following sequence: once a day for 20 days, no treatment for 15 days, once a day for 10 days, no treatment for 15 days, and lastly once a day for 10 days again.

ROS scavenger therapy consisted in intravenous high dose N-Acetylcysteine (12 g/die in continuous infusion) and low dosage of oral glucocorticoids (prednisone 25 mg/die).

Since the third session of HBOT, there was a significant improvement in her motor and cognitive skills: the patient

TABLE 1: Neuropsychological profile at different times after exposition.

Time after exposition (days)	30	45	100	540	Cut-off
Digit span Test	6	**4**	**4**	6	≥ 5
Immediate recall short story	12	**1**	16	16	≥ 8
Delayed recall short story	13	**3**	15	15	≥ 11
Brown-Peterson Interference Test after 10"	**3**	**0**	6	6	≥ 6
Brown-Peterson Interference Test after 30"	**2**	**0**	6	6	≥ 5
Trail making test -A	**91**	**N. E.**	**97"**	33"	≤ 45"
Trail making test - B	**N.E.**	**N. E.**	**342"**	107"	≤ 140"
Word fluency Phonemic	**3**	**0**	**7**	26	≥ 11
Verbal Abstraction Test	6	4	6	6	≥ 4
Superimposed Silhouettes Test	**20**	**0**	**31**	38	≥ 35
Drawing copy	**1**	**0**	**1**	2	≥ 2
Clock drawing test	**0**	**0**	**0**	9	≥ 8
Praxia Test	**5**	**4**	**5**	6	≥ 6
Token Test	5	5	5	5	≥ 5
Cognitive estimation task	5	**1**	5	5	≥ 4
Cognitive Quotient	***18/30***	***26/30***	***16/30***	*0/30*	

N.E. indicates that patient was not able to execute the test.
Bolded scores indicate a test under the normal performance range.
Cognitive Quotient: ratio between the number of tests under the normal performance range and the maximum obtainable score (two points for each).

became able to stand in upright position with arms on a surface. Her sustained attention began to last much longer and she became oriented in space and time. Language skills improved in both verbal comprehension and production.

After 100 days and 20 sessions of HBOT, she was able to walk for approximately 100 meters using a walker-rollator, however with some gait difficulties. MMSE raw score improved and reached the cut-off level for absence of cognitive impairment (24/30). Despite these improvements, the concurrent analytical neuropsychological evaluation showed performance deficits in several cognitive functions. For this reason, treatment was continued with 20 more sessions of HBOT, rehabilitation, and pharmacological therapy.

The neurological profile gradually improved until the time of discharge (i.e., at the end of the 40 HBOT sessions), when the patient appeared calm, lucid, and oriented and was able to relate to others. Complete motor recovery was observed within 150 days. DRS reached a score of 3/30, disclosing a partial residual disability.

At 18 months of follow-up, neuropsychological tests were all within normal range (see Table 1). The patient was now independent in her activities of daily living and was able to return to her previous job.

Figure 1 recapitulates the timeline of patient's clinical evolution.

The neuropsychological evaluation was carried out in multiple sessions, each lasting approximately 1 hour. The patient was sitting and relaxing in a room at a comfortable temperature and was required to perform tests included in the battery named "Esame Neuropsicologico Breve" [18], including a readapted version of the digit span test, trail-making test, word phonemic fluency, immediate and delayed recall of a short story, Brown-Peterson Interference Test, clock drawing test, verbal abstraction test, and Praxia test. To visually synthesize the cognitive skills' follow-up, we created a cognitive quotient (CQ) represented by the ratio between the number of tests under the normal performance range and the maximum obtainable score (two points for each).

MRI scans were performed on the 2nd, 30th, 45th, 60th, 150th, 180th, and 540th days after exposition. MRI images underwent a specific processing pipeline, aimed at improving the inspection and qualitative comparison of patient leukoencephalopathy across time-points. In brief, FLAIR images were first brain-extracted using the FSL brain extraction tool [19]. Afterwards, images were linearly transformed (FSL-flirt; 12 DOF affine registration [20]) to match a high-resolution MNI FLAIR template available at http://brainder.org, using sinc as interpolation method and a final resolution of 1x1x8mm (Hanning window, 7 voxels window width). Finally, to further reduce differences in intensity and contrast among different time-points, preprocessed images were imported in MATLAB v8.5.0, adjusted (imadjust) and filtered using Contrast-limited Adaptive Histogram Equalization algorithm (adapthisteq). The results of this processing pipeline are presented in Figure 2.

3. Discussion

We report the successful treatment of a 33-year-old woman suffering from DNS after accidental CO poisoning. Our patient showed a progressive and sustained clinical improvement in motor, cognitive, and behavioral symptoms, accompanied by a reduction on the extent of the white matter abnormalities in the follow-up MRI study.

To our knowledge, there are no reported cases of patients with DNS treated with HBOT and concurrent ROS scavenger

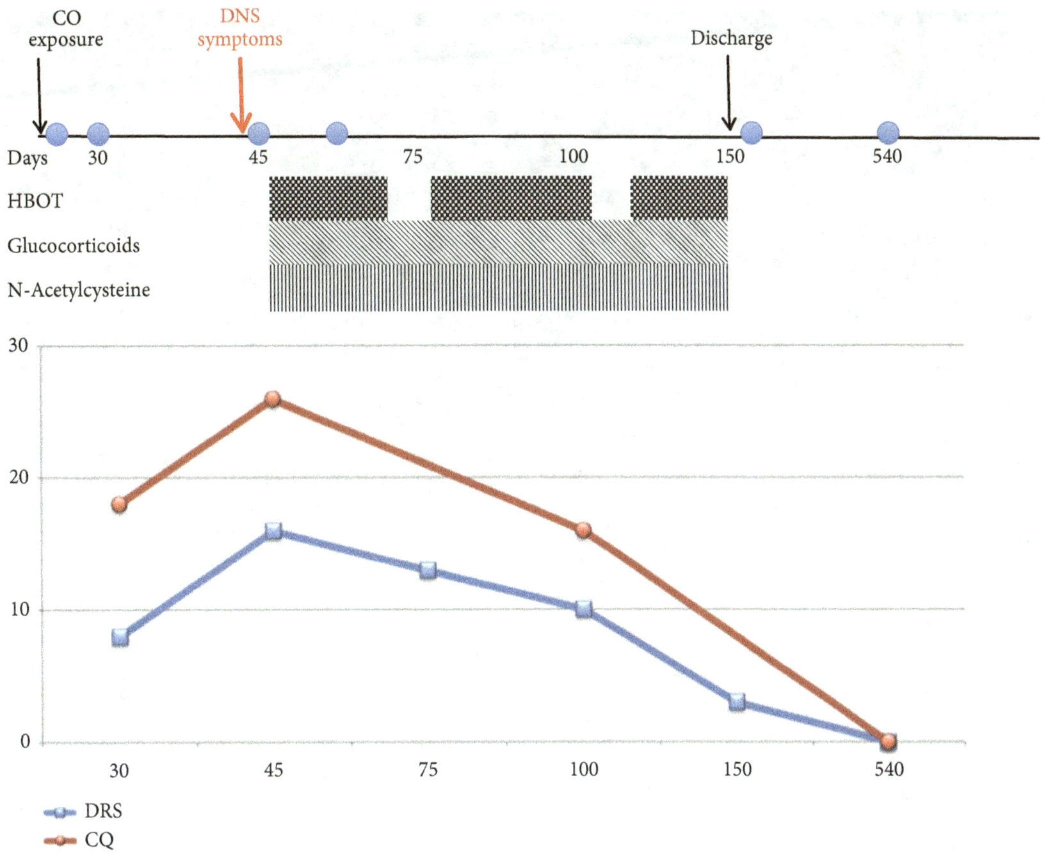

FIGURE 1: Timeline of clinical course. CO: carbon monoxide. HBOT: Hyperbaric Oxygen Therapy. DRS: Disability Rating Scale (Rappaport et al., 1992). CQ: cognitive quotient. Corresponding MRI scans are indicated as circles in the clinical course.

therapy. Moreover, our patient was periodically monitored with a comprehensive battery of neuropsychological tests aimed at characterizing her cognitive functions in detail.

Chang et al. [21] used MMSE as an outcome measure after CO poisoning and found a normalization of MMSE scores after the HBOT. In our patient, the normalization of MMSE score long predates the complete resolution of neuropsychological deficits in the different cognitive domains. This suggests the importance of using a battery of neuropsychological tests for the evaluation and follow-up after CO poisoning. There is still limited evidence on the efficacy of HBOT in the subacute phase of CO intoxication and/or DNS. HBOT has complex effects on immunity, oxygen transport, and hemodynamics. Mechanisms of neuroplasticity and cellular repair by HBOT have been suggested in many animal studies [22]. The ability of HBOT to induce angiogenesis was demonstrated in several different preclinical studies [23, 24]. HBOT may also promote neurogenesis of endogenous neural stem cells [25]. Efrati et al. [26] proved that HBOT can lead to significant neurological improvements in poststroke patients even at chronic late stages, implying that neuroplasticity can still be activated long after damage onset.

Furthermore, HBOT has been proposed for the treatment of some autoimmune diseases, given its immunosuppressive effect. HBOT produces changes in lymphocyte redistribution, suppression of antibody production, and suppression of leukocyte and macrophage function [27, 28]. Given the role of adaptive immunological response to chemically modified myelinic basic protein, HBOT could provide some beneficial effects in the treatment of CO-poisoned patients. Thom [29] reported reduced lipid peroxidation with HBOT in rats with CO poisoning. On the other hand, the therapeutic use of oxygen, particularly at supraphysiological pressures, might either increase systemic oxidative stress or cause an overproduction of oxygen free radicals [30]. An imbalance of free radical production has been known to result in deleterious modification of biological macromolecules [31]. ROS are known to mediate O2 toxicity, which for HBOT includes pulmonary injuries and central nervous system effects [32]. In addition, ROS formation may promote the inflammation via endothelial cells, chemotactic signals, and the release of products from the arachidonic acid cascade. In central nervous system, this results in progression of demyelinating lesions [33]. As consequence, the concurrent use of antioxidants and anti-inflammatory drugs may prevent the side effects of oxygen therapy at supraphysiological pressure due to oxidative stress. In this case, we administered low doses of glucocorticoids and high doses of N-Acetylcysteine (NAC). NAC is an antioxidant, used clinically to protect the liver from toxic effects of acetaminophen overdose and as mucolytic drugs. Moreover, in fibrosing alveolitis NAC prevent oxidative damage [34]. The effects of NAC are antioxidant because

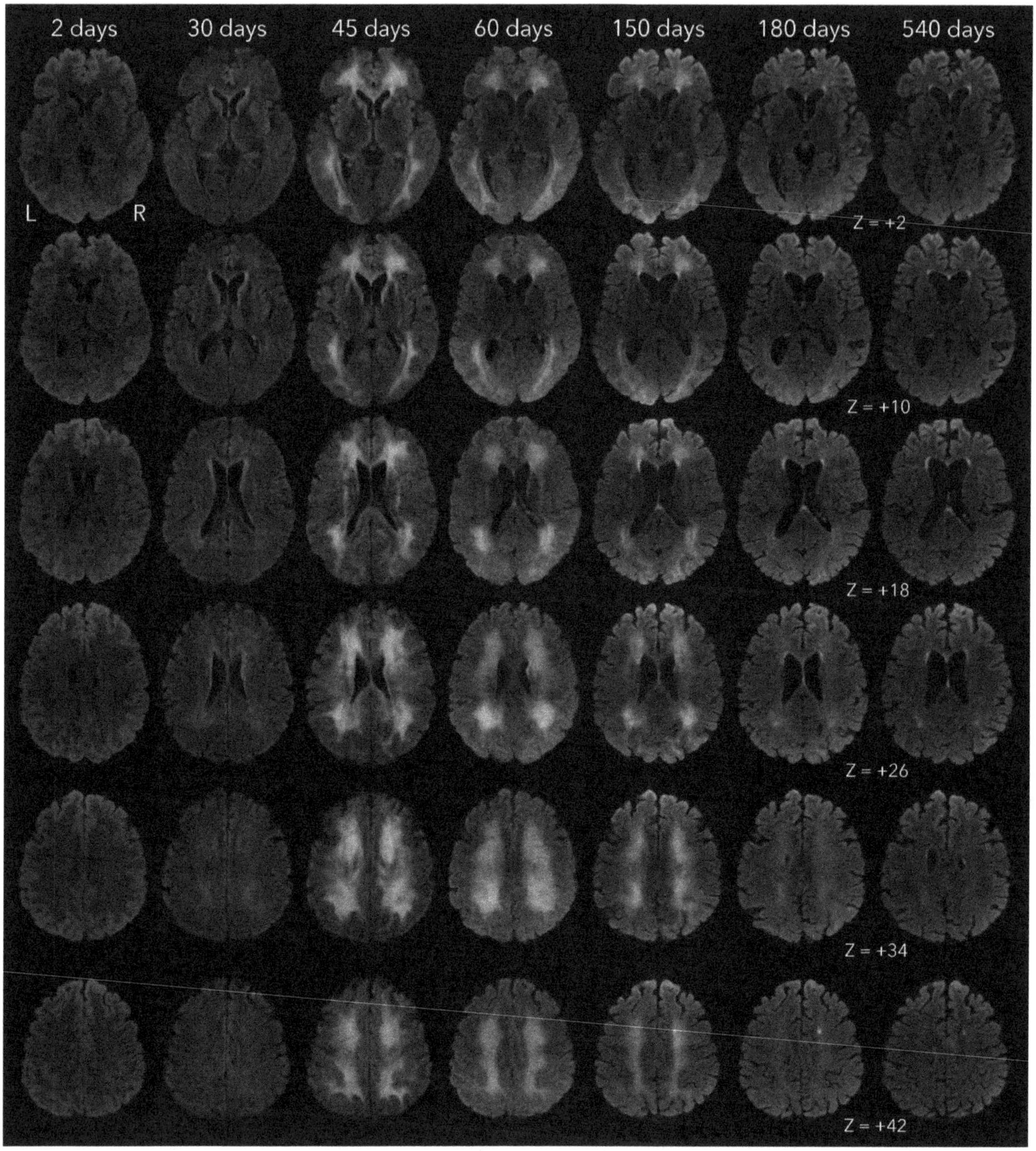

FIGURE 2: Comparison of MRI scans across different time-points after exposition. 30 and 45 days after initial event, FLAIR sequences show a diffuse and confluent hyperintensity involving predominantly the periventricular and deep white matter. Follow-up MRI scans (60, 150, 180, and 540 days after initial event) show gradual regression of the FLAIR hyperintensity.

it acts as a source of cysteine for the synthesis of glutathione [35]. NAC has also weak anti-inflammatory effects, by reducing Nuclear Factor-kB activation [36]. This same mechanism is responsible for powerful anti-inflammatory properties of glucocorticoids [37]. In a clinical study, Xiang [38] reported that the combined application of dexamethasone and HBOT, compared with HBOT alone, resulted in better functional recovery from DNS as assessed by means of MMSE score and National Institutes of Health Stroke Scale (NIHSS) [39] score. Therefore, NAC and glucocorticoids have synergic effects to counteract the supposed physiopathology of DNS and the putative HBOT-induced oxidative stress. Although spontaneous recovery cannot be excluded, our case suggests that a combination of HBOT and antioxidant and anti-inflammatory drugs may produce a positive synergistic effect, which could not be achieved when these therapies are applied independently. Further research is needed to clarify the role of antioxidants in the treatment and the time of complete recovery of DNS after CO poisoning.

Acknowledgments

The authors would like to thank Franco Ghelardoni, Stefano Bergamasco, Giuseppe De Iaco, and Roberta Bertolini from Intensive Care Unit of Pisa University Hospital for skillful technical assistance with Hyperbaric Oxygen Therapy.

References

[1] J. A. Raub, M. Mathieu-Nolf, N. B. Hampson, and S. R. Thom, "Carbon monoxide poisoning—a public health perspective," *Toxicology*, vol. 145, no. 1, pp. 1–14, 2000.

[2] C. Locatelli, I. Casagranda, D. Coern et al., "Gestione e trattamento del paziente con intossicazione acuta da monossido di carbonio: linee guida," *The Online Journal of Anesthesiology Italia*, vol. 6, 2000.

[3] C. G. Douglas, J. S. Haldane, and J. B. S. Haldane, "The laws of combination of hæmoglobin with carbon monoxide and oxygen," *The Journal of Physiology*, vol. 44, no. 4, pp. 275–304, 1912.

[4] J. D. Roderique, C. S. Josef, M. J. Feldman, and B. D. Spiess, "A modern literature review of carbon monoxide poisoning theories, therapies, and potential targets for therapy advancement," *Toxicology*, vol. 334, pp. 45–58, 2015.

[5] S. Choi, "Delayed neurologic sequelae in carbon monoxide intoxication," *JAMA Neurology*, vol. 40, no. 7, pp. 433–435, 1983.

[6] C.-P. Lo, S.-Y. Chen, K.-W. Lee et al., "Brain injury after acute carbon monoxide poisoning: early and late complications," *AJR. American journal of roentgenology*, vol. 189, no. 4, pp. W205–W211, 2007.

[7] P. O'donnell, P. J. Buxton, A. Pitkin, and L. J. Jarvis, "The magnetic resonance imaging appearances of the brain in acute carbon monoxide poisoning," *Clinical Radiology*, vol. 55, no. 4, pp. 273–280, 2000.

[8] S. R. Thom, V. M. Bhopale, D. Fisher, J. Zhang, and P. Gimotty, "Delayed neuropathology after carbon monoxide poisoning is immune-mediated," *Proceedings of the National Acadamy of Sciences of the United States of America*, vol. 101, no. 37, pp. 13660–13665, 2004.

[9] S. J. Wolf, E. J. Lavonas, E. P. Sloan, and A. S. Jagoda, "Clinical policy: critical issues in the management of adult patients presenting to the emergency department with acute carbon monoxide poisoning," *Annals of Emergency Medicine*, vol. 51, no. 2, pp. 138–152, 2008.

[10] N. A. Buckley, D. N. Juurlink, G. Isbister, M. H. Bennett, and E. J. Lavonas, "Hyperbaric oxygen for carbon monoxide poisoning.," *Cochrane Database of Systematic Reviews (Online)*, vol. 4, p. CD002041, 2011.

[11] Y.-T. Lin, S.-Y. Chen, C.-P. Lo et al., "Utilizing cerebral perfusion scan and diffusion-tensor MR imaging to evaluate the effect of hyperbaric oxygen therapy in carbon monoxide-induced delayed neuropsychiatric seqeulae-a case report and literature review," *Acta Neurologica Taiwanica*, vol. 24, no. 2, pp. 57–62, 2015.

[12] M. B. Hansen, D. Kondziella, E. R. Danielsen, V. A. Larsen, E. C. Jansen, and O. Hyldegaard, "Cerebral proton magnetic resonance spectroscopy demonstrates reversibility of N-acetylaspartate/creatine in gray matter after delayed encephalopathy due to carbon monoxide intoxication: A case report," *Journal of Medical Case Reports*, vol. 8, article no. 211, 2014.

[13] H. Kuroda, K. Fujihara, S. Takahashi, Y. Shinozawa, and Y. Itoyama, "A case of delayed encephalopathy after carbon monoxide poisoning longitudinally monitored by diffusion tensor imaging," *American Journal of Neuroradiology*, vol. 33, no. 4, pp. E52–E54, 2012.

[14] F. Spagnolo, M. Costa, M. Impellizzeri et al., "Delayed hyperbaric oxygen treatment after acute carbon monoxide poisoning," *Journal of Neurology*, vol. 258, no. 8, pp. 1553-1554, 2011.

[15] A. F. Geraldo, C. Silva, D. Neutel, L. L. Neto, and L. Albuquerque, "Delayed leukoencephalopathy after acute carbon monoxide intoxication," *Journal of Radiology Case Reports*, vol. 8, no. 5, pp. 1–8, 2014.

[16] M. Rappaport, K. M. Hall, K. Hopkins, T. Belleza, and D. N. Cope, "Disability rating scale for severe head trauma: coma to community," *Archives of Physical Medicine and Rehabilitation*, vol. 63, no. 3, pp. 118–123, 1982.

[17] M. F. Folstein, S. E. Folstein, and P. R. McHugh, ""Mini mental state". A practical method for grading the cognitive state of patients for the clinician," *Journal of Psychiatric Research*, vol. 12, no. 3, pp. 189–198, 1975.

[18] S. Mondini, D. Mapelli, A. Vestri, G. Arcara, and P. S. Bisiacchi, *L'esame Neuropsicologico Breve*, Raffaello Cortina Editore, Milan, Italy, 2011.

[19] S. M. Smith, "Fast robust automated brain extraction," *Human Brain Mapping*, vol. 17, no. 3, pp. 143–155, 2002.

[20] M. Jenkinson, P. Bannister, M. Brady, and S. Smith, "Improved optimization for the robust and accurate linear registration and motion correction of brain images," *NeuroImage*, vol. 17, no. 2, pp. 825–841, 2002.

[21] D. C. Chang, J. T. Lee, C. P. Lo et al., "Hyperbaric oxygen ameliorates delayed neuropsychiatrie syndrome of carbon monoxide poisoning," *The Undersea and Hyperbaric Medicine*, vol. 37, no. 1, pp. 23–33, 2010.

[22] A. Hadanny and S. Efrati, "Treatment of persistent post-concussion syndrome due to mild traumatic brain injury: current status and future directions," *Expert Review of Neurotherapeutics*, vol. 16, no. 8, pp. 875–887, 2016.

[23] K. Lin, K. Niu, K. Tsai et al., "Attenuating inflammation but stimulating both angiogenesis and neurogenesis using hyperbaric oxygen in rats with traumatic brain injury," *The Journal of Trauma and Acute Care Surgery*, vol. 72, no. 3, pp. 650–659, 2012.

[24] J. Mu, P. R. Krafft, and J. H. Zhang, "Hyperbaric oxygen therapy promotes neurogenesis: where do we stand?" *Medical Gas Research*, vol. 1, no. 1, p. 14, 2011.

[25] S. Efrati and E. Ben-Jacob, "Reflections on the neurotherapeutic effects of hyperbaric oxygen," *Expert Review of Neurotherapeutics*, vol. 14, no. 3, pp. 233–236, 2014.

[26] S. Efrati, G. Fishlev, Y. Bechor et al., "Hyperbaric oxygen induces late neuroplasticity in post stroke patients - randomized, prospective trial," *PLoS ONE*, vol. 8, no. 1, article no. e53716, 2013.

[27] N. Bitterman, N. Lahat, T. Rosenwald, A. Kinarty, Y. Melamed, and H. Bitterman, "Effect of hyperbaric oxygen on tissue distribution of mononuclear cell subsets in the rat," *Journal of Applied Physiology*, vol. 77, no. 5, pp. 2355–2359, 1994.

[28] K. M. McIntyre, P. S. Dixon, L. P. Krock, and E. H. Piepmeier Jr., "The influence of hyperbaric oxygenation on leukocyte

viability and surface protein expression," *Aviation, Space, and Environmental Medicine*, vol. 68, no. 12, pp. 1129–1133, 1997.

[29] S. R. Thom, "Antagonism of carbon monoxide-mediated brain lipid peroxidation by hyperbaric oxygen," *Toxicology and Applied Pharmacology*, vol. 105, no. 2, pp. 340–344, 1990.

[30] S. R. Thom, "Oxidative stress is fundamental to hyperbaric oxygen therapy," *Journal of Applied Physiology*, vol. 106, no. 3, pp. 988–995, 2009.

[31] J. P. Fessel and L. J. Roberts II, "Isofurans: Novel products of lipid peroxidation that define the occurrence of oxidant injury in settings of elevated oxygen tension," *Antioxidants & Redox Signaling*, vol. 7, no. 1-2, pp. 202–209, 2005.

[32] J. Clark, *Oxygen toxicity. Physiology and Medicine of Hyperbaric Oxygen Therapy*, T. S. Neuman and S. R. Thom, Eds., Saunders, Philadelphia, PA, USA, 2008.

[33] K. J. Smith, R. Kapoor, and P. A. Felts, "Demyelination: the role of reactive oxygen and nitrogen species," *Brain Pathology*, vol. 9, no. 1, pp. 69–92, 1999.

[34] J. Behr, K. Maier, B. Degenkolb, F. Krombach, and C. Vogelmeier, "Antioxidative and clinical effects of high-dose N-acetylcysteine in fibrosing alveolitis," *American Journal of Respiratory and Critical Care Medicine*, vol. 156, no. 6, pp. 1897–1901, 1997.

[35] I. Ziment, "Acetylcysteine: a drug that is much more than a mucokinetic," *Biomedicine & Pharmacotherapy*, vol. 42, no. 8, pp. 513–519, 1988.

[36] T. S. Blackwell, T. R. Blackwell, E. P. Holden, B. W. Christman, and J. W. Christman, "In vivo antioxidant treatment suppresses nuclear factor-kappa B activation and neutrophilic lung inflammation," *The Journal of Immunology*, vol. 157, no. 4, pp. 1630–1637, 1996.

[37] N. Auphan, J. A. DiDonato, C. Rosette, A. Helmberg, and M. Karin, "Immunosuppression by glucocorticoids: inhibition of NF-kB activity through induction of IkB synthesis," *Science*, vol. 270, no. 5234, pp. 286–290, 1995.

[38] W. Xiang, H. Xue, B. Wang et al., "Combined application of dexamethasone and hyperbaric oxygen therapy yields better efficacy for patients with delayed encephalopathy after acute carbon monoxide poisoning," *Drug Design, Development and Therapy*, vol. 11, pp. 513–519, 2017.

[39] T. Brott, H. P. Adams Jr., C. P. Olinger et al., "Measurements of acute cerebral infarction: a clinical examination scale," *Stroke*, vol. 20, no. 7, pp. 864–870, 1989.

28

Ipsilateral Limb Extension of Referred Trigeminal Facial Pain due to Greater Occipital Nerve Entrapment: A Case Report

Byung-Chul Son[1,2] **and Changik Lee**[1]

[1]*Department of Neurosurgery, Seoul St. Mary's Hospital, College of Medicine, The Catholic University of Korea, Seoul, Republic of Korea*
[2]*Catholic Neuroscience Institute, College of Medicine, The Catholic University of Korea, Seoul, Republic of Korea*

Correspondence should be addressed to Byung-Chul Son; sbc@catholic.ac.kr

Academic Editor: Dominic B. Fee

We report a very rare case of referred pain associated with entrapment of the greater occipital nerve (GON) occurring not only in the ipsilateral hemiface but also in the ipsilateral limb. There is an extensive convergence of cutaneous, tooth pulp, visceral, neck, and muscle afferents onto nociceptive and nonnociceptive neurons in the trigeminal nucleus caudalis (medullary dorsal horn). In addition, nociceptive input from trigeminal, meningeal afferents projects into trigeminal nucleus caudalis and dorsal horn of C1 and C2. Together, they form a functional unit, the trigeminocervical complex (TCC). The nociceptive inflow from suboccipital and high cervical structures is mediated with small-diameter afferent fibers in the upper cervical roots terminating in the dorsal horn of the cervical cord extending from the C2 segment up to the medullary dorsal horn. The major afferent contribution is mediated by the spinal root C2 that is peripherally represented by the greater occipital nerve (GON). Convergence of afferent signals from the trigeminal nerve and the GON onto the TCC is regarded as an anatomical basis of pain referral in craniofacial pain and primary headache syndrome. Ipsilateral limb pain occurs long before the onset of the referred facial pain. The subsequent severe hemifacial pain suggested GON entrapment. The occipital nerve block provided temporary relief from facial and extremity pain. Imaging studies found a benign osteoma in the ipsilateral suboccipital bone, but no direct contact with GON was identified. During GON decompression, severe entrapment of the GON was observed by the tendinous aponeurotic edge of the trapezius muscle, but the osteoma had no contact with the nerve. Following GON decompression, the referred trigeminal and extremity pain completely disappeared. The pain referral from GON entrapment seems to be attributed to the sensitization and hypersensitivity of the trigeminocervical complex (TCC). The clinical manifestations of TCC hypersensitivity induced by chronic entrapment of GONs are diverse when considering the occurrence of extremity pain as well as facial pain.

1. Introduction

Frequent pain referrals to the occipital region observed in patients with primary headache are attributed to the convergence of nociceptive afferents from the trigeminal and upper cervical structures to the trigeminocervical complex (TCC) [1]. The nociceptive input from dura mater is transmitted in the ophthalmic division of the trigeminal nerve by the trigeminal ganglion to nociceptive second-order neurons in the superficial and deep layers of the medullary dorsal horn of the TCC [2–4]. The TCC extends from the trigeminal nucleus caudalis to the segments of C2-C3 in the rat [5], cats [6], and monkeys [7]. These dural-sensitive trigeminal neurons show a high degree of convergent input from other afferent sources which typically show facial and corneal receptive fields [1, 8]. Meanwhile, the upper cervical spinal roots also contribute to the sensory innervation of occipital and suboccipital structures [9, 10].

Nociceptive inflow from these structures is mediated by small-diameter afferent fibers in the upper cervical roots terminating the dorsal horn of the cervical spinal cord extending from the C2 segment up to the medullary dorsal horn [9, 10]. The major afferent contribution is mediated by the C2 spinal root that is peripherally represented by the

GON [11, 12]. Similar to the trigeminal sensory neurons, these cervical neurons show a high convergence of input from neck muscles and the skin [1, 2]. ,In addition to an anatomical overlap of trigeminal and cervical nociceptive afferents throughout the TCC from the level of the trigeminal nucleus caudalis to at least the C2 segment, direct functional coupling between these afferents was described [3]. These trigeminocervical neurons showed convergent synaptic input from the supratentorial dura mater and from the ipsilateral and contralateral GONs [13, 14].

Occipital neuralgia is defined as paroxysmal stabbing pain arising from the distribution of the greater or lesser occipital nerves and is mostly primary in origin [15, 16]. However, several reports in the last decade suggested that the GON entrapment within the area where the aponeurotic edge of the trapezius muscle attached to the superior nuchal line (the so-called trapezial tunnel) is the most common cause of occipital neuralgia [17–21]. The GON originates in the medial branches of the dorsal rami of the second cervical nerve root and transmits nociceptive afferent information from the temporo-occipital area and vertex, as well as the suboccipital area [17, 18]. Therefore, the GON represents the main sensory afferent traversing through the C2 root, and this afferent information is transmitted directly to the high cervical dorsal horn where the TCC is located [3–5]. It is known that GON entrapment commonly causes aching, tightening, and pressure-like pain in the posterior head and neck, which are GON distributions, as well as occipital neuralgia [22–26]. Also, referred pain of the ipsilateral hemiface was frequently induced for occipital and neck pain due to GON entrapment [22–26]. The chronic, continuous, and noxious afferent inputs of the entrapped GON appear to be associated with sensitization and hypersensitivity of the second-order neurons in the TCC, resulting in referred pain in the trigeminal distribution [22–26].

We report a case of pain involving the ipsilateral extremity along with referred facial pain due to GON entrapment. The ipsilateral extremity pain disappeared along with the associated facial pain following GON decompression.

2. Case Report

A 49-year-old female patient presented with a three-month history of pain with a sudden onset, persistent tightness, and left-side facial pain, including periorbital, cheek, and jaw areas (Figure 1(a)). The patient's past history was characterized by chronic and persistent pain in the left neck, shoulder, and left leg. The tightening pain was similar to pulling of a rubber band on the left leg laterally and originated 5 years ago without specific antecedent events, including trauma. No pain was detected in the lower back or hip or numbness in the legs. Within a few days after the onset of pain in the left leg, the pain extended to the left arm (Figure 1(b)). This pain persisted throughout the day and was not exacerbated by changes in limb posture, including walking and straining. No abnormalities were found on X-rays and magnetic resonance imaging (MRI) of the lumbar spine and shoulder. The pain in the patient's left arm and leg did not improve despite months of medication and physical therapy. At that time, the pain intensity was evaluated as 2~4 out of 10 on the numerical rating scale (NRS-11). The pain did not interfere with daily life substantially, and the patient endured it with occasional physical therapies.

About 3 years ago, the patient's left neck and shoulder pain gradually got worse for no apparent reason (Figure 1(c)). The nature of pain was similar to that of the left leg and arm and was expressed as a feeling of persistent pulling and tightness. There was no limitation of motion (LOM) of the neck, and pain did not worsen with neck, arm, and shoulder movements. Repeated MRIs of the shoulder and cervical spine showed no abnormalities. The patient received long-term medications, physical therapy, tender injections, and nerve blocks for more than 6 months, but the pain persisted. The orthopedic surgeons, neurosurgeons, and pain doctors who treated her were unable to arrive at a specific diagnosis. Following months of ineffective medication and physical therapy, she opted for massage therapy for neck, shoulder, and extremity pain. When the pain in the left neck and shoulder was severe, the pain in the leg also worsened. While awake, pain in the left extremity, left neck, and shoulder continued and the intensity of the pain was 3~5/10, enabling daily life. Because of chronic pain, the patient received medication for 1 year following a provisional diagnosis of myofascial pain syndrome and fibromyalgia by the rheumatologist, without improvement in pain.

Three months before her visit, the pain in the left posterolateral neck suddenly worsened for several days (Figure 1(c)). One day, a tingling sensation and dullness appeared suddenly on her left hemiface (Figure 1(a)). In addition, the patient reports tightness and squeezing pain in the left periorbital and in the left cheek and jaw area. The left periorbital area was particularly painful, requiring pressure with a fist to suppress it (Figure 1(a)). The tightening pain persisted during waking, and its intensity was rated 5~6 out of 10 on the NRS-11. As the pain in her left hemiface developed, the intensity of pain in the left extremity, neck, and shoulder also increased (Figure 1(d)). Medications such as gabapentin, pregabalin, Ultracet®, and nonsteroidal anti-inflammatory drugs (NSAIDs) including indomethacin prescribed by the patient's rheumatologist were ineffective. She was referred to a neurologist, and neurological examination and MRI of the brain revealed no abnormalities. No organic cause was identified in the referral to ophthalmology and otolaryngology.

The patient's rheumatologist referred her to us for inexplicable left hemifacial and hemibody pain. Despite subjective dullness in her left hemiface, no objective sensory change was confirmed. No allodynia was found. A detailed interview revealed pain in the left ear canal and suboccipital area in addition to pain in the left eye, cheek, and jaw, but there was no pain in the left auricle. No neurological abnormalities were detected including masticatory function in the trigeminal nerve and other cranial nerves. There were no movement restrictions involving the neck, and no physical findings suggestive of cervical radiculopathy were found. There were no abnormal findings on laboratory

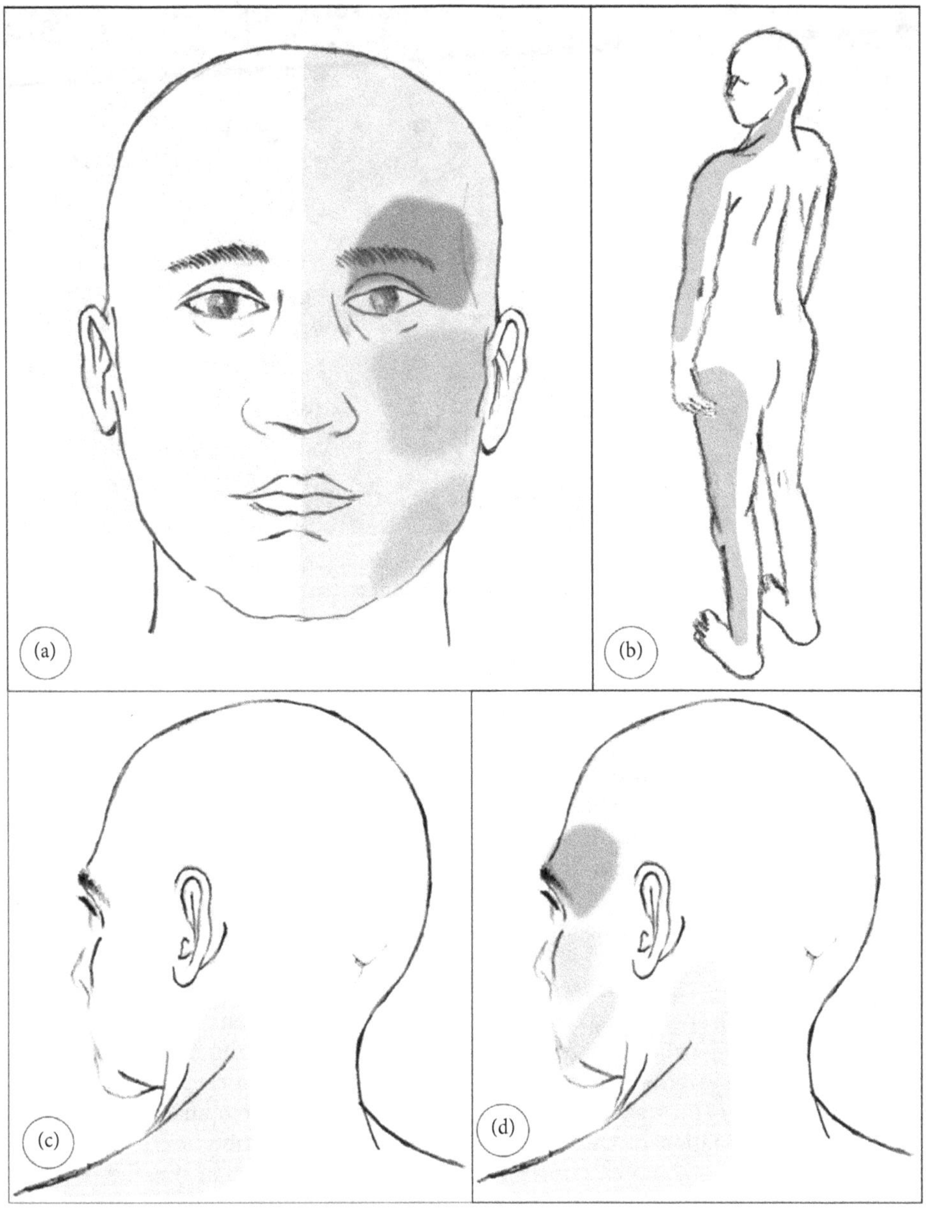

FIGURE 1: Schematic diagram showing the distribution and characteristics of chronic pain. (a) The gray areas over the left hemiface indicate the distribution of pain that occurred three months prior to the patient's visit. The pain was more severe in the left periorbital, cheek, and chin, and the periorbital area was the most painful. The nature of the pain was a feeling of tightness and pressure, which lasted all day. (b) The location (gray area) of tightening and squeezing pain on the side of the left leg that occurred 5 years ago. A few days after the onset of pain in the left leg, a similar pain occurred in the patient's left arm. (c) The location of the pain in the left posterolateral neck and shoulder that suddenly worsened 3 years before admission. (d) A drawing showing the distribution of pain in the left hemiface (gray area) that suddenly occurred as the existing left posterolateral neck pain worsened. This hemifacial pain was also described by the patient as a constant pulling and tightening pain.

examination, including the erythrocyte sedimentation rate, C-reactive protein, blood sugar, uric acid, and antinuclear bodies. There was no medical history including hypertension or diabetes other than extremity pain that started 5 years ago.

Physical examination revealed a small, nontender, immobile, hard mass, which was palpable in the left suboccipital area (Figure 2). She denied a relationship between the lump and facial pain. In fact, about three years ago, while receiving a neck massage, she heard from the therapist about the existence of a mass. However, she did not request further evaluation because there was no pain, tenderness, or discomfort at the site of the mass. A small calcified mass was observed under the left suboccipital bone during simple skull radiography (Figure 2(a)). Three-dimensional computed tomography and MRI of the brain confirmed a benign osteoma without intracranial extension (Figures 2(b) and 2(c)). Brain MRI showed no structural abnormalities in the cranium including the trigeminal nerve.

With the possibility of referred facial pain due to GON entrapment in mind, occipital nerve block (ONB) of the left GON was performed using 2 mL of 2% lidocaine, which relieved the intensity of the left hemifacial pain by 80% for

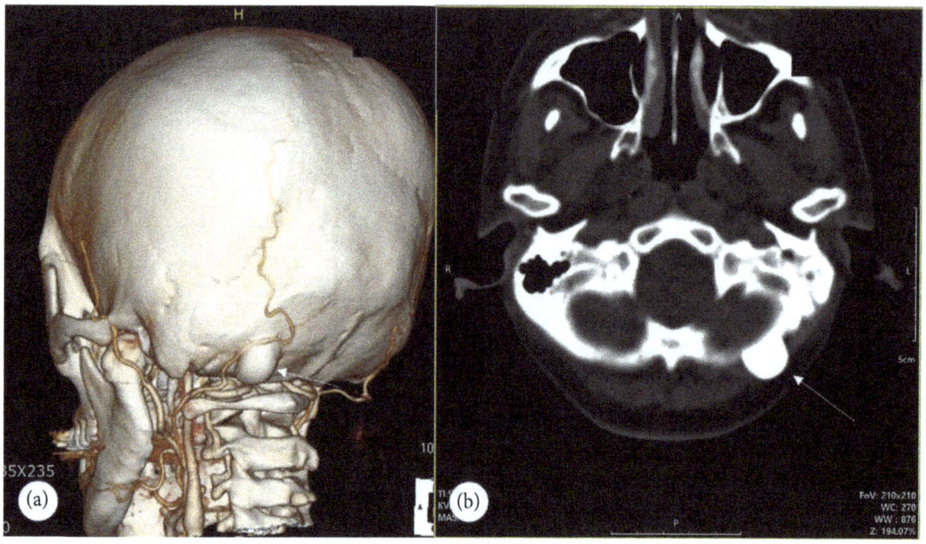

FIGURE 2: Computed tomographic (CT) scan images showing a single incidental suboccipital osteoma (arrow). A three-dimensional CT scan (a) and an axial CT image (b) of the osteoma. No association was found between osteoma and the greater occipital nerve.

2 hours. The same temporary improvement was confirmed at the second ONB, which was performed two weeks later. The second ONB temporarily alleviated the pain in the left neck, shoulder, and left limb for 1 to 2 hours. Three hours after receiving ONB, pain in the left face, neck, and arm continued to persist with the same intensity as before. Due to chronicity and refractoriness of the pain and the possibility of referred facial pain due to chronic entrapment of GON, exploration and decompression of the left GON in addition to excision of the osteoma were recommended after obtaining written informed consent.

In order to expose both the osteoma and the left GON, a 6 cm straight incision was made at an angle in the center of both structures (Figure 3). The incision then involved the trapezius fascia. The GON was found severely entrapped by the fibro-tendinous aponeurotic edge of the trapezius muscle (trapezial tunnel), showing an indentation of chronic entrapment (Figure 3(a)). After the circumferential release of the GON from the tendinous aponeurotic arch, the proximal and distal courses of the left GON were dissected (Figure 3(b)). After retracting the decompressed left GON using a vascular loop, the underlying superior oblique muscle was incised to expose the protruding osteoma (Figure 3(c)). As expected, the osteoma had no direct contact with the GON. The protruding part was removed by drilling (Figure 3(d)).

The effects of GON decompression appeared from the day after surgery. The patient reported that the persistent pain and discomfort in the left eye, cheek, jaw, and half face were reduced by about 70% compared with previous conditions. Simultaneously, it was reported that the tightening pain in the left neck, shoulder, and left arm and leg was no longer felt. Two weeks after the operation, the pain in her left face, neck, shoulder, and limbs disappeared, and the patient did not feel any difficulty in daily life. The patient's occipital discomfort due to the incision was not great either. She refused medications such as gabapentin and Ultracet®. Six months after surgery, the patient reported that she was doing well with no discomfort in her left face and neck. The tightening pain involving her left arm and leg that had lasted for 5 years disappeared.

3. Discussion

3.1. Convergence and Sensitization in the Trigeminocervical Complex. Nociceptive second-order neurons in the spinal cord can be subjected to transient or long-lasting hyper-excitability in response to afferent stimuli, such as strong noxious stimuli [3, 27]. Increased afferent barrage from primary nociceptive afferents, especially C-fibers, onto second-order neurons is known to be critical in the development of central hypersensitivity in the spinal cord [27–29]. Central hypersensitivity in the nociceptive second-order neurons in the spinal cord was found to be more easily evoked by stimulation of afferents from visceral and deep somatic tissues, such as muscles and joints than cutaneous input [30–32]. The clinical correlates of this central hypersensitivity include the development of spontaneous pain, hyperalgesia, and allodynia [28, 33].

In line with this finding in the spinal cord, central sensitization in the nociceptive neurons in the trigeminal nucleus caudalis, the V homologue of the spinal dorsal horn [34], was demonstrated with the application of a small fiber irritant [35, 36]. Chemical activation and sensitization of meningeal sensory neurons induced a central sensitization of trigeminal second-order neurons in the caudal trigeminal nucleus with a subsequent increased responsiveness to dural and cutaneous facial stimulation [2]. In a population of nociceptive neurons in the laminae V/VI layers of the C2 dorsal horn with convergent input from the supratentorial dura, innervated by the trigeminal nerve, and cervical skin and muscle that are innervated by the GON, stimulation of dural afferent C-fibers increased the background activity, extended the size of cutaneous trigeminal and cervical receptive fields, and decreased the thresholds to mechanical dural stimulation [3, 27]. Furthermore, stimulation of the

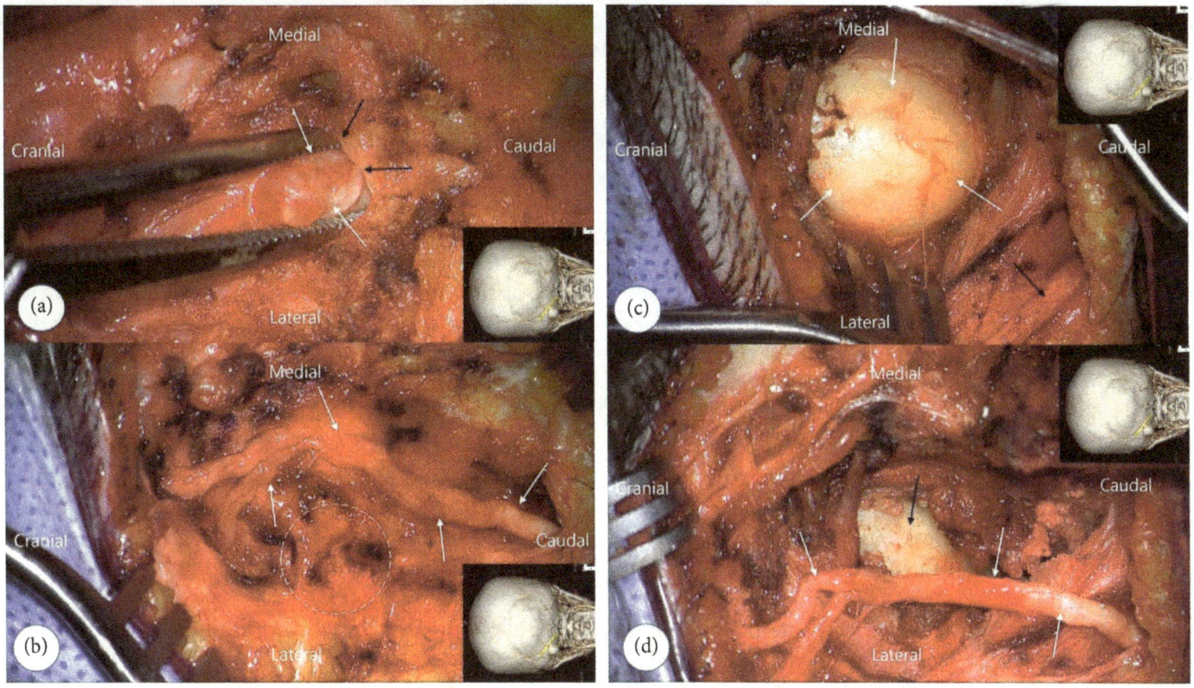

FIGURE 3: Intraoperative photographs of decompression of the greater occipital nerve (GON) and osteoma removal. (a) GON (white arrows) entrapment at the trapezial tunnel. The GON entrapment is observed by lifting the trapezial aponeurotic edge (black arrows). The inset shows the direction of the image and the location of the incision. The skull reconstruction image in the inset represents the position of the head and skin incision in the surgical field. (b) Complete decompression of the GON (arrows) around the trapezial tunnel. The white circle indicates the location of the osteoma. The GON had no direct contact with the osteoma. (c) Osteoma (white arrow) exposed after retraction of the GON (black arrow). (d) Intraoperative photograph showing the decompressed GON (white arrow) after removal of the osteoma (black arrow). The patient's left hemiface, posterolateral neck, and shoulder pain, as well as pain in the left extremity, had completely improved by 2 weeks after surgery.

dura mater led to a sensitization of these convergent neurons with a subsequent increased excitability to neck muscle and GON stimulation [3, 27]. This demonstrates that dural afferents and GON afferents make anatomic connections and these connections are functionally relevant in terms of mutual changes in excitability [1]. Convergence and sensitization in the nociceptive second-order neurons were suggested to be involved in the spread and referral of pain in the trigeminal and cervical area in craniofacial pain and primary headache syndromes [1, 3, 27].

3.2. Entrapment of the Greater Occipital Nerve and Pain Referral. The GON originates in the medial branch of the dorsal rami of the second cervical nerve root [17, 18]. It also receives a branch from the dorsal rami of the C3 root [17, 18]. It ascends through the semispinalis capitis muscle and runs rostrolaterally before entering the scalp by piercing the aponeurotic fibrous sling between the trapezius and the sternocleidomastoid muscle near their attachment to the superior nuchal line [17–21]. This aperture (trapezial tunnel) is a frequent site of GON entrapment [19–21]. Compared with other peripheral nerves, the GON widens towards its course to the periphery after piercing the aponeurotic sling between the trapezius and the sternocleidomastoid [18]. This anatomical finding is regarded as relevant to GON entrapment, as widening of the nerve increases the risk of entrapment, especially in the firm trapezius muscle aponeurosis [18].

There is no electrophysiologic evidence from animal experiments on whether entrapment of the GON induces hyperactivity of the nociceptive secondary neurons in the TCC. However, acute stimulation of cervical roots and structures innervated by upper cervical roots in humans, such as the dura mater, vessels, and tumors of the posterior fossa, lead to pain referred to the front of the head [1, 37, 38]. Structures in the back of the head are mainly innervated by the GON that is a branch of the C2 spinal root [39]. The GON constitutes the main sensory afferent nerve through the C2 root, and this afferent input is transmitted directly to the TCC.

"Entrapment neuropathies" refer to isolated peripheral nerve injuries that occur at specific locations where a nerve is mechanically constricted in a fibrous or fibro-osseous tunnel or deformed by a fibrous band [39]. The trapezial tunnel is an anatomical passageway through which the GON must pass and is known as a site where entrapment can occur [17–21]. Entrapment of the peripheral nerve is known to be associated with nerve inflammation and result in pain and headache [40]. Compression injury of the peripheral nerve in a rat model showed inflammation, both local and remote, from the site of peripheral nerve compression [41, 42]. Therefore, it is thought that chronic entrapment of GON induces inflammatory changes, possibly leading to sensitization and hypersensitivity of secondary neurons in the TCC. Although chronic GON entrapment itself is an individual's constitutional problem, the degree of compression seems to vary from person to person [25].

Indeed, referred trigeminal pain caused by GON entrapment in the trapezial tunnel has been reported in several recent reports. Pain referral to the facial trigeminal distribution triggered by GON entrapment occurred not only in the *V*1 region but also in the *V*2 and *V*3 regions and even caused hemifacial pain and sensory changes [22–26]. We frequently found immediate disappearance of the referred trigeminal facial pain after GON decompression [22–24]. These reports are considered direct clinical evidence that the chronic, continuous, noxious afferent input of GON entrapment may be associated with sensitization and hypersensitivity of the second-order neurons in the TCC.

The patient's left hemifacial pain was presumed to be a sudden onset of referred facial trigeminal pain due to chronic GON entrapment. The authors have already experienced many cases of referred trigeminal pain manifesting suddenly in the facial half in many patients with GON entrapment [14–18]. In addition, pain within the ipsilateral ear canal and lateral neck was frequently reported by patients with GON entrapment [15, 16]. In addition, pain in the suboccipital area was noted along with posterolateral neck pain. By the ONBs, which was performed with the possibility of GON entrapment in mind, not only neck pain but also ipsilateral facial and extremity pain were improved temporarily.

3.3. Referred Pain to the Extratrigeminal Area. The current case is unique in that the referred pain due to GON entrapment extended not only to the face, where it occurs frequently, but also to the extremities. The nondermatomal pain in the limbs was not accompanied by objective neurological or musculoskeletal abnormalities. The pain in the left arm and leg disappeared promptly along with the referred pain involving the left hemiface with GON decompression. Considering the pathogenesis of referred trigeminal facial pain due to chronic GON entrapment based on the convergence of trigeminocervical afferents and subsequent sensitization of secondary neurons in TCC [1, 3, 27], the neuroanatomical basis of pain referral to the extremities is attributed to GON distribution and connectivity. The fact that hemifacial pain, which occurred additionally in chronic neck, shoulder, and limb pain, disappeared due to GON decompression means that GON entrapment caused hypersensitivity of the TCC.

It has been shown that caudal trigeminal nucleus (Sp5C) trigeminovascular neurons receiving convergent input from the dura and periorbital area not only increase their responses following the application of inflammatory agents to the dura but also become sensitized for several hours [43, 44]. Sp5C-sensitized neurons have lower thresholds to both dural and periocular skin stimulation and show a significant increase in the size of their dural and cutaneous receptive fields [2]. Based on these findings, it was proposed that the referred, cutaneous allodynia observed in migraine patients is due to central sensitization of Sp5C neurons following peripheral sensitization of meningeal nociceptors [2]. Moreover, the ophthalmic region of Sp5C, which contains neurons that receive convergent input from the dura and periorbital skin, sends projections to the ophthalmic primary afferent projection area of the contralateral trigeminal brain stem sensory complex [44]. These projections are somatotopically organized and extend rostrocaudally from the caudal spinal trigeminal nucleus to the upper cervical dorsal horn C2–3 segments [44, 45]. Contralateral projections could provide input that specifically modulates the activity of medullary and spinal dorsal horn cells driven from the ophthalmic division of the trigeminal nerve [43]. Such input could become effective following long-lasting noxious stimulation of meningeal nociceptors and thus contribute to the central sensitization that occurs after long-lasting migraine attacks [46]. Sp5C also projects to the ipsilateral junction of Sp5C and interpolaris (Sp5I), oralis (Sp5O), and principal sensory (Pr5) nuclei over their whole caudal-rostral extent [47]. Ipsilateral input from Sp5C neurons to rostral trigeminal nuclei could contribute to the amplification of nociceptive output to supramedullary structures via the interpolar, oral, and principal subdivisions since these regions convey orofacial input to the brain stem and thalamic areas [48].

Following trigeminal nerve injury (or inflammation), the changes in the excitability of afferents may not be limited to the damaged afferents [49]. The excitability of undamaged afferents may also be altered. Changes may also occur in the peripheral innervation patterns of afferents spared from the nerve injury. As a result, an increased pain sensitivity reflected in extraterritorial secondary hyperalgesia may occur [49]. The interactions between satellite glia cells and neurons involve the release of chemical mediators and changes in signaling mechanisms that can result in the spread of hyperexcitability throughout the different trigeminal divisions of the trigeminal ganglion [49, 50]. For example, injury to primary afferents in the infraorbital nerve, a branch of the maxillary division of the trigeminal nerve, may increase the excitability of not only primary afferent neurons in the maxillary division but also neurons in the other two trigeminal divisions of the ganglion [49]. Meanwhile, transection of the upper cervical spinal nerves in rats resulted in mechanical allodynia and thermal hyperalgesia in the facial skin, phosphorylated extracellular signal-regulated kinase (pERK) expression, and astroglial cell activation in the rats [51]. This suggested that extraterritorial facial pain can occur in the upper cervical nerve injury [51]. Therefore, the convergence of cervical and trigeminal afferents onto caudal trigeminal nucleus and upper cervical dorsal horns is thought to be a mechanism in orofacial pain related to neck injury. Chronic entrapment of the GON does not cause the same nerve damage such as nerve transection, but it is thought to have the potential to induce nerve inflammation, leading to hypersensitivity of the TCC.

Nociceptive transmission from the central endings of the nociceptive primary afferents to neurons in trigeminal brainstem sensory nuclear complex (TBSNC) may take place in the rostral components of the TBSNC (e.g., Sp5O) but is especially evident in its more caudal components (Sp5C), the medullary dorsal horn, also known as caudal trigeminal nucleus and caudalis-interpolaris transition zone, and in the upper cervical dorsal horns [47, 49]. The nociceptive transmission process involves the release of several neurochemicals, such as glutamatergic, neurokinin (e.g., substance P and CGRP), and purinergic mediators, from the central endings of the primary afferents. In the situation where there are abnormal hyperexcitable or ectopic afferent inputs, neuroplastic and glioplastic changes may be produced in the TBSNC [49].

Central sensitization of the TBSNC, along with peripheral sensitization reflecting hyperexcitability of afferent inputs, is thought to be consistent with the sensory experiences of human subjects under acute or chronic experimental orofacial pain conditions [49, 52]. A typical example is temporomandibular disorders (TMDs). They typically displayed allodynia an hyperalgesia and complicated by one or more comorbidities such as depression, anxiety, stress, sleep disturbance, and comorbid pain, as well as extraterritorial sensory abnormalities and spread of sensitivity (ETSS) to widespread areas innervated by the trigeminal nerve or even tissues supplied by upper cervical nerves [49, 52]. Unilateral transection of the medial branch of the infraorbital nerve supplying the medial upper lip and anterior teeth induced hypersensitivity in not only ipsilateral face but also ETSS lasting several weeks in extraterritorial trigeminal areas (e.g., contralateral ear and upper lip and ipsilateral lower lip) and even in nontrigeminal regions such as the hindpaw [49, 52, 53]. Therefore, ETSS can occur in different body regions in some chronic orofacial pain conditions. These clinical features are thought to be related to neuroplasticity and glioplasticity expressed as central sensitization occurring in the TBSNC and other brainstem areas (e.g., rostral ventromedial medulla and reticular formation) that receive trigeminal nociceptive inputs and send modulatory influences to areas of the spinal cord (e.g., spinal dorsal horn) [49]. Sensitized neurons of TBSNC may influence spinal nociceptive circuits and related behavior [49, 54].

The rostral ventromedial medulla (RVM) plays a major role in the endogenous modulation of nociceptive transmission in the spinal and trigeminal nociceptive pathways in the central nervous system [55]. It receives spinal and trigeminal somatosensory afferent inputs that include nociceptive inputs relayed through the spinal dorsal horn, medullary dorsal horn (also known as Sp5C), parabrachial nucleus, locus coeruleus, and subnucleus reticularis dorsalis and receives descending projections from higher brain centers such as midbrain periaqueductal gray (PAG) and hypothalamus [54, 55]. The major projection sites of the RVM include spinal and medullary dorsal horns, and stimulation of the RVM modulates nociceptive behavior and the activity of the spinal dorsal horn and nociceptive neurons in the medullary dorsal horn [54, 55]. Noxious thermal stimulation of the tail or perioral skin in the rat evoked the tail-flick response (TF) and jaw-motor response (JMR), and the latency of the JMR was significantly shorter than that of the TF. Heating at either tail or perioral skin caused an increase in ON-cell activity and a decrease in OFF-cell activity before the occurrence of the TF and JMR [54]. The activity of RVM is closely related to the activity of the medullary dorsal horn and plays an important role in the elaboration of diverse nociceptive behaviors evoked by noxious stimulation of widely separated regions of the body [56]. In connection with the central sensitization of Sp5C by trigeminal and high cervical excitatory inputs, it is likely that systemic pain may be caused by changes in RVM activity, which is closely related to the nociception processing of Sp5C.

Meanwhile, headache-related extracephalic pain referral to the upper and lower extremities has already been observed for a long time in migraine, a primary headache [56]. In fact, central sensitization and hyperactivity caused by noxious peripheral input have been demonstrated to occur not only in secondary neurons in the TCC but also in the third-order thalamic neurons that receive convergent information from the head and forearms [57, 58]. It has been confirmed that cutaneous allodynia during migraine attacks occurs not only in the referred pain area of the ipsilateral head but also in the nonreferred pain area in the ipsilateral head and extracephalic arm during migraine attacks [58]. Hypersensitivity of the third-order thalamic neurons can occur with stimulation of the large skin areas on both sides of the body following a small unilateral injury [59]. Thus, in migraine headaches, the importance of peripheral sensitization, as well as central sensitization, is emphasized [60, 61]. The extremity pain observed in the present case can also be interpreted as the occurrence of hypersensitivity of the thalamic third neurons, which is thought to be the pathophysiology of extension of cutaneous allodynia observed in migraine patients.

4. Conclusions

We report a case of referred extremity pain due to chronic GON entrapment that preceded referred trigeminal facial pain. The unexplained pain in the extremities lasted for 5 years without any specific cause identified via multiple tests. It was impossible to suspect an association with GON until later neck and facial pain appeared. This case presents diverse clinical manifestations of referred pain triggered by the sensitization of the TCC following chronic entrapment of the GON. GON entrapment may induce sensitization of TCC, which may affect brainstem and thalamus activity involved in nociceptive information processing in the central nervous system, resulting in associated pain in the extremities and ipsilateral face.

References

[1] T. Bartsch and P. J. Goadsby, "The trigeminocervical complex and migraine: current concepts and synthesis," *Current Pain and Headache Reports*, vol. 7, no. 5, pp. 371–376, 2003.

[2] R. Burstein, H. Yamamura, A. Malick, and A. M. Strassman, "Chemical stimulation of the intracranial dura induces enhanced responses to facial stimulation in brain stem trigeminal neurons," *Journal of Neurophysiology*, vol. 79, no. 2, pp. 964–982, 1998.

[3] T. Bartsch and P. J. Goadsby, "Stimulation of the greater occipital nerve induces increased central excitability of dural afferent input," *Brain*, vol. 125, no. 7, pp. 1496–1509, 2002.

[4] D. Levy and A. M. Strassman, "Mechanical response properties of A and C primary afferent neurons innervating the rat intracranial dura," *Journal of Neurophysiology*, vol. 88, no. 6, pp. 3021–3031, 2002.
[5] A. M. Strassman, Y. Mineta, and B. P. Vos, "Distribution of fos-like immunoreactivity in the medullary and upper cervical dorsal horn produced by stimulation of dural blood vessels in the rat," *Journal of Neuroscience*, vol. 14, no. 6, pp. 3725–3735, 1994.
[6] H. Kaube, K. A. Keay, K. L. Hoskin, R. Bandler, and P. J. Goadsby, "Expression of c-Fos-like immunoreactivity in the caudal medulla and upper cervical spinal cord following stimulation of the superior sagittal sinus in the cat," *Brain Research*, vol. 629, no. 1, pp. 95–102, 1993.
[7] P. J. Goadsby and K. L. Hoskin, "The distribution of trigeminovascular afferents in the non-human primate brain *Macaca nemestrina* a c-fos immunocytochemical study," *Journal of Anatomy*, vol. 190, no. 3, pp. 367–375, 1997.
[8] N. Bogduk, "Cervicogenic headache: anatomic basis and pathophysiologic mechanisms," *Current Pain and Headache Reports*, vol. 5, no. 4, pp. 382–386, 2001.
[9] D. A. Bakker, F. J. R. Richmond, and V. C. Abrahams, "Central projections from cat suboccipital muscles: a study using transganglionic transport of horseradish peroxidase," *The Journal of Comparative Neurology*, vol. 228, no. 3, pp. 409–421, 1984.
[10] W. L. Neuhuber and W. Zenker, "Central distribution of cervical primary afferents in the rat, with emphasis on proprioceptive projections to vestibular, perihypoglossal, and upper thoracic spinal nuclei," *The Journal of Comparative Neurology*, vol. 280, no. 2, pp. 231–253, 1989.
[11] N. Becser, G. Bovim, and O. Sjaastad, "Extracranial nerves in the posterior part of the head: anatomic variations and their possible clinical significance," *Spine*, vol. 23, no. 13, pp. 1435–1441, 1998.
[12] S. Scheurer, J. Gottschall, and V. Groh, "Afferent projections of the rat major occipital nerve studied by transganglionic tansport of HRP," *Anatomy and Embryology*, vol. 167, no. 3, pp. 425–438, 1983.
[13] K. Pfaller and J. Arvidsson, "Central distribution of trigeminal and upper cervical primary afferents in the rat studied by anterograde transport of horseradish peroxidase conjugated to wheat germ agglutinin," *The Journal of Comparative Neurology*, vol. 268, no. 1, pp. 91–108, 1988.
[14] J. Ellrich and K. Messlinger, "Afferent input to the medullary dorsal horn from the contralateral face in rat," *Brain Research*, vol. 826, no. 2, pp. 321–324, 1999.
[15] Headache Classification Committee of the International Headache Society (His), "The international classification of headache disorders," *Cephalalgia*, vol. 381, pp. 1–211, 2018.
[16] P. Vanelderen, A. Lataster, R. Levy, N. Mekhail, M. van Kleef, and J. Van Zundert, "Occipital neuralgia," *Pain Practice*, vol. 10, no. 2, pp. 137–144, 2010.
[17] R. S. Tubbs, E. G. Salter, J. C. Wellons, J. P. Blount, and W. J. Oakes, "Landmarks for the identification of the cutaneous nerves of the occiput and nuchal regions," *Clinical Anatomy*, vol. 20, no. 3, pp. 235–238, 2007.
[18] K. Natsis, X. Baraliakos, H. J. Appell, P. Tsikaras, I. Gigis, and J. Koebke, "The course of the greater occipital nerve in the suboccipital region: a proposal for setting landmarks for local anesthesia in patients with occipital neuralgia," *Clinical Anatomy*, vol. 19, no. 4, pp. 332–336, 2006.
[19] I. Ducic, M. Moriarty, and A. Al-Attar, "Anatomical variations of the occipital nerves: implications for the treatment of chronic headaches," *Plastic and Reconstructive Surgery*, vol. 123, no. 3, pp. 859–863, 2009.
[20] S. W. Mosser, B. Guyuron, J. E. Janis, and R. J. Rohrich, "The anatomy of the greater occipital nerve: implications for the etiology of migraine headaches," *Plastic and Reconstructive Surgery*, vol. 113, no. 2, pp. 693–697, 2004.
[21] A. Cesmebasi, M. A. Muhleman, P. Hulsberg et al., "Occipital neuralgia: anatomic considerations," *Clinical Anatomy*, vol. 28, no. 1, pp. 101–108, 2015.
[22] B. C. Son and J. G. Choi, "Hemifacial pain and hemisensory disturbance referred from occipital neuralgia caused by pathological vascular contact of the greater occipital nerve," *Case Reports in Neurological Medicine*, vol. 2017, Article ID 3827369, 5 pages, 2017.
[23] B. C. Son, "Referred trigeminal facial pain from occipital neuralgia occurring much earlier than occipital neuralgia," *Case Reports in Neurological Medicine*, vol. 2020, Article ID 8834865, 6 pages, 2020.
[24] B. C. Son, "Entrapment of the greater occipital nerve with chronic migraine and severe facial pain: a case report," *Journal of Neurological Surgery Part A: Central European Neurosurgery*, vol. 82, no. 05, pp. 494–499, 2021.
[25] C. I. Lee and B. C. Son, "Decompression of the greater occipital nerve for persistent headache attributed to whiplash accompanying referred facial trigeminal pain," *World Neurosurgery*, vol. 155, pp. e814–e823, 2021.
[26] B. C. Son, "Decompression of the greater occipital nerve for occipital neuralgia and chronic occipital headache caused by entrapment of the greater occipital nerve," *Journal of Neurological Surgery Part A: Central European Neurosurgery*, vol. 83, 2022.
[27] T. Bartsch and P. J. Goadsby, "Increased responses in trigeminocervical nociceptive neurons to cervical input after stimulation of the dura mater," *Brain*, vol. 126, no. 8, pp. 1801–1813, 2003.
[28] S. B. McMahon, G. R. Lewin, and P. D. Wall, "Central hyperexcitability triggered by noxious inputs," *Current Opinion in Neurobiology*, vol. 3, no. 4, pp. 602–610, 1993.
[29] C. J. Woolf and M. W. Salter, "Neuronal plasticity: increasing the gain in pain," *Science*, vol. 288, no. 5472, pp. 1765–1768, 2000.
[30] B. J. Sessle and J. W. Hu, "Mechanisms of pain arising from articular tissues," *Canadian Journal of Physiology and Pharmacology*, vol. 69, no. 5, pp. 617–626, 1991.
[31] H. G. Schaible and B. D. Grubb, "Afferent and spinal mechanisms of joint pain," *Pain*, vol. 55, no. 1, pp. 45–54, 1993.
[32] S. Mense, "Nociception from skeletal muscle in relation to clinical muscle pain," *Pain*, vol. 54, no. 3, pp. 241–289, 1993.
[33] M. Koltzenburg, "Neural mechanisms of cutaneous nociceptive pain," *The Clinical Journal of Pain*, vol. 16, pp. S131–S138, 2000.
[34] B. J. Sessle, "Invited review: the neurobiology of facial and dental pain: present knowledge, future directions," *Journal of Dental Research*, vol. 66, no. 5, pp. 962–981, 1987.
[35] J. W. Hu, B. J. Sessle, P. Raboisson, R. Dallel, and A. Woda, "Stimulation of craniofacial muscle afferents induces prolonged facilitatory effects in trigeminal nociceptive brain-stem neurones," *Pain*, vol. 48, no. 1, pp. 53–60, 1992.
[36] X. M. Yu, B. J. Sessle, and J. W. Hu, "Differential effects of cutaneous and deep application of inflammatory irritant on mechanoreceptive field properties of trigeminal brain stem nociceptive neurons," *Journal of Neurophysiology*, vol. 70, no. 4, pp. 1704–1707, 1993.

[37] F. W. L. Kerr, "A mechanism to account for frontal headache in cases of posterior fossa tumors," *Journal of Neurosurgery*, vol. 18, no. 5, pp. 605–609, 1961.
[38] E. J. Piovesan, P. A. Kowacs, C. E. Tatsui, M. C. Lange, L. C. Ribas, and L. C. Werneck, "Referred pain after painful stimulation of the greater occipital nerve in humans: evidence of convergence of cervical afferences on trigeminal nuclei," *Cephalalgia*, vol. 21, no. 2, pp. 107–109, 2001.
[39] J. D. England, "Entrapment neuropathies," *Current Opinion in Neurology*, vol. 12, no. 5, pp. 597–602, 1999.
[40] P. Blake and R. Burstein, "Emerging evidence of occipital nerve compression in unremitting head and neck pain," *The Journal of Headache and Pain*, vol. 20, no. 1, p. 76, 2019.
[41] A. B. Schmid, M. W. Coppieters, M. J. Ruitenberg, and E. M. McLachlan, "Local and remote immune-mediated inflammation after mild peripheral nerve compression in rats," *Journal of Neuropathology & Experimental Neurology*, vol. 72, no. 7, pp. 662–680, 2013.
[42] S. E. Berini, R. J. Spinner, M. E. Jentoft et al., "Chronic meralgia paresthetica and neurectomy: a clinical pathologic study," *Neurology*, vol. 82, no. 17, pp. 1551–1555, 2014.
[43] L. Villanueva and R. Noseda, "Trigeminal mechanisms of nociception," in *Wall and Melzack's Textbook Of Pain*, S. R. McMahon, M. Koltzenburg, T. Tracey, and D. C. Turk, Eds., Elsevier Saunders, Philadelphia, PA, USA, 6th edition, 2013.
[44] M. F. Jacquin, M. R. Wiegand, and W. E. Renehan, "Structure-function relationships in rat brain stem subnucleus interpolaris. VIII. Cortical inputs," *Journal of Neurophysiology*, vol. 64, no. 1, pp. 3–27, 1990.
[45] R. Noseda, L. Monconduit, L. Constandil, M. Chalus, and L. Villanueva, "Central nervous system networks involved in the processing of meningeal and cutaneous inputs from the ophthalmic branch of the trigeminal nerve in the rat," *Cephalalgia*, vol. 28, no. 8, pp. 813–824, 2008.
[46] R. Burstein, M. F. Cutrer, and D. Yarnitsky, "The development of cutaneous allodynia during a migraine attack: clinical evidence for the sequential recruitment of spinal and supraspinal nociceptive neurons in migraine," *Brain*, vol. 123, no. 8, pp. 1703–1709, 2000.
[47] A. Woda, J. L. Molat, and P. Luccarini, "Low doses of N-methyl-D-aspartate antagonists in superficial laminae of medulla oblongata facilitate wind-up of convergent neurones," *Neuroscience*, vol. 107, no. 2, pp. 317–327, 2001.
[48] M. F. Jacquin, M. Barcia, and R. W. Rhoades, "Structure-function relationships in rat brainstem subnucleus interpolaris: IV. Projection neurons," *The Journal of Comparative Neurology*, vol. 282, no. 1, pp. 45–62, 1989.
[49] B. J. Sessle, "Chronic orofacial pain: models, mechanisms, and genetic and related environmental influences," *International Journal of Molecular Sciences*, vol. 22, no. 13, p. 7112, 2021.
[50] K. Iwata and B. J. Sessle, "The evolution of neuroscience as a research field relevant to dentistry," *Journal of Dental Research*, vol. 98, no. 13, pp. 1407–1417, 2019.
[51] A. Kobayashi, M. Shinoda, B. J. Sessle et al., "Mechanisms involved in extraterritorial facial pain following cervical spinal nerve injury in rats," *Molecular Pain*, vol. 77-12 pages, 2011.
[52] J. D. Greenspan, G. D. Slade, N. Rathnayaka, R. Fillingim, R. Ohrbach, and W. Maixner, "Experimental pain sensitivity in subjects with temporomandibular disorders and multiple other chronic pain conditions: the OPPERA prospective cohort study," *Journal of Oral & Facial Pain and Headache*, vol. 34, pp. s43–s56, 2020.
[53] I. Suzuki, Y. Tsuboi, M. Shinoda et al., "Involvement of ERK phosphorylation of trigeminal spinal subnucleus caudalis neurons in thermal hypersensitivity in rats with infraorbital nerve injury," *PLoS One*, vol. 8, no. 2, Article ID e57278, 2013.
[54] J. S. Tang, C. Y. Chiang, J. O. Dostrovsky, D. Yao, and B. J. Sessle, "Responses of neurons in rostral ventromedial medulla to nociceptive stimulation of craniofacial region and tail in rats," *Brain Research*, vol. 1767, Article ID 147539, 2021.
[55] H. Fields H and A. Basbaum, "Central nervous system mechanisms of pain modulation," in *Textbook of Pain*, P. Wall and R. Melzack, Eds., Churchill Livingstone, Edinburgh, Scotland, 2010.
[56] R. J. Guiloff and M. Fruns, "Migrainous limb pain. A historical note," *Headache*, vol. 30, no. 3, pp. 138–141, 1990.
[57] R. Burstein, D. Yarnitsky, I. Goor-Aryeh, B. J. Ransil, and Z. H. Bajwa, "An association between migraine and cutaneous allodynia," *Annals of Neurology*, vol. 47, no. 5, pp. 614–624, 2000.
[58] A. M. Strassman, S. A. Raymond, and R. Burstein, "Sensitization of meningeal sensory neurons and the origin of headaches," *Nature*, vol. 384, no. 6609, pp. 560–564, 1996.
[59] G. Guilbaud, J. M. Benoist, F. Jazat, and M. Gautron, "Neuronal responsiveness in the ventrobasal thalamic comp; lex of rats with an experimental peripheral mononeuropathy," *Journal of Neurophysiology*, vol. 64, no. 5, pp. 1537–1554, 1990.
[60] J. Olsen, R. Burnstein, M. Ashina, and P. Tfelt-Hansen, "Origin of pain in migraine: evidence for peripheral sensitization," *The Lancet Neurology*, vol. 8, no. 7, pp. 679–690, 2009.
[61] R. Burstein, P. Blake, A. Schain, and C. Perry, "Extracranial origin of headache," *Current Opinion in Neurology*, vol. 30, no. 3, pp. 263–271, 2017.

29

Bithalamic Infarction (Artery of Percheron Occlusion) after Anterior Cervical Discectomy and Fusion

Hatem B. Afana[1], **Nidal M. M. Abuhadrous**[2] and **Alaa Eldin Elsharkawy**[3,4]

[1] *Orthopaedic Department, European Gaza Hospital, Gaza Strip, State of Palestine*
[2] *Neurosurgery Department, European Gaza Hospital, Gaza Strip, State of Palestine*
[3] *Neurosurgery Department, Bonifatius Hospital, Lingen, Germany*
[4] *Neurosurgery Teaching Program, University of Traditional Medicine, Yerevan, Armenia*

Correspondence should be addressed to Hatem B. Afana; hatembafana@gmail.com
and Alaa Eldin Elsharkawy; alaa.elsharkawy@googlemail.com

Academic Editor: Jacqueline A. Pettersen

Bithalamic infarction resulting from occlusion of the artery of Percheron after cervical spine surgery is a rare pathological entity. Diagnosis and early detection are challenging. Prompt management may help to improve the outcome. We present a case of a 39-year-old male patient, smoker, diagnosed with multiple cervical disc herniations, who underwent Anterior Cervical Discectomy and Fusion (ACDF) for C3-C4, C4-C5, and C5-C6. During the 2-hour and 50-minute surgery, the patient was lying supine with his neck hyperextended. The intraoperative procedure was uneventful. During surgery, blood pressure ranged around 110 mmHg\50 mmHg. At the end of surgery, the patient's recovery from general anesthesia was normal with no delaying or complication; on next the day, patient developed a sudden loss of consciousness. Urgent brain computed tomography (CT) was normal; two days later, follow-up CT and CT Angiography (CTA) revealed bilateral thalamic infarction with right vertebral artery occlusion from its origin. Intraoperative surgical manipulation, hypotensive anesthesia, and prolonged neck hyperextension might have contributed to stroke in this patient. ACDF carries a potential risk for posterior circulation stroke. Artery of Percheron infarction should be considered in the differential diagnosis of patients developing a sudden loss of consciousness after ACDF. Vertebral artery thrombosis should be taken into account as an important possible cause of embolism.

1. Introduction

Anterior cervical discectomy with fusion (ACDF) is an established intervention for cervical degenerative disease [1]. ACDF is a relatively safe procedure with a very low morbidity and mortality rate [2]. However, this procedure may be associated with serious postoperative complications like strokes. Several case reports have described patients suffering strokes following ACDF [3–5]. Published data showed that patients with carotid artery stenosis have a greater incidence of postoperative stroke [5].

A postoperative stroke of the posterior circulation in a previously asymptomatic patient is a rare neurological event [6]. Thalamic infarction is relatively uncommon, it accounts for about 11% of all vertebrobasilar infarcts [7].

Bithalamic infarction after ACDF is a very rare presentation of stroke. A combination of predisposing factors and anatomic variations may be responsible for this type of stroke [7].

One of the vascular variations of the brain where a cerebral blood vessel supplies structures on both sides is the artery of Percheron. The artery of Percheron (AOP) is a rare anatomic variation in the posterior circulation of the brain in which a single arterial trunk arises from the first part of the posterior cerebral artery (PCA) and supplies the medial region of both thalami. The occlusion of the artery of Percheron results in bilateral infarctions in the middle aspects of thalami and brainstem [8, 9]. We report a case of bithalamic infarction due to embolic occlusion of the artery of Percheron as a consequence of vertebral artery (VA) thrombosis.

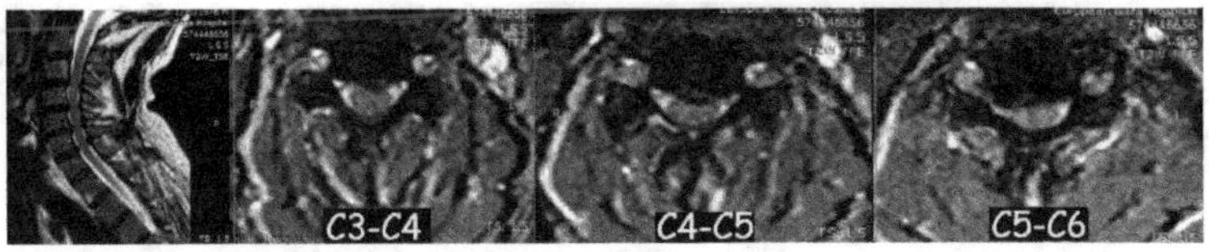

FIGURE 1: Preoperative cervical magnetic resonance image (MRI) demonstrated multilevel cervical disc with myelopathy C3-C4, C4-C5, C5-C6.

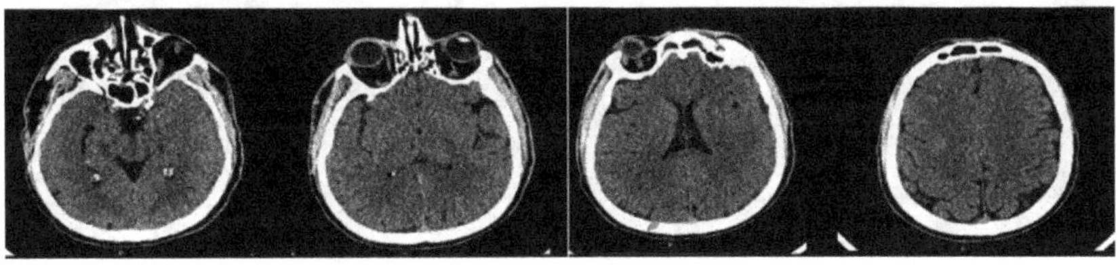

FIGURE 2: Normal finding postoperative brain CT.

2. Case Presentation

A 39-year-old male patient, smoker, presented in the outpatient clinic with chronic neck pain radiating to the right upper limb. The patient had no history of chronic disease and no previous surgeries. Cervical magnetic resonance image (MRI) demonstrated multilevel cervical disc herniation (C3-C4, C4-C5, C5-C6) with T2 high signal intensity changes (Figure 1). The patient examination was normal except for cervical muscle spasm and tenderness. Preoperative laboratory examination was within normal range. After the failure of standard conservative treatment, anterior 3-level ACDF was recommended.

Standard microscopic anterior ACDF approach in general anesthesia with endotracheal tube was carried out. During surgery, the patient was in supine position with the extension of the neck by the support of the shoulders with a pillow, plaster traction of both shoulders, and Fixation of the head with plaster. For the interbody spaces, PEEK cages of size 5.0 mm were used. Interpretatively there were no complications or bleeding. Surgery duration was 2 hours and 50 minutes. The patient recovery from general anesthesia was smooth with no delaying or complication. The first 18 hours after surgery were uneventful with normal postoperative cervical X-ray.

However, 18 hours after surgery, he developed a sudden loss of consciousness. Clinical examination showed 8-9/15 score on Glasgow Coma Score (GCS), blood pressure 110/70 mmHg, temperature 37 degrees, pulse 84 beats per minute, oxygen saturation 98%, and blood glucose 113 mg/dl by glucometer with normal ECG. Urgent brain and cervical CT was done (Figure 2); no abnormality was detected in brain and cervical spine.

CT Angiography and MRI were not available at this time. Bilateral carotid Duplex ultrasound revealed normal blood flow in both carotid arteries. Full laboratory investigations were done and were within normal. Provisional diagnosis as stroke was done and the patient was transported emergently to the intensive care unit (ICU) for observation under heparin 1000 IU infusion/hour.

In the second postoperative day, the patient showed some improvement in level of consciousness with slurred speech, hypersomnia and loss of interest, right sided ptosis with vertical gaze palsy and diminished light reflex, memory impairment (amnesia), and right upper limb paralysis.

On the 3rd day, CT brain and angiography revealed a bilateral thalamic with upper brainstem ischemic infarction (Figure 3), with total occlusion of Rt vertebral artery from its origin and normal flow in both carotid arteries. On the same day, the patient shifted back to neurosurgery department. Heparin infusion was stopped and shifted to clexane 80mg SC bid with the addition of cerebrolysin, ginkgo biloba+Mg, Trental, and a multivitamin.

On the 7th day after operation, patient was shifted to rehabilitation, with the improvement of the upper arm paralysis and cerebellar ataxia.

After 2 weeks, brain and cervical MRI showed a bilateral thalamic infarction with no compression on the spinal cord (Figure 4). Clinical examination after two weeks showed GCS 15/15 with normal speech, no cerebellar ataxia, no upper limb paralysis, but continuing to have hypersomnia and loss of interest with aggressive response (behavior changes), amnesia (mainly short memory amnesia), and downward gaze palsy.

At 3 months of follow-up, CT Angiography revealed a bilateral hypodense area in both thalami with no recanalization of right vertebral artery (Figure 5). The patient was conscious and oriented, full motor power, normal gait, no speech, sleep, and behavior deficiency. Intermittent short memory amnesia and downward gaze palsy were still present.

3. Discussion

ACDF is a relatively safe procedure, with ischemic stroke following Anterior Cervical Discectomy and Fusion (ACDF) being a very rare complication [2, 10]. Higher risk of postoperative stroke was reported in patients with carotid artery stenosis [5].

Stroke due to one vertebral artery occlusion has also been reported. Posterior circulation stroke and AOP occlusion are a serious complication with a higher risk of mortality and

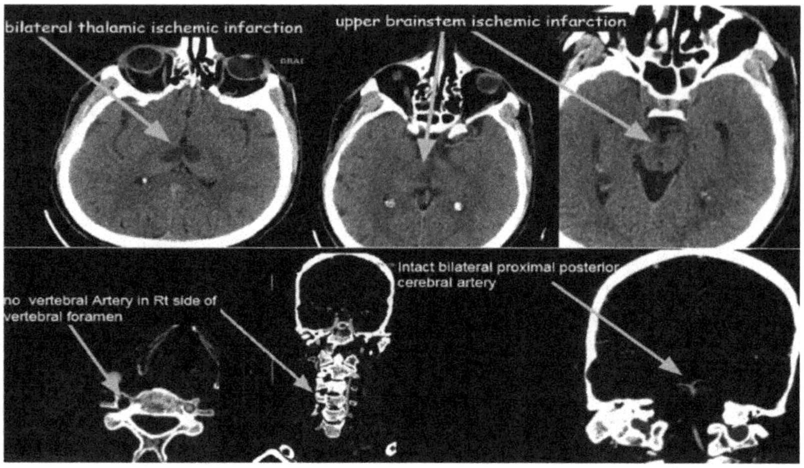

FIGURE 3: Brain and cervical CT Angiography (3rd day Post Op) revealed bilateral thalamic with upper brainstem ischemic infarction, with total occlusion of right vertebral artery from its origin and patent bilateral carotid artery with a normal flow.

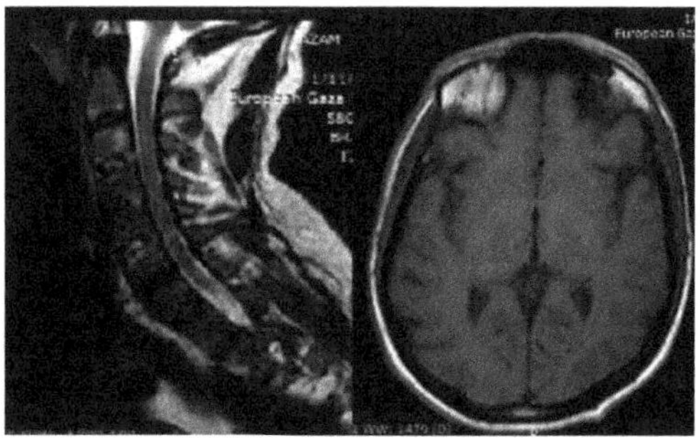

FIGURE 4: Brain and cervical MRI (after 2 weeks) show bilateral thalamic infarction with no compression on the spinal cord.

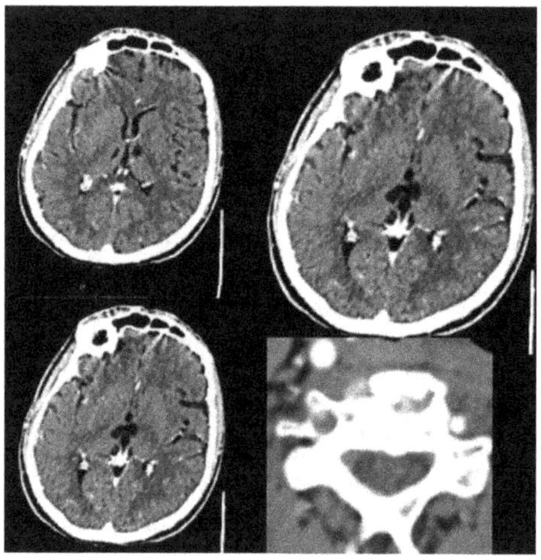

FIGURE 5: Brain and cervical CT Angiography (after 3 months) revealed a bilateral hypodense area in the site of both thalami with no recanalization of right vertebral artery.

morbidity [6, 9, 11]. Yunoki et al., 2017, reported a case of right cerebellar infarction in a 50-year-old woman due to vertebral artery occlusion after ACDF [6].

A bilateral thalamic stroke is an unusual event; it raises the suspicion of the presence of the anatomical variation with the artery of Percheron, because both sides of the thalamus are supplied by the same blood supply, despite the fact that bilateral infarcts due to osculation of artery Percheron has not been established [7].

Several pathological processes may cause occlusion of VA leading to stroke. The common predisposing factor is atherosclerotic disease, dissection, fibrous banding in the neck, extrinsic compression in its second and third parts due to trauma of the cervical vertebrae or osteophyte impingement and compression, vasculitis, and arthritis [12]. Extracranial vertebral artery stenosis of the first part may account for up to 20% of posterior circulation ischemic strokes. Left side vertebral stenosis occurs more frequently [12]. Choi et al. reported a case of cerebellar infarction in 38-year-old man originating from vertebral artery stenosis caused by a hypertrophied uncovertebral joint after ACDF [13]. VA occlusion after ACDF [6], cervical fracture [14], chiropractic manipulation [15], or even after abrupt head movement [15] has been reported.

A potential mechanism of VA occlusion in such cases is intimal disruption followed by thrombus formation and, thus, clots occlusion of the vessel lumen. The reason why VA occlusion occurred, in this case, is unknown; however, repeated use of a spreader with forced distortion and/or stretching in three consecutive intervertebral spaces may have triggered this sequence of events [6, 16].

In the case of AOP, an embolism is the most frequent cause of occlusion [9]. In our case, there was vertebral artery occlusion on Rt side thrombosis from the origin. Embolus from vertebral artery to the AOP is most probably the case of the occlusion of AOP.

Interpretation of the case is challenging due to the limited evidence regarding bilateral thalamic infarction because of AOP. The scenario in our case as we assume is hyperextension injuries of the vertebral artery during the surgery. The hyperextension injury leads to disruption of intima and gradual development of thrombus. Hours after trauma, an embolism to AOP was the cause of symptoms. Our assumption is supported with published data which showed that hyperextension injuries are one mechanism of closed injury to the vertebral artery and that artery is at risk, especially in the mid-cervical region and that the fibro-osseous tunnel does not offer adequate protection [17].

López-Serna et al. reported a similar case of bilateral thalamic stroke due to occlusion of the artery of Percheron in a patient with patent foramen ovale; the outcome was similar to the outcome in our case [7].

Clinical outcome is not poor, but the initial recovery phase is crucial. If the patient does not improve in the initial phase, the chance for further recovery appears to be low; hence, in the appropriate patient, thrombolytic therapy should be considered [9].

The published cases show that the state of consciousness may spontaneously resolve during the first 3 weeks [7] with some patients without persistent neurological symptoms [6]. The outcome in our case is in agreement with published data which showed that unilateral vertebral artery occlusion seldom results in a permanent neurological deficit. However, transient neurological symptoms are not uncommon [17]. Published data showed that memory deficits, vertical gaze paresis, and hypersomnia considerably subsided in the majority of patients [18].

Our experience demonstrates the need for surgeons performing ADCF procedures to be aware of this potential complication. There are many other prophylactic treatments of this complication such as maintaining appropriate cervical positioning during surgery or prevention of postoperative dehydration; however, care should be taken to avoid intimal disruption of the VA by overly dilating the intervertebral space.

Consent

Written informed consent was obtained from the patient for publication of this case report and any accompanying images. A copy of the written consent is available for review by the Editor-in-Chief of this journal.

References

[1] T. Sugawara, "Anterior cervical spine surgery for degenerative disease: a review," *Neurologia Medico-Chirurgica*, 2015.

[2] A. Nanda, M. Sharma, A. Sonig, S. Ambekar, and P. Bollam, "Surgical complications of anterior cervical diskectomy and fusion for cervical degenerative disk disease: a single surgeon's experience of 1576 patients," *World Neurosurgery*, vol. 82, no. 6, pp. 1380–1387, 2014.

[3] Y.-C. Yeh, W.-Z. Sun, C.-P. Lin, C.-K. Hui, I.-R. Huang, and T.-S. Lee, "Prolonged retraction on the normal common carotid artery induced lethal stroke after cervical spine surgery.," *The Spine Journal*, vol. 29, no. 19, pp. E431–434, 2004.

[4] K. R. Chin, J. Seale, V. Butron, and V. Cumming, "Postoperative cervical haematoma complicated by ipsilateral carotid thrombosis and aphasia after anterior cervical fusion: a case report," *Case Reports in Medicine*, vol. 2013, Article ID 590639, 2013.

[5] M. Chughtai, A. A. Sultan, J. Padilla et al., "Postoperative stroke after anterior cervical discectomy and fusion in patients with carotid artery stenosis: a statewide database analysis," *The Spine Journal*, 2018.

[6] M. Yunoki, K. Suzuki, and A. Uneda, "Vertebral artery occlusion after anterior cervical discectomy with fusion," *Iranian Journal of Neurology*, 2017.

[7] R. López-Serna, P. González-Carmona, and M. López-Martínez, "Bilateral thalamic stroke due to occlusion of the artery of Percheron in a patient with patent foramen ovale: a case report," *Journal of Medical Case Reports*, vol. 3, no. 1, article 7392, 2009.

[8] M. Karcaaltincaba, J. Strottman, and L. Washington, "Multidedector-row CT angiography findings in the bilateral aortic arch origin of the vertebral arteries," *American Journal of Neuroradiology*, vol. 24, no. 1, article 157, pp. 2005–2008, 2003.

[9] S. Aaron, S. Mani, A. T. Prabhakar et al., "Stuck with a drowsy patient, evoke the Percheron," *Neurology India*, vol. 63, no. 4, pp. 542–547, 2015.

[10] C. S. Graffeo, R. C. Puffer, E. F. M. Wijdicks, and W. E. Krauss, "Delayed cerebral infarct following anterior cervical diskectomy and fusion," *Surgical Neurology International*, vol. 7, no. 1, 2016.

[11] Y. F. Tsai, A. G. Doufas, C. S. Huang, F. C. Liou, and C. M Lin, "Postoperative coma in a patient with complete basilar syndrome after anterior cervical discectomy," *Canadian Journal of Anesthesia*, vol. 53, no. 2, pp. 202–207, 2006.

[12] G. C. Cloud and H. S. Markus, "Diagnosis and management of vertebral artery stenosis," *QJM: An International Journal of Medicine*, vol. 96, no. 1, pp. 27–34, 2003.

[13] J. M. Choi, H. J. Hong, S. K. Chang, and S. H. Oh, "Cerebellar infarction originating from vertebral artery stenosis caused by a hypertrophied uncovertebral joint," *Journal of Stroke and Cerebrovascular Diseases*, vol. 21, no. 8, pp. 908.e7–908.e9, 2012.

[14] H. Taneichi, K. Suda, T. Kajino, and K. Kaneda, "Traumatically induced vertebral artery occlusion associated with cervical spine injuries: prospective study using magnetic resonance angiography," *The Spine Journal*, vol. 30, no. 17, pp. 1955–1962, 2005.

[15] M. J. Haynes, K. Vincent, C. Fischhoff, A. P. Bremner, O. Lanlo, and G. J. Hankey, "Assessing the risk of stroke from neck manipulation: A systematic review," *International Journal of Clinical Practice*, vol. 66, no. 10, pp. 940–947, 2012.

[16] M. Komatsu, K. Suda, M. Takahata, S. Matsumoto et al., "Delayed bilateral vertebral artery occlusion after cervical spine injury: a case report," *Spinal Cord Series and Cases*, vol. 2, no. 1, article 16031, 2016.

[17] J. A. Louw, N. A. Mafoyane, B. Small, and C. P. Neser, "Occlusion of the vertebral artery in cervical spine dislocations," *Journal of Bone and Joint Surgery-British*, vol. 72, no. 4, pp. 679–681, 1990.

[18] M. Gentilini, E. De Renzi, and G. Crisi, "Bilateral paramedian thalamic artery infarcts: report of eight cases," *Journal of Neurology, Neurosurgery & Psychiatry*, vol. 50, no. 7, pp. 900–909, 1987.

30

Manganese Neurotoxicity as a Complication of Chronic Total Parenteral Nutrition

Alisha Khan,[1] **Jonathan Hingre,**[2] **and Amit S. Dhamoon**[1]

[1]*Department of Medicine, SUNY Upstate Medical University, Syracuse, NY, USA*
[2]*College of Medicine, SUNY Upstate Medical University, Syracuse, NY, USA*

Correspondence should be addressed to Alisha Khan; khanali@upstate.edu

Academic Editor: Abbass Amirjamshidi

Manganese accumulation in the central nervous system creates clinical symptoms of cognitive dysfunction, behavioral changes, and movement disorders resembling Parkinson's disease. Radiographic features of this rare clinical entity include symmetric T1 hyperintensities in the bilateral globus pallidi, with corresponding hypointensities on T2-weighted images. Total parenteral nutrition (TPN) is an increasingly used potentially lifesaving therapy for patients who cannot tolerate enteral nutrition. However, when used over a period of several weeks to months, its associated risks and complications carry significant morbidity and mortality. One of the more rare complications of TPN use is manganese toxicity. We provided care for a 38-year-old female on chronic TPN who presented to the hospital with Parkinsonian features, confusion, falls, and lethargy. MRI brain showed T1 hyperintensities in the bilateral globus pallidi, which were attributed to manganese toxicity from chronic TPN use. Supporting evidence for this rare entity included decreased signal intensity in the bilateral globus pallidi on T2-weighted images and T1 hyperintensities in the substantia nigra. With antifungal treatment and permanent cessation of TPN, her mentation and neurological symptoms began to improve within a week. Repeat MRI brain performed one month after discontinuation of TPN revealed improvement of the T1 hyperintensities in the bilateral globus pallidi. Our objective in presenting this case is to highlight manganese neurotoxicity as a rare complication of TPN in a patient without known hepatic dysfunction and to emphasize the importance of routinely monitoring patients for the possible adverse effects of chronic TPN. Our case is among the handful of published cases in which a patient without known liver dysfunction, which is the primary organ responsible for manganese elimination from the body, developed manganese neurotoxicity.

1. Introduction

Total parenteral nutrition (TPN) is a short-term potentially lifesaving therapy for patients who cannot tolerate enteral nutrition. TPN also has several risks and patients need to be monitored closely while on therapy. One of the more rare complications of TPN is manganese toxicity. Manganese is an essential dietary mineral tightly regulated in humans through the control of absorption, distribution, storage, and excretion. Elevated tissue levels of manganese can occur from excessive exposure, often through inhalation or parenteral exposures [1]. Parenteral exposure to manganese has high bioavailability because normal regulatory mechanisms in the gastrointestinal tract are bypassed. Manganese is cleared through the liver, increasing the risk for overload in patients with hepatic dysfunction [2]. Manganese accumulation in the central nervous system creates clinical symptoms of cognitive dysfunction, behavioral changes, and movement disorders resembling Parkinson's disease. Clinical features include bradykinesia, tremor, weakness, muscle rigidity, mask-like facies, postural instability, gait disturbances, headaches, confusion, and somnolence [3]. In this report, we will further describe the clinical presentation and corresponding imaging results of manganese toxicity due to TPN.

2. Case Presentation

Our patient is a 38-year-old woman with a past medical history most significant for a Roux-en-Y gastric bypass surgery in March 2017, complicated by a marginal ulcer at the anastomosis site with subsequent perforation. The patient could not tolerate oral nutrition and became severely malnourished, and a PICC line was placed for TPN in December 2017. Chronic TPN use led to recurrent candidemia with blood cultures growing *Candida albicans* resistant to fluconazole and voriconazole. Over several months, her PICC line was replaced thrice, and she was ultimately treated with micafungin. The patient had multiple admissions over the past few months for workup of altered mental status and unsteady gait. Her other past medical history included systemic lupus erythematosus treated with mycophenolate mofetil and hydroxychloroquine, left portal vein branch thrombosis on enoxaparin therapy, type 2 diabetes mellitus not on insulin, fibromyalgia, depression, and anxiety. She presented to our hospital in July 2018 with complaints of tremors, impaired mobility, confusion, gait instability, falls, and lethargy.

On admission, she was noted to be confused, with horizontal nystagmus and dilated pupils as well as bradypnea. Dilated fundus examination was indicative of candida retinitis. She was lethargic but arousable. Her speech was difficult to understand, and the history of presenting illness was provided primarily by the patient's mother who relayed to the team that she had been having tremors, episodes of confusion, and numerous falls for the past several months. Her mother also noticed that she had increased irritability and emotional lability during this time. She was initially admitted to the intensive care unit for airway management due to her acute encephalopathy. Due to a lack of meningeal signs, a lumbar puncture was not performed.

The infectious disease service was consulted, and she was started on liposomal amphotericin B and flucytosine for a total of 6 weeks. MRI brain showed worsening T1 hyperintensities from June 2018 to July 2018 in the bilateral globus pallidi, as evidenced by the arrows in Figures 1(a) and 1(b), which were thought to be secondary to manganese toxicity from chronic TPN use. Furthermore, a repeat MRI brain was performed in August 2018, one month after discontinuation of TPN, which showed improvement of the T1 hyperintensities in the bilateral globus pallidi, as evidenced by the white arrows in Figure 1(c), approaching the intensity level noted in June 2018. Other supporting findings included T1 hyperintensities in the substantia nigra, as evidenced by the arrows in Figure 2, and decreased signal in the bilateral globus pallidi on T2-weighted images, as evidenced by the arrows in Figure 3. With antifungal treatment and cessation of TPN, her mentation and neurological symptoms improved within 3-4 days of cessation of TPN.

General surgery was consulted for gastrostomy tube placement in her remnant stomach, as the patient was unable to consume more than 500 calories by mouth per day due to complaints of nausea and vomiting. Although our patient presented to the hospital seven months after initiation of TPN therapy, her Parkinsonian symptoms had begun to manifest after three months on TPN.

3. Investigations

Her MRI brain, shown in Figure 1, showed symmetric T1 hyperintensities in the bilateral globus pallidi, a finding compatible with manganese toxicity. A serum manganese (Mn) level was elevated at 4.0 μg/L (reference range <2.5 μg/L), collected 1 day after TPN was permanently discontinued. Relevant laboratory investigations revealed a copper level of 22 μg/dL, zinc level of 44 μg/dL, vitamin B1 level of 149.8 nmol/L, vitamin B12 level of 703 ng/L, and 1,25-dihydroxyvitamin D level of 7.3 ng/mL, for which she was started on weekly supplementation. CBC on admission showed a WBC count of $7.5 \times 10^3/\mu$L, haemoglobin level of 9.2 g/dL, haematocrit level of 27.6%, platelet level of $453 \times 10^3/\mu$L, MCV of 79.9 fL, and red cell distribution width of 18.2%. CMP on admission showed the following levels: sodium 146 mmol/L, potassium 4.8 mmol/L, chloride 107 mmol/L, bicarbonate 26 mmol/L, blood urea nitrogen 27 mg/dL, creatinine 0.94 mg/dL, glucose 228 mg/dL, calcium 8.5 mg/dL, ALT 40 U/L, AST 28 U/L, albumin 3.3 g/dL, alkaline phosphatase 159 IU/L, anion gap 13 mEq/L, total bilirubin <0.2 mg/dL, direct bilirubin <0.1 mg/dL, and osmolality 314 mmol/kg.

The composition of the TPN solution she received from December 2017 to July 2018 was as follows: 40 g of 15% amino acids solution, 120 g of 70% dextrose solution, 15 g of 30% fat emulsion, 21.1 g of 4 mEq/mL sodium chloride solution, 10 mmol of 45 mmol/15 mL sodium phosphate solution, 45.5 mEq of 4 mEq/mL sodium acetate solution, 2.15 g of 10% calcium gluconate solution, 70 mEq of 2 mEq/mL potassium chloride solution, 2.22 g of 50% magnesium sulfate solution, 10 mL of adult multivitamin solution, 100 mg of 100 mg/mL thiamine solution, and 978.96 mL of sterile water solution. Importantly, a 1 mL injection of a solution containing trace elements (Cr-Cu-Mn-Se-Zn: 10-1000-500-60 mcg/mL) was added to each bag of TPN. In other words, each bag of TPN contained 500 mcg of manganese.

4. Differential Diagnosis

(i) T1 hyperintensities in the globus pallidus and clinical features of Parkinson's have been noted in individuals with inherited mutations of SLC30A10, a Mn transporter gene.

(ii) Bilateral pallidal hyperintensity can also be seen in patients with ischemic or hypoxic encephalopathy, hypoparathyroidism or pseudohypoparathyroidism, hamartomas of neurofibromatosis type 1, and cerebral haemorrhage due to Japanese encephalitis; however, these conditions would not present with Parkinsonism.

(iii) Ephedrone abuse is an emerging cause of Mn-induced Parkinsonism.

(iv) Both inherited and acquired hypermanganesemia have similar presentations and lead to Mn deposition in the basal ganglia and hyperintense signalling on T1-weighted images.

(v) Prior to brain imaging, infective causes of her presentation would have included encephalitis, fungemia, and bacteremia; however, these were less likely as the patient was afebrile and did not have an

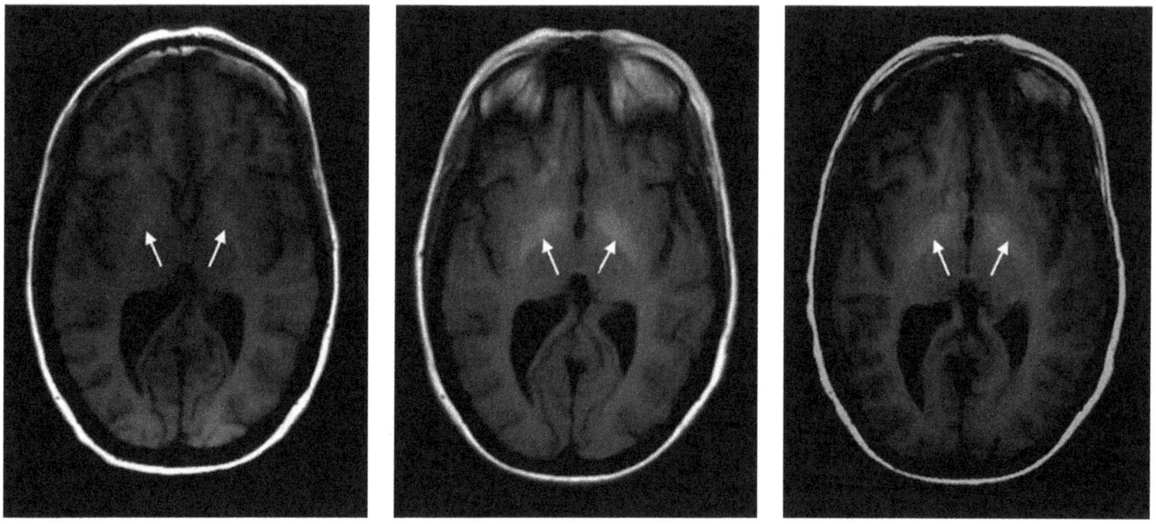

June 2018 (a) July 2018 (b) August 2018 (c)

Figure 1: Axial T1-weighted MRI brain performed serially over three months, showing the progression of the T1 hyperintensities in the globus pallidi from June 2018 to July 2018, followed by the improvement of the T1 hyperintensities in August 2018, one month after discontinuation of TPN. (a) Evidence of developing T1 hyperintensities in the bilateral globus pallidi on a previous hospital admission in June 2018. (b) Further increase in signal in the bilateral globus pallidi on T1-weighted images in July 2018, corresponding to her pronounced Parkinsonian features on clinical presentation. (c) Improvement in the T1 hyperintensities in the globus pallidi, collected one month after cessation of TPN use and corresponding to near-resolution of her Parkinsonism.

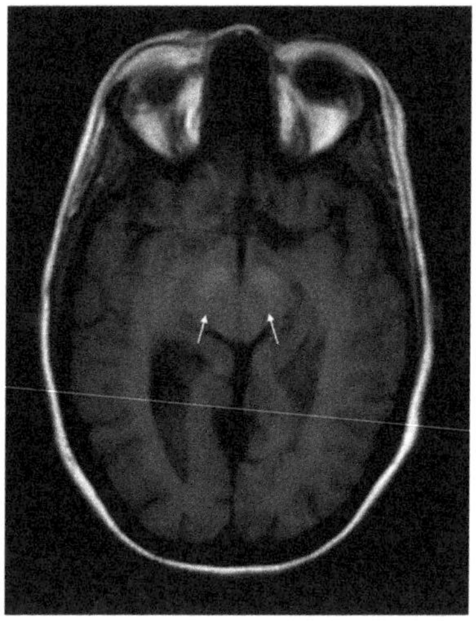

July 2018

Figure 2: Axial T1-weighted MRI brain from July 2018 showing hyperintensities in the substantia nigra, as evidenced by the two white arrows.

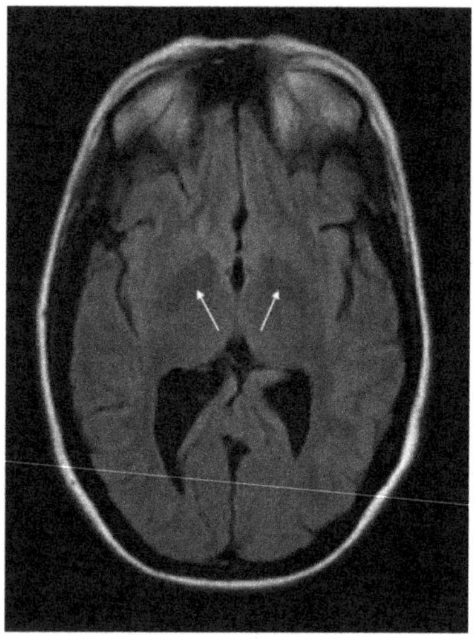

July 2018

Figure 3: Supporting evidence for manganese neurotoxicity includes decreased signal intensity in the bilateral globus pallidi on axial T2-weighted images of the MRI brain from July 2018.

abnormal white cell count or localizing neurological signs. Noninfective causes would include drug intoxication, aseptic meningitis, and autoimmune meningitis with her history of SLE.

5. Discussion

Manganese (Mn) is a metal that is essential for the human body. It is a requirement for the maintenance of the nervous and immunological systems, acts as a cofactor for many enzymes, and participates in the regulation of blood sugar levels and vitamin metabolism [4–7]. In particular, Mn is a required component of Mn metalloproteins, which function as oxidoreductases, transferases, hydrolases, lyases, isomerases, and ligases [8]. Mn is also required for the functioning of enzymes such as arginase, glutamine synthetase, phosphoenolpyruvate decarboxylase, pyruvate carboxylase, and Mn superoxide dismutase [9]. These are some of the reasons why Mn is a component of nutritional support formulas such as TPN, as well as infant and neonatal formulas. Mn has a propensity to form tight complexes with other molecules normally leading to low free plasma and tissue concentrations [10, 11].

A metal's concentration in various parts of the body depends on its absorption, distribution, storage, and excretion. Despite the fact that there are over a dozen proteins involved in maintaining Mn homeostasis, including the divalent metal transporter, transferrin and transferrin receptor, superoxide dismutase, ceruloplasmin, and ferroportin [12], among various others, manganese toxicity develops relatively rapidly due to the mechanisms by which our bodies regulate Mn as discussed below.

5.1. Absorption. Enteric absorption in the small intestine and absorption from the pulmonary system following airborne, usually occupational exposure, are the most common ways through which Mn enters our bodies [4]. Water contaminated with Mn from nonpublic sources can also lead to toxicity [13]. Inhaled Mn can bypass first-pass metabolism by the liver as well as the blood-brain barrier to enter the nervous system via the olfactory tract [4, 14, 15]. Intravenous injection of illicit narcotics is an emerging cause of Mn toxicity [16]. A less common mechanism for manganese toxicity is prolonged TPN use, as well as prolonged use of infant and neonatal formulas.

5.2. Distribution and Storage. Mn accumulates mainly in the liver, brain, and bone; however, the brain is the organ most likely to be affected by Mn toxicity. It is postulated that the choroid plexus transports Mn into the nervous system, as Mn is detectable in the cerebrospinal fluid before it is detected in the brain tissue [17]. Mn can also enter the brain through the capillary endothelial cells of the blood-brain barrier or directly by the way of the olfactory nerve [7]. In rat brains, the globus pallidi, followed by the substantia nigra pars compacta, thalamus, caudate putamen, axon bundles, and cortex, accumulate the highest concentrations of Mn [4, 18]. In humans, the superior and inferior colliculi, amygdala, stria terminalis, and hippocampus are additional susceptible areas [4]. In these areas, the half-life of Mn is 5–7 days, which is longer than in other organs [19]. In rat models, even when Mn reaches a steady-state concentration in the blood, the CSF concentration of Mn continues to rise due to its slower elimination rate, which likely contributes to the fact that the brain is the organ most susceptible to Mn toxicity [4, 20]. In addition, iron deficiency can also precipitate Mn toxicity, as both Mn and Fe compete for similar transport proteins [21].

5.3. Excretion. The fecal hepatobiliary system is the primary route of Mn elimination, accounting for 80% of Mn elimination, followed by the urinary system [4, 22]. Sweat and breast milk also serve as the minor routes of elimination [4, 23]. Therefore, in individuals with liver failure, due to the decreased excretion of Mn in bile, Mn toxicity becomes more likely. Mn hepatic encephalopathy is a term that has been coined to specifically identify individuals in whom hepatic dysfunction is the primary cause of Mn neurotoxicity.

5.4. Manganese Toxicity. Although idiopathic Parkinson's disease and Mn-induced neurotoxicity both present with extrapyramidal symptoms, their target areas in the brain differ, resulting in similar but differing clinical presentations. Mn primarily affects the globus pallidus and the striatum of the basal ganglia, whereas idiopathic Parkinson's disease affects the substantia nigra [7]. Mn preferentially deposits in the dopaminergic cells of the basal ganglia, notably the globus pallidus, resulting in extrapyramidal motor disturbances presenting similarly to Parkinson's disease. In fact, Mn has been found to upregulate histone deacetylase (HDAC) and downregulate histone acetyltransferase (HAT) in neuronal cells, which damages dopaminergic neurons [24].

Mn has been found to disrupt the signalling of dopamine, serotonin, and glutamine, as evidenced by synchrotron X-ray fluorescent imaging, which provides insight into Mn toxic kinetics and its neural distribution. High levels of Mn exposure have also been noted to decrease the copper levels in the subventricular and subgranular zones of the brain, which have been postulated to be responsible for the nonmotor symptoms of Mn-induced Parkinsonism [4, 25, 26].

Our patient's TPN solution contained 500 mcg of Mn, which we would argue is an excessive amount, even though many commercial TPN formulas contain up to 800 mcg of Mn. Takagi et al. performed a study in which patients received 0, 55, 110, and 1100 mcg of Mn/day using an on/off design [27]. Elevated blood Mn levels were noted when patients received 110 or 1100 mcg of Mn/day, but not when receiving 55 mcg of Mn/day [27]. Takagi et al., therefore, concluded that the recommended dose of Mn for stable patients receiving TPN at home is 55 mcg/day [27]. As a result, the American Society for Parenteral and Enteral Nutrition (ASPEN) has adopted the recommendation that parenteral nutrition formulas should contain 40 to 100 mcg of Mn/day, with a daily requirement set at 55 mcg/day.

5.5. Treatment. Treatment of Mn toxicity is dependent on eliminating the source of Mn exposure. However, methods such as chelation with intravenous EDTA, which increase urinary excretion of Mn, do not seem to improve the symptoms of Mn toxicity [4, 7, 26] but can still be used in an emergency setting to decrease the blood concentration of Mn [4]. For this reason, in the case of our patient, chelation therapy was not attempted. In addition, her symptoms improved within a few days of TPN discontinuation, which is the cornerstone of treatment. Of note, in cases of normal serum or urine manganese levels, noting an abnormally elevated urinary excretion of manganese following chelation therapy can also be indicative of manganese toxicity. When chelation therapy is used in conjunction with iron supplementation, however, a significant improvement of neurological symptoms can be expected [28].

Following Mn toxicity, internal organs themselves, particularly bones which house 40% of the body's total Mn stores [29] and where Mn has been found to have a half-life of 8-9 years, serve as a continuous internal source of Mn exposure [4]. However, cases have been described in the literature in which the characteristic MRI findings and clinical Parkinsonian symptoms have resolved following elimination of the Mn source or after hepatic transplantation [30, 31]. As the liver is the organ primarily responsible for the elimination of Mn, liver dysfunction can precipitate Mn toxicity. Liver transplantation has thus been shown to reduce the Mn burden on the brain on repeat T1-weighted MRI imaging performed months after the surgery [32].

In the past, it was hypothesized that treatment with levodopa may improve the extrapyramidal symptoms of Mn-induced neurotoxicity; however, response to levodopa is short-lived, lasting only two to three years, and even ten years after eliminating the source of Mn, the severity of patients' symptoms continued to progress [7, 33, 34].

6. Conclusion

Total parenteral nutrition should not be used as a chronic source of nutrition. Fungemia, fungal retinitis, and manganese toxicity are complications of TPN that may develop with long-term therapy. Parkinsonian features of manganese toxicity were visible in our patient approximately three months after initiation of TPN although the time frame can be highly variable depending on individual patient characteristics, particularly liver function and individual pharmacokinetic mechanisms regulating manganese absorption, distribution, storage, and excretion. One may expect the Parkinsonian features of manganese toxicity to develop even sooner than three months in patients with liver dysfunction. Current guidelines recommend monitoring patients for manganese toxicity if TPN is administered for greater than 30 days. In addition, being mindful of the fact that the recommended daily dose of Mn in TPN formulations is 55 mcg/day is essential, as many TPN formulations contain more than the recommended amount. Both providers and patients should be vigilant and educated about monitoring for complications of TPN, especially in patients with liver disorders.

References

[1] J. L. Aschner and M. Aschner, "Nutritional aspects of manganese homeostasis," *Molecular Aspects of Medicine*, vol. 26, no. 4-5, pp. 353–362, 2005.

[2] T. V. Peres, M. R. C. Schettinger, P. Chen et al., "Manganese-induced neurotoxicity: a review of its behavioral consequences and neuroprotective strategies," *BMC Pharmacology & Toxicology*, vol. 17, no. 1, p. 57, 2016.

[3] G. Alves, J. Thiebot, A. Tracqui, T. Delangre, C. Guedon, and E. Lerebours, "Neurologic disorders due to brain manganese deposition in a jaundiced patient receiving long-term parenteral nutrition," *Journal of Parenteral and Enteral Nutrition*, vol. 21, no. 1, pp. 41–45, 1997.

[4] S. L. O'Neal and W. Zheng, "Manganese toxicity upon overexposure: a decade in review," *Current Environmental Health Reports*, vol. 2, no. 2, pp. 315–328, 2015.

[5] M. Aschner, T. R. Guilarte, J. S. Schneider, and W. Zheng, "Manganese: recent advances in understanding its transport and neurotoxicity," *Toxicology and Applied Pharmacology*, vol. 221, no. 2, pp. 131–147, 2007.

[6] T. R. Guilarte, "Manganese and Parkinson's disease: a critical review and new findings," *Environmental Health Perspectives*, vol. 118, no. 8, pp. 1071–1080, 2010.

[7] J. Crossgrove and W. Zheng, "Manganese toxicity upon overexposure," *NMR in Biomedicine*, vol. 17, no. 8, pp. 544–553, 2004.

[8] M. Aschner and K. Erikson, "Manganese," *Advances in Nutrition: An International Review Journal*, vol. 8, no. 3, pp. 520-521, 2017.

[9] K. J. Horning, S. W. Caito, K. G. Tipps, A. B. Bowman, and M. Aschner, "Manganese is essential for neuronal health," *Annual Review of Nutrition*, vol. 35, no. 1, pp. 71–108, 2015.

[10] G. C. Cotzias, K. Horiuchi, S. Fuenzalida, and I. Mena, "Chronic manganese poisoning clearance of tissue manganese concentrations with persistence of the neurological picture," *Neurology*, vol. 18, no. 4, p. 376, 1968.

[11] A. P. Neal and T. R. Guilarte, "Mechanisms of lead and manganese neurotoxicity," *Toxicology Research*, vol. 2, no. 2, pp. 99–114, 2013.

[12] P. Chen, S. Chakraborty, S. Mukhopadhyay et al., "Manganese homeostasis in the nervous system," *Journal of Neurochemistry*, vol. 134, no. 4, pp. 601–610, 2015.

[13] K. Khan, P. Factor-Litvak, G. A. Wasserman et al., "Manganese exposure from drinking water and children's classroom behavior in Bangladesh," *Environmental Health Perspectives*, vol. 119, no. 10, pp. 1501–1506, 2011.

[14] R. G. Lucchini, D. C. Dorman, A. Elder, and B. Veronesi, "Neurological impacts from inhalation of pollutants and the nose-brain connection," *Neurotoxicology*, vol. 33, no. 4, pp. 838–841, 2012.

[15] S. Zoni, G. Bonetti, and R. Lucchini, "Olfactory functions at the intersection between environmental exposure to manganese and Parkinsonism," *Journal of Trace Elements in Medicine and Biology: Organ of the Society for Minerals and Trace Elements (GMS)*, vol. 26, no. 2-3, pp. 179–182, 2012.

[16] K. Sikk, S. Haldre, S. M. Aquilonius, and P. Taba, "Manganese-induced parkinsonism due to Ephedrone abuse," *Parkinson's Disease*, vol. 2011, Article ID 865319, 8 pages, 2011.

[17] C. Schmitt, N. Strazielle, P. Richaud, A. Bouron, and J. F. Ghersi-Egea, "Active transport at the blood-CSF barrier contributes to manganese influx into the brain," *Journal of Neurochemistry*, vol. 117, no. 117, pp. 747–756, 2011.

[18] G. Robison, T. Zakharova, S. Fu et al., "X-ray fluorescence imaging: a new tool for studying manganese neurotoxicity," *PLoS One*, vol. 7, no. 11, Article ID e48899, 2012.

[19] B. Grünecker, S. F. Kaltwasser, A. C. Zappe et al., "Regional specificity of manganese accumulation and clearance in the mouse brain: implications for manganese-enhanced MRI," *NMR in Biomedicine*, vol. 26, no. 5, pp. 542–556, 2013.

[20] S. L. O'Neal, L. Hong, S. Fu et al., "Manganese accumulation in bone following chronic exposure in rats: steady-state concentration and half-life in bone," *Toxicology Letters*, vol. 229, no. 229, pp. 93–100, 2014.

[21] I. Mena, K. Horiuchi, K. Burke, and G. C. Cotzias, "Chronic manganese poisoning: individual susceptibility and absorption of iron," *Neurology*, vol. 19, no. 10, p. 1000, 1969.

[22] C. D. Klaassen, "Biliary excretion of metals," *Drug Metabolism Reviews*, vol. 5, no. 2, pp. 165–196, 1976.

[23] F. O. Omokhodion and J. M. Howard, "Trace elements in the sweat of acclimatized persons," *Clinica Chimica Acta*, vol. 231, no. 1, pp. 23–28, 1994.

[24] Z. Guo, Z. Zhang, Q. Wang et al., "Manganese chloride induces histone acetylation changes in neuronal cells: its role in manganese-induced damage," *Neurotoxicology*, vol. 65, pp. 255–263, 2018.

[25] S. Fu, S. O'Neal, L. Hong, W. Jiang, and W. Zheng, "Elevated adult neurogenesis in brain subventricular zone following in vivo manganese exposure: roles of copper and DMT1," *Toxicological Sciences*, vol. 143, no. 2, pp. 482–498, 2015.

[26] Y.-M. Jiang, X.-A. Mo, F.-Q. Du et al., "Effective treatment of manganese-induced occupational Parkinsonism with p-aminosalicylic acid: a case of 17-year follow-up study," *Journal of Occupational and Environmental Medicine*, vol. 48, no. 6, pp. 644–649, 2006.

[27] Y. Takagi, A. Okada, K. Sando, M. Wasa, H. Yoshida, and N. Hirabuki, "Evaluation of indexes of in vivo manganese status and the optimal intravenous dose for adult patients undergoing home parenteral nutrition," *The American Journal of Clinical Nutrition*, vol. 75, no. 1, pp. 112–118, 2002.

[28] K. Tuschl, P. B. Mills, and P. T. Clayton, "Manganese and the brain," *International Review of Neurobiology*, vol. 110, pp. 277–312, 2013.

[29] H. A. Schroeder, J. J. Balassa, and I. H. Tipton, "Essential trace metals in man: manganese," *Journal of Chronic Diseases*, vol. 19, no. 5, pp. 545–571, 1966.

[30] T. F. Barron, A. G. Devenyi, and A. C. Mamourian, "Symptomatic manganese neurotoxicity in a patient with chronic liver disease: correlation of clinical symptoms with MRI findings," *Pediatric Neurology*, vol. 10, no. 2, pp. 145–148, 1994.

[31] H.-W. Shin, S.-W. Ahn, Y. C. Youn, and S.-H. Han, "Reversal of pallidal magnetic resonance imaging T1 hyperintensity in a welder presenting as reversible parkinsonism," *Neurology India*, vol. 62, no. 1, pp. 117-118, 2014.

[32] L.-L. Long, X.-R. Li, Z.-K. Huang, Y.-M. Jiang, S. X. Fu, and W. Zheng, "Relationship between changes in brain MRI and 1H-mrs, severity of chronic liver damage, and recovery after liver transplantation," *Experimental Biology and Medicine*, vol. 234, no. 9, pp. 1075–1085, 2009.

[33] C.-C. Huang, N.-S. Chu, C.-S. Lu, R.-S. Chen, and D. B. Calne, "Long-term progression in chronic manganism: ten years of follow-up," *Neurology*, vol. 50, no. 3, pp. 698–700, 1998.

[34] C.-C. Huang, C.-S. Lu, N.-S. Chu et al., "Progression after chronic manganese exposure," *Neurology*, vol. 43, no. 8, p. 1479, 1993.

31

Recovering Voiding and Sex Function in a Patient with Chronic Complete Spinal Cord Injury by Olfactory Ensheathing Cell Transplantation

Di Chen,[1] Haitao Xi,[2] Ke Tan,[3] and Hongyun Huang[1]

[1]*Beijing Hongtianji Neuroscience Academy, Beijing 100143, China*
[2]*Department of Neurorehabilitation, Capital Medical University Affiliated Beijing Rehabilitation Hospital, Beijing 100144, China*
[3]*Department of Neurosurgery, Capital Medical University Affiliated Beijing Chaoyang Hospital, Beijing 100020, China*

Correspondence should be addressed to Hongyun Huang; huanghongyun001@126.com

Academic Editor: Dominic B. Fee

Spinal cord injury (SCI) is life-altering damage for patients, their family, and society. Transplantation of olfactory ensheathing cells has demonstrated neurorestoration effects for many neurological conditions, including SCI. But voiding and sex dysfunction in patients with chronic complete SCI is still a major issue even though neurorestorative therapies can restore their partial neurological functions. Here we report a case with traumatic complete SCI at the level of C6-C7 one year ago, who received OEC transplantation with intensive neurorehabilitation. The patient started to show clinical improvements within a few days after cell treatment. Six-year follow-up demonstrated his American Spinal Injury Association (ASIA)-Impairment Scale change from ASIA A to become ASIA C. The scores of International Association of Neurorestoratology Spinal Cord Injury Functional Rating Scale changed from 14 (prior to cell therapy) to 31 + 3 (six years after cell therapy). His main improvements in activity of daily life included eating, dressing and writing by himself, standing and walking, and urine control or voiding. His sex function recovered to be normal. He married and had a son through natural sex life. His improving functions and activities of daily life stayed stable in subsequent phone call follow-up. This was one individual case report. In the future, the deep mechanisms of why he got positive results, but other patients with similar condition did not get so much benefits from OEC transplantation should be explored.

1. Introduction

Spinal cord injury (SCI) is life-altering damage for patients, their family, and society. Olfactory ensheathing cells (OECs) were transplanted for patients with SCI to restore injured cord functions and structures 20 years ago [1]. Cellular therapies have been found to have many benefits in clinical studies. Most patients with SCI got various benefits from OEC therapy [2–16], but voiding and sex dysfunction in patients with chronic complete SCI is still a major issue. Here we present a case report in which an adult young male with one year completes SCI received OEC transplantation. Besides improvements of motor function, sensation, and activity of daily life, he recovered his voiding and sex function during long-term follow-up.

2. Case Presentation

2.1. A Case Report. A 21-year-old man was injured in a car accident one year ago, causing trauma to the spinal cord. His lower limbs and hands were paralyzed after the accident. Magnetic resonance imaging (MRI) showed focal cord compression and injury by fractured bone and protruded disc in C6 (see Figure 1). He suffered spinal cord decompression and spinal stabilization. After extensive rehabilitation, his hand functions partially recovered. However, his functional recovery reached plateau and stopped recovering losing functions for half year before requesting for our treatment.

Prior to cell transplantation, his sensory level intact was at C6 for pinprick and light touch bilaterally, abnormal sensation at C7, and no sensation in other dermatomes below T1.

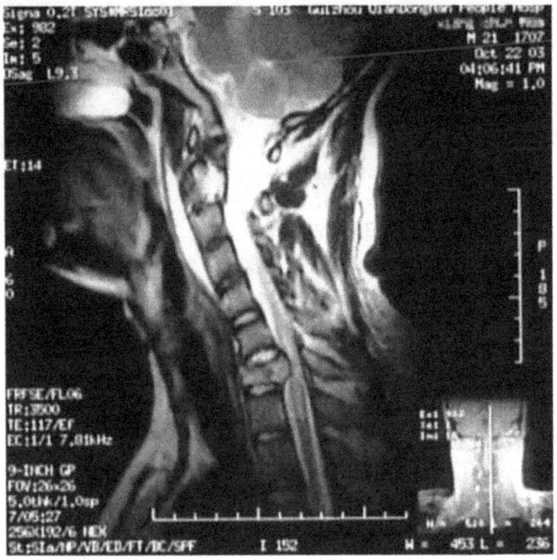

FIGURE 1: The spinal cord was compressed by fracture vertebral body.

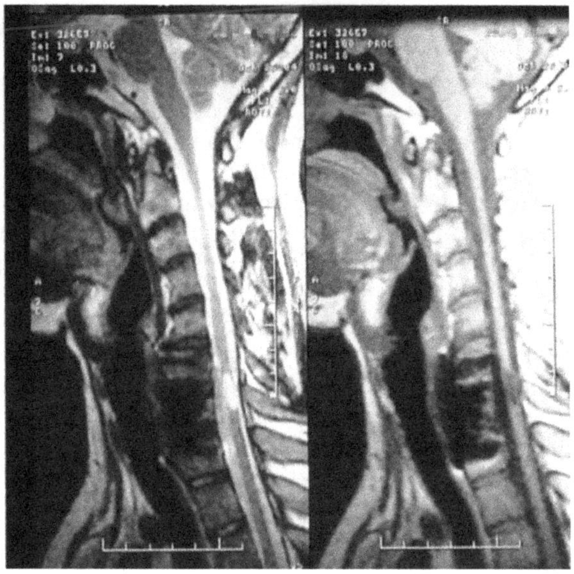

FIGURE 2: The cavitation volume is about $1 \times 0.5 \times 0.5\,cm^3$ in cervical vertebral 6.

Both sides' muscle testing showed grade 4 at C7 function and no voluntary muscle movement below the T1 level. The rectal exam indicated no sensory or motor function preserved in sacral segments S4/5. Therefore, the deficit was classified as American Spinal Injury Association (ASIA)-Impairment Scale was at level C7 ASIA A motor and sensory complete tetraplegia. The scores of International Association of Neurorestoratology Spinal Cord Injury Functional Rating Scale (IANR-SCIFRS) were 14 out of 48. His activities of daily living were difficult, such as eating, dressing, standing, walking, and poor trunk control. He had urinary incontinence with poor urine control. MRI showed focal myelomalacia from C6 to C7 with altered signals at these two levels (see Figure 2).

2.2. Cell Preparation and Transplantation. Olfactory ensheathing cells (OECs) were isolated from aborted human fetal olfactory bulbs (received approval and signed donation consent form). The OECs were cultured in Dulbecco's modified Eagle's medium/Ham's F12 (DMEM/F12; Hyclone, Logan, UT, USA) with 10% fetal bovine serum (FBS; Hyclone) and the neurotrophic factors and then propagated for 2-3 weeks. The cells were characterized by immunostaining with antibodies against p75 (Sigma, St. Louis, MO, USA).

A signed informed consent was obtained from the patient and his family member. The protocol of cell therapy was approved by the ethics committee. Under general anaesthesia, the patient underwent cervical posterior approach surgery to expose injured cord in C6 and 7. OECs (1×10^6 in 0.06 ml DMEM liquid) were transplanted into the spinal cord parenchyma in adjacent upper and lower injured site (the injecting OEC amount and delivery vehicle was referred to our pre-clinical research in rats [17]). Cell injection procedure is under microscopy, injection points are in the middle of the upper and lower injured cord borders with normal tissue, injection rate is slowly (each injection takes about 10 seconds), the depth of injection is about 3-4 mm within cord parenchyma. After cell injection is completed, the needle is kept for 2-3 seconds. The gauge size of this needle is $4.5^{\#}$ thin needle (Chinese product specifications). The patient recovered well after the surgery and cell transplantation without using immunosuppression. Then, he continued intensive neurorehabilitation as before.

3. Results

He started to show some clinical recoveries of lost neurological functions in a few days after cell transplantation, including sensory and motor improvement in hands, trunk, and lower limbs.

Assessments were conducted at three weeks after cell transplantation. His sensation, motor functions, and activity of daily life improved. His ASIA AIS was A. ASIA motor scores were 42; ASIA pin prick scores were 34; ASIA light touch scores were 40. IANR-SCIFRS were 17.

Assessments conducted in six-year follow-up showed improving sensation, motor functions, and activity of daily life. His ASIA AIS changed from Grade A to Grade C; ASIA motor scores were 54; ASIA pin prick scores were 66; ASIA light touch scores were 82. IANR-SCIFRS were 31 + 3 (sex function)/48. The main recoveries took in upper limb, trunk, and lower limb movement. He could finish eating, dressing, and writing by himself. With brace and walker support, he could stand and walk. His rectal function had improved. He was able to hold urine and void almost normally without any assistance. His sex function recovered to be normal (married and had a son through natural sex). His improving functions and activities of daily life remained stable in subsequent phone call follow-up.

4. Discussion

4.1. Managing Voiding and Sex Dysfunction in Clinic. Condom drainage for voiding remains the most frequent bladder method for male patients with spinal cord injury

[18]. Clean intermittent catheterization is also a preferred method of bladder management for many patients with SCI, but long-term adherence is low [19]. Patients could undergo neurorestorative treatments, such as nerve bridging, neurostimulation/neuromodulation, cell therapy, and so on, for their voiding [20]. There are some methods for ejaculation in SCI patients with sex dysfunction. Electroejaculation is suitable for the injured level at caudal to T10. Ejaculation in penile vibratory stimulation is appropriate for men with SCI at T10 or rostral [21]. In vitro fertilization/intracytoplasmic sperm injection is for male patients with SCI, who want to have children [22]. So far, there are no reported methods for man with chronic complete SCI to recover their natural sex function and have children except this report.

4.2. OEC Transplantation for Patients with Spinal Cord Injury. Our team first transplanted OEC into the spinal cord parenchyma in adjacent injured site for SCI patients in 2002. Twenty-three patients with chronic SCI (most complete) improved their neurological functions and quality of life and still kept the improving trend after OEC transplantation during follow-up [1]. Later, the study of long-term follow-up by our team proved the safety and effects of OEC transplantation for patients with SCI [3]. Important finding was that chronic complete SCI patients with intensive neurorehabilitation received more benefits than patients with poor neurorehabilitation [3]. Simultaneously, more clinical studies of OECs or their combination with other cells had been reported, in which patients with acute, subacute and chronic, complete, and incomplete SCI at different injured levels demonstrated neurological functional improvements including sensation, motor, urine and rectal control, and activities of daily life [2, 4–16].

4.3. Neurorestorative Mechanisms of OECs. OECs are special glial cells sharing the characteristic of Schwann cell and astrocyte properties. Their neurorestorative mechanisms include neuroprotection, axonal regeneration, remyelination, neural network or circuitry reconstruction, neuroplasticity, neuromodulation, anti-inflammatory response or immunomodulation, promoting neurogenesis, stimulating angiogenesis, and so on [23]. There is no barrier for OECs between the central nervous system and peripheral nervous system. They can easily migrate into the injured spinal cord after being transplanted and restore injured nerves which are responsible for voiding and sex function. This patient's voiding and sex function may be restored through those mechanisms.

4.4. Limitation and Unsolved Questions. Among our treated patients with chronic complete SCI, one third of them recovered more or less voiding and rectal functions. Also male patients recovered partially sex function, but few patients could recover to be normal state like this reported patient. The reasons puzzle us, which need further exploration.

5. Conclusion

OEC transplantation with intensive neurorehabilitation showed favorable effects in improving neurological function in this patient with chronic complete SCI, especially in recovering his voiding and sex function. His improving functions and activities of daily life remained stable in subsequent phone call follow-up. Since this was a single case report, not all patients could attain positive results like this patient. In the future, the deep mechanisms, and the reason why some patients received more benefits and some received fewer benefits from OEC transplantation, should be explored.

Authors' Contributions

Di Chen and Haitao Xi contributed equally to this study.

Acknowledgments

The authors thank Mr. Daqian Huang for his language polishing.

References

[1] H. Huang, L. Chen, H. Wang et al., "Influence of patients' age on functional recovery after transplantation of olfactory ensheathing cells into injured spinal cord injury," *Chinese Medical Journal*, vol. 116, no. 10, pp. 1488–1491, 2003.

[2] J. Guest, L. P. Herrera, and T. Qian, "Rapid recovery of segmental neurological function in a tetraplegic patient following transplantation of fetal olfactory bulb-derived cells," *Spinal Cord*, vol. 44, no. 3, pp. 135–142, 2006.

[3] H. Huang, H. Xi, L. Chen, F. Zhang, and Y. Liu, "Long-term outcome of olfactory ensheathing cell therapy for patients with complete chronic spinal cord injury," *Cell Transplantation*, vol. 21, pp. S23–S31, 2012.

[4] S. S. Rabinovich, V. I. Seledtsov, O. V. Poveschenko et al., "Transplantation treatment of spinal cord injury patients," *Biomedicine & Pharmacotherapy*, vol. 57, no. 9, pp. 428–433, 2003.

[5] G. V. Seledtsova, S. S. Rabinovich, S. N. Belogorodtsev, O. V. Parlyuk, V. I. Seledtsov, and V. A. Kozlov, "Delayed results of transplantation of fetal neurogenic tissue in patients with consequences of spinal cord trauma," *Bulletin of Experimental Biology and Medicine*, vol. 149, no. 4, pp. 530–533, 2010.

[6] J. Wu, T. Sun, C. Ye, J. Yao, B. Zhu, and H. He, "Clinical observation of fetal olfactory ensheathing glia transplantation (OEGT) in patients with complete chronic spinal cord injury," *Cell Transplantation*, vol. 21, pp. S33–S37, 2012.

[7] Z. Zheng, C. Liu, L. Zhang et al., "Olfactory ensheathing cell transplantation in 106 patients with old spinal cord injury. differences in ages, sexes, disease courses, injured types and sites," *Neural Regeneration Research*, vol. 2, no. 6, pp. 380–384, 2007.

[8] Z. Zheng, G. Liu, Y. Chen, and S. Wei, "Olfactory ensheathing cell transplantation improves sympathetic skin responses in chronic spinal cord injury," *Neural Regeneration Research*, vol. 8, no. 30, pp. 2849–2855, 2013.
[9] N. Kuang, X. Wang, Y. Chen et al., "Olfactory ensheathing cell transplantation for chronic spinal cord injury: a long-term follow-up study," *Journal of Neurorestoratology*, vol. 9, no. 2, pp. 94–105, 2021.
[10] G. F. Bao, Z. M. Cui, W. D. Li et al., "Olfactory ensheathing cell transplantation in the treatment of spinal cord injury in 5 cases," *Journal of Clinical Rehabilitative Tissue Engineering Research*, vol. 11, no. 3, pp. 512–514, 2007.
[11] Y. Rao, W. Zhu, H. Liu, C. Jia, Q. Zhao, and Y. Wang, "Clinical application of olfactory ensheathing cells in the treatment of spinal cord injury," *Journal of International Medical Research*, vol. 41, no. 2, pp. 473–481, 2013.
[12] Y. Rao, W. Zhu, Y. Guo et al., "Long-term outcome of olfactory ensheathing cell transplantation in six patients with chronic complete spinal cord injury," *Cell Transplantation*, vol. 22, pp. S21–S25, 2013.
[13] Y. J. Rao, W. X. Zhu, Z. Q. Du et al., "Effectiveness of olfactory ensheathing cell transplantation for treatment of spinal cord injury," *Genetics and Molecular Research*, vol. 13, no. 2, pp. 4124–4129, 2014.
[14] P. Tabakow, W. Jarmundowicz, B. Czapiga et al., "Transplantation of autologous olfactory ensheathing cells in complete human spinal cord injury," *Cell Transplantation*, vol. 22, no. 9, pp. 1591–1612, 2013.
[15] P. Tabakow, G. Raisman, W. Fortuna et al., "Functional regeneration of supraspinal connections in a patient with transected spinal cord following transplantation of bulbar olfactory ensheathing cells with peripheral nerve bridging," *Cell Transplantation*, vol. 23, no. 12, pp. 1631–1655, 2014.
[16] Z. Cheng, R. Wang, K. Cao et al., "Ten years of clinical observation of olfactory ensheathing cell transplantation in patients with spinal cord injury," *Journal of Neurorestoratology*, vol. 9, no. 2, pp. 106–116, 2021.
[17] H. Huang, K. Liu, W. Huang, Z. Liu, and W. Young, "Olfactory ensheathing cells promoting neuroregeneration and functional recovery after spinal cord contusion," *Journal of the Navy General Hospital*, vol. 14, no. 2, pp. 65–67, 2001.
[18] G. Savic, H. L. Frankel, M. A. Jamous, B. M. Soni, and S. Charlifue, "Long-term bladder and bowel management after spinal cord injury: a 20-year longitudinal study," *Spinal Cord*, vol. 56, no. 6, pp. 575–581, 2018.
[19] I. M. Crescenze, J. B. Myers, S. M. Lenherr et al., "Predictors of low urinary quality of life in spinal cord injury patients on clean intermittent catheterization," *Neurourology and Urodynamics*, vol. 38, no. 5, pp. 1332–1338, 2019.
[20] X. Guo, Y. Feng, T. Sun et al., "Clinical guidelines for neurorestorative therapies in spinal cord injury (2021 China version)," *Journal of Neurorestoratology*, vol. 9, no. 1, pp. 31–49, 2021.
[21] E. Ibrahim, T. C. Aballa, N. L. Brackett, and C. M. Lynne, "Electroejaculation in men with spinal cord injury: a step-by-step video demonstration," *Fertility and Sterility*, vol. 115, no. 5, pp. 1344–1346, 2021.
[22] A. S. Kathiresan, E. Ibrahim, T. C. Aballa et al., "Comparison of in vitro fertilization/intracytoplasmic sperm injection outcomes in male factor infertility patients with and without spinal cord injuries," *Fertility and Sterility*, vol. 96, no. 3, pp. 562–566, 2011.
[23] H. Huang, "Why is olfactory neuroepithelium?" *Journal of Neurorestoratology*, vol. 9, no. 4, pp. 211–218, 2021.

32

Successful Extracorporeal Membrane Oxygenation (ECMO) use without Systemic Anticoagulation for Acute Respiratory Distress Syndrome in a Patient with Aneurysmal Subarachnoid Hemorrhage

Amanda L. Faulkner,[1] James David Bacon,[1] Brian A. Fischer,[1] Stephen L. Grupke,[2] and Kevin W. Hatton[1]

[1]*Department of Anesthesiology, N-202 UKMC, 800 Rose Street, Lexington, KY 40536, USA*
[2]*Department of Neurosurgery, 800 Rose Street, Lexington, KY 40536, USA*

Correspondence should be addressed to Kevin W. Hatton; kevin.hatton@uky.edu

Academic Editor: Norman S. Litofsky

Extracorporeal membrane oxygenation (ECMO) is an important life-saving technology for patients with severe acute respiratory distress syndrome (ARDS). Unfortunately, ECMO has been traditionally contraindicated in patients with hemorrhagic neurologic diseases. The recent improvement in ECMO devices, increased utilization and experience with venovenous ECMO technologies among healthcare teams, and the use of ECMO without anticoagulation has expanded the potential populations that may benefit from ECMO. We present a case of successful utilization of venovenous ECMO for severe respiratory failure secondary to ARDS in a patient with aneurysmal subarachnoid hemorrhage and severe, episodic cerebral vasospasm. We also discuss important limitations and considerations for future successful use of ECMO in hemorrhagic stroke. This case report highlights the potential for this life-saving technology in patients with hemorrhagic stroke.

1. Introduction

Acute respiratory distress syndrome (ARDS) is a life-threatening respiratory system clinical presentation resulting in severe hypoxemia that frequently requires mechanical ventilation and adjunctive respiratory therapies to support respiratory function [1]. Venovenous extracorporeal membrane oxygenation (VV-ECMO) is an evolving therapy that is sometimes used as rescue in patients with severe ARDS to stabilize gas exchange until lung recovery occurs [2–6]. VV-ECMO was developed from cardiopulmonary bypass (CPB) technologies and its use has historically required complicated CPB devices, surgical and perfusion technical expertise, and systemic anticoagulation [6–8]. For these reasons, the use of VV-ECMO has been contraindicated in hemorrhagic neurologic diseases, such as aneurysmal subarachnoid hemorrhage (aSAH) [8–10]. The development of less-complicated VV-ECMO devices, the increased experience with VV-ECMO technologies among critical care specialists, critical care nurses, and other support staff, and the growing expertise in the use of VV-ECMO without anticoagulation have expanded the potential populations that may benefit from VV-ECMO. We present a case of successful utilization of VV-ECMO without systemic anticoagulation for severe respiratory failure in a patient with aSAH. The patient has provided written consent to publish this case report.

2. Case Report

A 44-year-old female with history of asthma, tobacco abuse, intravenous drug abuse, schizophrenia, and chronic hepatitis C infection was transferred to our hospital after computed tomography (CT) scan at an outside hospital demonstrated aSAH. During transport, she had an acute decline in her mental status and was emergently intubated after several failed attempts on arrival to our emergency department. Additional imaging revealed an anterior communicating artery aneurysm with surrounding subarachnoid hemorrhage, intraventricular extension, and hydrocephalus. An extraventricular drain (EVD) was placed emergently and she underwent uncomplicated endovascular coiling of her aneurysm that same day.

Following her coiling procedure, she developed worsening oxygenation and vasodilatory shock, presumed to be from aspiration pneumonitis as she had negative respiratory cultures, a negative procalcitonin analysis, and mildly hyperdynamic left ventricular function on cardiac echocardiography. On post-bleed day (PBD) 1, she remained on mechanical ventilation, her chest x-ray demonstrated bilateral infiltrates, her PaO2/FiO2 ratio was less than 100, and her clinical course was consistent with severe Acute Respiratory Distress Syndrome (ARDS) [11]. Lung-protective ventilation was initiated with increased oxygen (FiO2), positive end-expiratory pressure (PEEP), and inhaled epoprostenol therapy as per protocol [12]. On PBD 2, despite neuromuscular blockade, inhaled epoprostanol, and maximal ventilator support (FiO2=100%, PEEP=15 cmH20) which was limited by her hemodynamic response to additional PEEP, the patient developed refractory hypoxemic respiratory failure and VV-ECMO was proposed to support her worsening lung function. After a multidisciplinary discussion that included the patient's family, neurosurgery (NS), critical care medicine (CCM), and mechanical circulatory support (MCS) teams, the decision was made to proceed with bedside cannulation for VV-ECMO to facilitate respiratory support.

In the Neuroscience Intensive Care Unit (NSICU), the MCS team placed a 25 French ECMO access cannula in the right femoral vein (outflow to ECMO) and an 18 French ECMO return cannula in the left subclavian vein (inflow from ECMO) without difficulty. The internal jugular vein was not utilized for this cannulation due to concern for obstruction to intracranial venous outflow. VV-ECMO was then initiated using a CARDIOHELP ECMO System (Maquet Cardiovascular, Wayne, NJ). Due to concern for additional subarachnoid hemorrhage, routine heparin bolus was not administered at the time of ECMO initiation and therapeutic anticoagulation was not administered at any time during her VV-ECMO therapy. After VV-ECMO initiation, her hypoxemia and hypercarbia rapidly stabilized and ventilator settings were reduced to provide additional lung protection. This was accomplished by converting mechanical ventilation from a volume-control mode to a pressure-control mode with target tidal volume maintained between 4 mL/kg and 6 mL/kg and measured plateau pressure less than 30 cm H2O (Table 1). She was then transported to the Cardiovascular Intensive Care Unit (CVICU) for treatment and monitoring during VV-ECMO therapy. Daily multidisciplinary rounds with NS, CCM, and MCS teams evaluated her neurologic and other organ system injuries and codeveloped a daily plan of care. Daily evaluation of plasma free hemoglobin and routine evaluation for the development of thrombosis in the oxygenator and tubing were performed by perfusion, nursing, and physician MCS specialists. VV-ECMO blood flow rate was maintained greater than 3 LPM to reduce the risk of thrombosis and VV-ECMO FiO2 and VV-ECMO sweep gas settings were titrated to maintain systemic pH > 7.25, PaO2 55-80 mmHg, and PaCO2 35-50 mmHg.

Unfortunately, on PBD 5, she developed acute kidney injury that required initiation of continuous renal replacement therapy (CRRT) via her femoral VV-ECMO cannula. On PBD 6, her transcranial Doppler (TCD) values significantly increased and, following a multidisciplinary conversation, she was transported to the angiography suite where CV was identified and treated with intra-arterial verapamil. During angiography, she developed significant hypoxemia requiring increased ventilator and ECMO support to maintain adequate oxygenation (Table 1). Her hypoxemia improved on return to the CVICU and her ECMO and ventilator support were returned to minimal settings after approximately 24 hours. Because of the risk for additional CV and the potential for recurrent hypoxemia during angiography and vasodilator administration, the multidisciplinary team decided to continue ECMO therapy through at least PBD 10. On PBD 9, her TCD values again increased and she was transported back to the angiography suite for additional diagnostic angiography and intra-arterial vasodilator administration. No hypoxemia occurred during this second procedure.

On PBD 10, after a seven-day course of VV-ECMO, her respiratory status had significantly improved, she had not developed additional hypoxemia after angiography, and she required only minimal VV-ECMO and ventilator settings. After another multidisciplinary conversation, she was successfully separated from VV-ECMO and her venous cannulae were removed. Importantly, there was no evidence of enlargement of her subarachnoid hemorrhage. On PBD 11, she underwent percutaneous tracheostomy, percutaneous enterogastrostomy (PEG) tube, and tunneled dialysis catheter placement. On PBD 22, she underwent placement of a permanent ventriculoperitoneal shunt. On PBD 36, she was transferred from the NSICU to a long-term acute care hospital for continued ventilator weaning and aggressive neurorehabilitation. At the time of her transfer, she opened her eyes spontaneously, followed verbal commands with all four extremities and attempted phonation during tracheostomy collar trials. At her 90-day clinic followup, her tracheostomy had been removed and she was alert, oriented, and able to converse with appropriate syntax and content and was independently ambulatory without assistance. Her venous cannulation sites, arterial angiography access sites, and ventriculoperitoneal shunt surgery wounds were well-healed.

3. Discussion

In this case report, we highlight the successful use of VV-ECMO to support respiratory failure with severe ARDS, likely resulting from aspiration pneumonitis, in a patient with aneurysmal subarachnoid hemorrhage. In this case, we learned the importance of a multidisciplinary approach to this complicated technology in a high-risk patient, the necessity to plan for transport throughout the hospital during

Table 1: Extracorporeal Life Support (ECMO) and Mechanical Ventilation Parameters. ECMO was initiated on PBD 2 and discontinued on PBD 10. PBD = Post-bleed day. PEEP = Positive end-expiratory pressure.

PBD	ECMO FiO2 (%)	ECMO Sweep (L/min)	ECMO Flow (L/min)	Ventilator FiO2 (%)	Ventilator Mode	Pressure Above PEEP/PEEP (cm H2O)	pH	PaO2	PaCO2
2	100	3	3.9	100	PCV	15/10	7.30	244	54
3	100	6	4.1	50	PCV	15/10	7.45	152	36
4	70	6	3.9	50	PCV	15/10	7.47	124	34
5	30	1	3.7	50	PCV	12/8	7.43	97	36
6	21	0	3.8	50	PCV	20/5	7.34	84	38
7	60	3	6.5	60	PCV	18/10	7.42	76	46
8	21	0	3.5	40	PSV	10/10	7.36	117	46
9	21	0	3.6	40	PSV	12/8	7.38	95	42
10	21	0	3.5	40	PSV	10/5	7.43	84	36

ECMO therapy, especially to areas not traditionally used by patients with ECMO, such as the angiography suite, and the potential to use VV-ECMO for a prolonged period of time without systemic anticoagulation.

Despite significant preclinical and clinical research to develop new therapies for ARDS, the management of patients with ARDS remains largely supportive. [1]. Current ARDS support therapies include lung protective ventilation strategies, prone positioning, meticulous attention to fluid balance, and early recognition and reduction of secondary injuries, including malnutrition, pneumonia, and deep venous thrombosis [13, 14]. The use of VV-ECMO to support the failing respiratory system in ARDS remains controversial [15]. While early studies of ECMO, primarily as a rescue therapy in severe ARDS, failed to demonstrate significant benefit to patients, the development of technical improvements and strategies that leaned toward earlier initiation of ECMO support improved clinical outcomes of ECMO in ARDS [16]. In 2009, the CESAR trial demonstrated, for the first time, that the use of ECMO as an early rescue therapy provided the potential for benefit in patients with severe ARDS [17]. Subsequent studies, including the recently-published EOLIA trial, have continued to refine our knowledge and clinical experience V-V ECMO in populations with ARDS [18]. While research is ongoing, it is increasingly apparent that V-V ECMO can be a viable option for many patients with ARDS, including populations that may have, traditionally, been excluded from this life-saving therapy.

aSAH is a devastating acute hemorrhagic neurologic disease affecting approximately 30,000 Americans every year. Between 30 and 50% of these patients will have significant long-term neurologic disability. aSAH occurs when an intracranial arterial aneurysm ruptures, releasing oxygenated blood into the subarachnoid space. Immediate complications from aneurysm rupture include severe neurologic injury with frequent loss of consciousness, hydrocephalus, seizure and neurocardiogenic shock. The primary goal of immediate therapy includes aneurysm obliteration, stabilization of cardiopulmonary status, and extracranial drainage of cerebrospinal fluid (CSF). Cerebral vasospasm (CV) is a secondary neurologic insult that occurs 3-10 days after aneurysm rupture and results in delayed cerebral ischemia, cerebral infarction and additional neurologic disability. Patients with aSAH are monitored closely for CV for approximately 2 weeks after their aneurysm rupture and undergo digital subtraction angiography with injection of intra-arterial vasodilators to spastic arteries when CV is detected.

In patients with aSAH, as is true of many critically ill patients with neurologic injury, ventilator management consists of balancing support of the failing lungs and the injured brain. Treatments for hypoxemia, including increasing FiO2, PEEP, and diuresis, may all be associated with negative consequences in patients with aSAH. Treatments for hypercarbia, including increasing respiratory rate and tidal volume, may also be associated with negative consequences in patients with aSAH. Likewise, permissive hypercapnia may not be possible in patients with elevated intracranial pressure. Given these potential problems, the decision to pursue alternatives to mechanical ventilation, such as VV-ECMO therapy, may be desirable to balance the management of respiratory and neurologic injury in these critically ill patients.

In our institution, our neurocritical care team is staffed by anesthesiology critical care specialists who also rotate their clinical service in the cardiovascular intensive care unit (CVICU) and surgical intensive care unit (SICU). Because of this "cross-training" across the NSICU, the CVICU, and the SICU, the critical care team has developed significant expertise in team-based management of VV-ECMO for patients with various cardiac, pulmonary, and cardiopulmonary diseases. This expertise was utilized to facilitate shared decision-making among the care teams and to bridge physician, nursing, respiratory therapy, and other healthcare worker knowledge gaps in the care of patients with aSAH and the utilization of VV-ECMO.

In addition to the multidisciplinary approach, our team also learned to plan for patient transport throughout the hospital, including to the angiography suite. In our institution, the angiography suite is in a different, but connected, hospital building. To transport the patient from the ICU to angiography, the patient traveled via an elevator and several hallways. This process took up to 30 minutes, depending on the time of day, and utilized physician, nursing, perfusion, and respiratory therapist expertise to safely transport this patient back and forth from the angiography suite. Prior to transport, contingency plans were developed and additional staff and resources were prepositioned along the route to assist with unexpected problems that may have occurred during transport. Because of these actions, the patient did not have any significant issues or problems during any of transports to or from angiography.

Finally, in this case we were able to utilize VV-ECMO for approximately 1 week without systemic anticoagulation. The major concerns with this strategy were increased risk of clot formation in the oxygenator and venous thromboembolism in the patient [10]. To reduce these risks, short lengths of heparin-bonded VV-ECMO tubing was used for this patient [1]. In addition, the VV-ECMO pump speed was maintained at a slightly higher than normal speed for increased flow throughout the VV-ECMO circuit. Fortunately, routine evaluation of the oxygenator did not demonstrate clot formation during VV-ECMO therapy, there were no significant changes in daily plasma free hemoglobin levels, and the patient did not exhibit signs of venous thromboembolism.

While it is not the first reported use of VV-ECMO in a patient with aSAH, our case was substantially different from the previously reported case and significantly adds to the overall experience of the use of VV-ECMO in patients with aSAH [19]. In the original case, the patient deteriorated within a few hours of aneurysm rupture from apparent neurogenic pulmonary edema, underwent VV-ECMO cannulation in the operating room immediately prior to a surgical clipping procedure, suffered severe intracranial hypertension, required pharmacologic coma, and was not monitored or treated for CV during hospitalization. Unlike our case, the patient was placed on nafamostat mesylate, a serine protease inhibitor most frequently used as an anticoagulant during hemodialysis.

In summary, we report the successful use of VV-ECMO to support severe respiratory failure secondary to ARDS in a patient with aSAH who underwent endovascular coiling and developed multiple episodes of CV during her hospitalization. Our report highlights the importance of a multidisciplinary approach among physician, nursing, pharmacy, perfusion, respiratory therapy, and many other experts, as well as, the importance of understanding transportation issues for these complex medical patients. In addition, it further highlights the growing experience with the use of VV-ECMO without systemic anticoagulation in patients with hemorrhagic neurologic disease. Future cases should consider these lessons and apply ECMO in appropriate patients with multidisciplinary support to achieve maximum patient benefit.

References

[1] S. Wang, Y. Chen, W. Ko, and S. Chu, "Extracorporeal membrane oxygenation support for postcardiotomy cardiogenic shock," *Artificial Organs*, vol. 20, no. 12, pp. 1287–1291, 1996.

[2] K. Shekar, D. V. Mullany, B. Thomson, M. Ziegenfuss, D. G. Platts, and J. F. Fraser, "Extracorporeal life support devices and strategies for management of acute cardiorespiratory failure in adult patients: a comprehensive review," *Critical Care*, vol. 18, no. 3, article 219, 2014.

[3] G. Lafçı, A. B. Budak, A. Ü. Yener, and O. F. Cicek, "Use of extracorporeal membrane oxygenation in adults," *Heart, Lung and Circulation*, vol. 23, no. 1, pp. 10–23, 2014.

[4] A. Wallinder, V. Pellegrino, J. F. Fraser, and D. C. McGiffin, "ECMO as a bridge to non-transplant cardiac surgery," *Journal of Cardiac Surgery*, vol. 32, no. 8, pp. 514–521, 2017.

[5] S. F. Marasco, G. Lukas, M. McDonald, J. McMillan, and B. Ihle, "Review of ECMO (extra corporeal membrane oxygenation) support in critically ill adult patients," *Heart, Lung and Circulation*, vol. 17, no. 4, pp. S41–S47, 2008.

[6] J. B. Zwischenberger and H. T. Pitcher, "Extracorporeal membrane oxygenation management: techniques to liberate from extracorporeal membrane oxygenation and manage post-intensive care unit issues," *Critical Care Clinics*, vol. 33, no. 4, pp. 843–853, 2017.

[7] J. Jones-Akhtarekhavari, T. A. Tribble, and J. B. Zwischenberger, "Developing an extracorporeal membrane oxygenation program," *Critical Care Clinics*, vol. 33, no. 4, pp. 767–775, 2017.

[8] Extracorporeal Life Support Organization (ELSO). Guidelines for adult respiratory failure. 2017 July 11, 2018]; https://www.elso.org/Portals/0/ELSO%20Guidelines%20For%20Adult%20Respiratory%20Failure%201_4.pdf.

[9] R. Lango, Z. Szkulmowski, D. Maciejewski, A. Sosnowski, and K. Kusza, "Revised protocol of extracorporeal membrane oxygenation (ECMO) therapy in severe ARDS. Recommendations of the Veno-venous ECMO Expert Panel appointed in February 2016 by the national consultant on anesthesiology and intensive care," *Anaesthesiology Intensive Therapy*, vol. 49, no. 2, pp. 88–99, 2017.

[10] A. Sen, H. E. Callisen, C. M. Alwardt et al., "Adult venovenous extracorporeal membrane oxygenation for severe respiratory failure: current status and future perspectives," *Annals of Cardiac Anaesthesia*, vol. 19, no. 1, pp. 97–111, 2016.

[11] A. D. T. Force, V. M. Ranieri, G. D. Rubenfeld et al., "Acute respiratory distress syndrome: the Berlin definition," *The Journal of the American Medical Association*, vol. 307, no. 23, pp. 2526–2533, 2012.

[12] T. Bein, S. Grasso, O. Moerer et al., "The standard of care of patients with ARDS: ventilatory settings and rescue therapies for refractory hypoxemia," *Intensive Care Medicine*, vol. 42, no. 5, pp. 699–711, 2016.

[13] M. D. Howell and A. M. Davis, "Management of ARDS in adults," *Journal of the American Medical Association*, vol. 319, no. 7, pp. 711-712, 2018.

[14] V. Fielding-Singh, M. A. Matthay, and C. S. Calfee, "Beyond low tidal volume ventilation: treatment adjuncts for severe respiratory failure in acute respiratory distress syndrome," *Critical Care Medicine*, vol. 46, no. 11, pp. 1820–1831, 2018.

[15] L. Gattinoni, F. Vasques, and M. Quintel, "Use of ECMO in ARDS: Does the EOLIA trial really help?" *Critical Care*, vol. 22, no. 1, article 171, 2018.

[16] J. B. Zwischenberger and J. E. Lynch, "Will CESAR answer the adult ECMO debate?" *The Lancet*, vol. 374, no. 9698, pp. 1307-1308, 2009.

[17] G. J. Peek, M. Mugford, R. Tiruvoipati et al., "Efficacy and economic assessment of conventional ventilatory support versus extracorporeal membrane oxygenation for severe adult respiratory failure (CESAR): a multicentre randomised controlled trial," *The Lancet*, vol. 374, no. 9698, pp. 1351–1363, 2009.

[18] A. Combes, D. Hajage, G. Capellier et al., "Extracorporeal membrane oxygenation for severe acute respiratory distress syndrome," *The New England Journal of Medicine*, vol. 378, no. 21, pp. 1965–1975, 2018.

[19] G. J. Hwang, S. H. Sheen, H. S. Kim et al., "Extracorporeal membrane oxygenation for acute life-threatening neurogenic pulmonary edema following rupture of an intracranial aneurysm," *Journal of Korean Medical Science*, vol. 28, no. 6, p. 962, 2013.

33

Acute Confusional Migraine: Unusual Great Masquerader—Case Report and Literature Review

Bashar Tanous,[1] Raad Tahtouh,[1] Sundus Sardar,[1] Sara Mohamed,[1] Aseel Sukik,[1] Mhd-Baraa Habib,[1] Jamal Sajid,[2] and Mouhand F. H. Mohamed[2]

[1]Internal Medicine Residency Program, Internal Medicine Department, Hamad Medical Corporation, Doha, Qatar
[2]Internal Medicine Department, Hamad Medical Corporation, Doha, Qatar

Correspondence should be addressed to Mouhand F. H. Mohamed; dr.m.oraiby@hotmail.com

Academic Editor: Abbass Amirjamshidi

Background. Acute confusional migraine (ACM) is a rare variant of migraine, mainly prevalent in children and adolescents. It is not currently indexed as a distinct variant of migraine likely since only a few cases were reported in the adult population. We report a case of delayed ACM diagnosis in a young man and present a concise-related literature review. *Case Presentation.* A thirty-eight-year-old man with a past medical history of migraine, not on any treatment, presented with headaches accompanied by confusion. Over a two-year period before the current presentation, he experienced two episodes of confusion, which required hospital admission for evaluation: once mislabeled as a psychiatric illness and diagnosed as a migrainous infarct in the second hospitalization. In the current presentation, he reported a similar history of headache accompanied by confusion. The examination was remarkable for disorientation; otherwise, no focal deficit was elicited. Laboratory testing, cerebrospinal fluid, and neurological imaging were all unremarkable. His symptoms improved spontaneously within less than twenty-four hours, similar to his previous presentations. After two-year history of episodic confusion and after excluding other plausible causes of confusion, guided by proposed diagnostic criteria, we diagnosed him as a case of ACM. The patient remains well at the follow-up of two months after discharge. *Discussion and Conclusion.* ACM is a rare variant of migraine and is often a challenge for clinicians to diagnose appropriately. Until recent years, the disease was thought to be limited to children and adolescents. However, recently few reports also expanded the incidence of this entity to the adult population. There is a significant gap in knowledge about proper identification and treatment of this condition, leading to delayed or overlooked ACM diagnosis. Moreover, the recent edition of the International Classification of Headache Disorders (ICHD-3) does not account for this entity, thereby further adding to physicians' lack of awareness regarding this migraine subtype. The authors emphasize that clinicians be aware of this entity and adequately utilize the existing proposed diagnostic criteria for ACM until standardized and validated tools are available. We also believe that this entity should be acknowledged in the subsequent migraine guidelines and classifications.

1. Introduction

Migraine is a widespread disease affecting over one billion individuals worldwide [1]. It leads to increased morbidity and adds to the global healthcare burden, with more than twenty million years of life lost in disability (YLD) in 2016 [1]. It is a primary headache disorder characterized by moderate-to-severe unilateral headaches, usually lasting up to 72 hours and is more common in females [2]. Migraine can occur either with aura (transient focal neurological symptoms preceding or accompanying the headache) or without aura [3].

There are numerous well-characterized subtypes of migraine mentioned in the third edition of the International Classification of Headache Disorders (ICHD-3), including, but not limited to, hemiplegic migraine, retinal migraine, menstrual migraine, vestibular migraine, chronic migraine, and migraine with brainstem aura. The ICHD-3 failed to index acute confusional migraine (ACM), a rare and highly disabling distinct subtype of migraine [4, 5]. It has been described in the pediatrics population for the last fifty years. Since its description, very few reports documented this subtype, especially in adults, deeming ACM an infrequent entity. We report a case of delayed diagnosis of ACM in a young adult man. Additionally, we present an updated literature review highlighting the typical presenting features, diagnosis, and management of ACM to enable clinicians to identify and treat this condition properly.

2. Case Presentation

We present the case of a 38-year-old previously healthy man who was admitted to our hospital three times over the last two years. The first encounter was in early 2018 when the patient presented with a severe headache associated with photophobia, nausea, and vomiting with subsequent slurred speech and disorientation to time, place, and person. During hospitalization, the patient could not follow commands; thus, a formal neuropsychiatric evaluation was limited. Laboratory tests' results were unremarkable (white blood cells, hemoglobin, electrolytes, toxicology screening, kidney and liver functions, etc.).

Furthermore, a computed tomography (CT) scan of the head was normal. His confusion settled within a few hours with no specific treatment. He was then discharged from the emergency with psychiatry follow-up as a case of a functional confusional state. The patient did not attend his scheduled follow-up. One year later, he presented again with headache and confusion, resembling his earlier presentation. Examination, laboratory testing, and CT head were yet unremarkable. Magnetic resonance imaging (MRI) head revealed a left occipital tiny acute to subacute lacunar infarct, which was the only positive finding (Figure 1). The patient's symptoms resolved completely within twenty-four hours. At this time, the patient reported a fifteen-year history of migraine for which he is not on any specific therapy. Although the MRI finding did not explain the patient presentation, he was assessed to be a case of migrainous infarction (proved later to be an incorrect diagnosis) and started a short course of aspirin and statins.

In January 2020, the patient was admitted with the third episode of headache and confusion. The patient was brought to our hospital by his roommates, who stated he initially experienced severe headaches associated with photophobia, nausea, and three vomiting episodes. Soon thereafter, he developed incomprehensible slurred speech, and he became unaware of his surroundings. There was no history of head trauma, seizure, loss of sphincter control, or loss of consciousness.

On admission, his temperature was 36.8°C, heart rate, 90 beats/min, and blood pressure, 108/60 mmHg. He was confused, not following commands, restless, and disoriented. His uncooperative status limited thorough neuropsychiatric assessment. Nonetheless, there were no gross focal neurological deficits. Systemic examination was otherwise unremarkable. Laboratory blood test results were normal (Table 1). Cerebrospinal fluid (CSF) analysis was unremarkable. MRI head was normal. The remaining workup, including carotid-doppler ultrasonography, Holter monitoring, and echocardiography, was unremarkable.

The patient's hospital course was similar to his previous admissions as he returned to his baseline status within a few hours. At this stage, the information available for us was three hospitalizations (mimicking psychiatric disease and stroke) with headache and confusion settling within a few hours. All investigations were unremarkable, including MRI head. Given the exclusion of other organic causes and his stable course between his symptoms, we diagnosed him as a case of acute confusional migraine (ACM)—a rare migraine variant. The patient is well at the follow-up upon two months after discharge, occasionally taking analgesics for headache relief.

3. Discussion

Gascon and Barlow in 1969 described a unique confusional state that accompanied juvenile migraine [6]. Eight years later, Ehayi and Fenichel reported additional cases of five children with migraine and confusion along with their outcome, and they further coined the term "acute confusional migraine" (ACM) [7]. The prevalence of this rare condition was estimated from focused studies on pediatric migraine patients and ranged as low as 0.45% (most extensive survey of 1106 migraine patients), up to 7% (the retrospective study of 280 children and adolescents) [8, 9]. Till recently, it was thought that this rare entity is limited to children and adolescents. However, few recent reports described its occurrence in adults, suggesting expanding this entity to the adult population. The exact prevalence of this entity in the adult cohort is yet unclear. This is likely owing to the scarcity of data describing ACM in the adult population. A recent review by Farooqi et al. estimated that only 20 cases of ACM were reported in adults, making this condition extremely rare in this population [10].

The clinical presentation is variable. Personal or family history of migraine is usually present in 54% and 62% of the cases, respectively. The distinctive features are headaches, accompanied by confusion, agitation, or disorientation. These patients may also develop speech or memory disturbances, numbness, or even blindness. The neurological symptoms and the confusion usually resolve within less than 24 hours; however, the confusion may last for a few minutes up to 72 hours [10]. Laboratory workup and imaging are often unremarkable, but occasional abnormalities were previously reported. Nezu et al. reported transient cerebral hypoperfusion in the posterior cerebral artery (PCA) territory, as demonstrated by single-photon emission computerized tomography in a child with ACM [11]. Using magnetic resonance angiogram (MRA), Fujita et al. described the same phenomenon only during acute ACM attack in a child with migraine [12]. EEG demonstrated generalized slowing during ACM attacks in some cases [12], and a typical slow pattern of frontal intermittent rhythmic delta activity (FRIDA) was shown by Pietrini et al. [13]. There is no specific therapy as the condition is usually self-limiting; however, sodium valproate and topiramate have

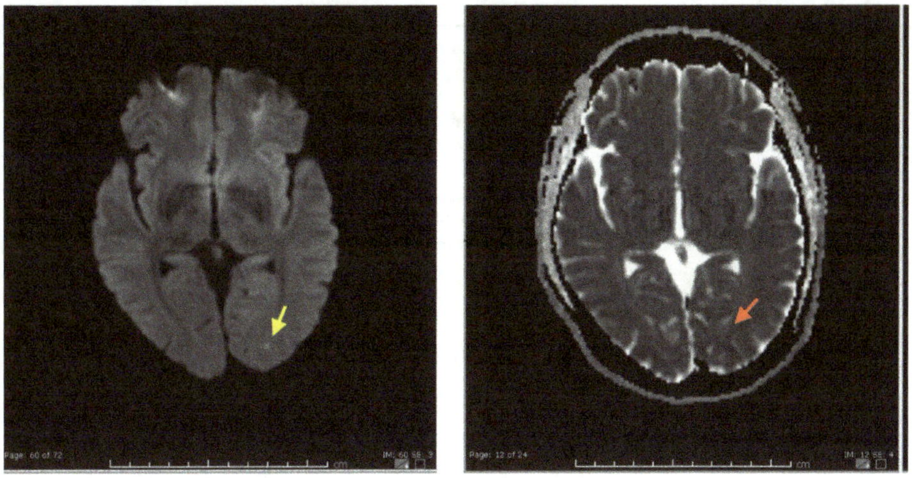

(a) (b)

Figure 1: (a) Diffusion-weighted imaging (DWI) MRI head showing a tiny occipital subcortical hyperintense lesion. (b) The same lesion appearing faintly hypodense on apparent diffusion coefficient (ADC) MRI head. These findings of diffusion restriction were keeping with acute to early subacute lacunar infarction. Notably, these findings were not present on the new MRI done in the third admission (index admission).

Table 1: The patient's laboratory test results.

Test (normal range/unit)	Result
WBC (4–11 x 10^3/ul)	H 13.4
RBC (2.8–4.8 x 10^6/ul)	5.1
Hb (12–15 gm/dL)	14.9
Platelets (150–400 x 10^3/ul)	235
Urea (2.7–8 mmol/L)	3.20
Creatinine (44–80 umol/L)	68
Sodium (135–145 mmol/L)	138
Potassium (mmol/L 3.5–5.1)	3.7
Glucose (3.3–5.5 mmol/L)	8.1
ALT (05–5 U/L)	25
AST (04–0 U/L)	25
TSH (0.3–4.2 IU/L)	0.18
Free T3 (3.7–6.4 pmol/L)	5.2
Free T4 (11.6–21.9 pmol/L)	18.8
Acetaminophen (66.0-199.0)	Below level of detection
Ethanol <10,9 mmol/L	<2.2
Salicylate (150–300 mg/L)	Below level of detection
Cholesterol (<5.2 mmol/L)	4.0
Triglyceride (<1.7 mmol/L)	0.5
HDL (>1.0 mmo/L)	0.9
LDL-calc <3.36 mmol/L	2.9 mmol/L
HbA1C % 4.8-5.9	5.6 %
Lactic acid (0.5–2.2 mmol/L)	1.0
CRP (0–5 mg/L)	<5
CSF glucose (2.22–3.89 mmol/L)	3.84
CSF protein (0.15–0.45 gm/L)	0.32
CSF color	Colorless
CSF appearance	Clear
CSF WBC (0–5 uL)	1

Table 1: Continued.

Test (normal range/unit)	Result
CSF RBC* (0–2 uL)	460
Protein C activity (70–140%)	73.2%
Protein S activity (72–126%)	96%
Factor V	Negative factor V Leiden mutation
Anticardiolipin ab IgM/IgG	Negative
ANA	Negative

*RBCs in the CSF were likely traumatic given the difficulty encountered while performing the lumbar puncture. WBC = white blood cells, RBC = red blood cells, Hb = hemoglobin, ALT = alanine aminotransferase, AST = aspartate aminotransferase, TSH = thyroid stimulating hormone, T3 = triiodothyronine, T4 = thyroxine, HDL = high-density lipoprotein, LDL = low-density lipoprotein, CRP = C-reactive protein, CSF = cerebrospinal fluid.

Table 2: Proposed criteria for the diagnosis of acute confusional migraine (By Farooqi et al. [9]).

At least one attack, fulfilling criteria A to F
A: at least one of the following: decreased attention/altered awareness/impaired cognition
B: at least one of the following: agitation or combativeness/perception disturbances/slowing or FRIDA pattern on EEG resolving within less than a week/aura lasting less than an hour
C: complete resolution in less than 24 hours or after sleep, additionally partial or complete amnesia of the event
D: normal neurological exam following the attack (no persistence of acquired neurologic deficit)
E: at least one of the following: personal history of migraine or family history of migraine or headache occurring before/during or after the confusion.
F: not attributed to another disorder (medical disorder or intoxication).

Adapted from Farooqi et al [9].

been attempted with variable efficacy for ACM treatment and prevention, respectively [10, 12].

The diagnosis can be overlooked, delayed, or missed as with our patient. Our patient presented to the emergency department on three occasions: first being misdiagnosed as a psychiatric illness; secondly, managed as migrainous infarct, another migraine variant; and lastly, as the clinical picture became apparent, the diagnosis of ACM was established (after more than two years from the initial encounter). The latest edition of the International Classification of Headache Disorders (ICHD-3) involves many rare migraine variants. Despite the knowledge of ACM for half a century, it remains unclassified. [5, 9] This, in part, contributes to the lack of awareness among front-line clinicians about this condition and its proper management. Although there are no standardized and validated criteria for ACM diagnosis, Farooqi et al. recently suggested proposed criteria that are practical and straightforward to implement in clinical practice (Table 2) [10]. We used it as a guide in establishing the diagnosis in our case. An essential pillar of these diagnostic criteria is that ACM diagnosis remains that of exclusion.

4. Conclusion

We presented the unusual case of confusional migraine. Our review revealed that this entity is infrequent in adults. It also showed the lack of standardized diagnostic criteria or recognizing this entity as a distinct migraine variant. Our case also highlighted the lack of proper knowledge about this entity among clinicians, which results in unnecessary overinvestigation and treatments and, thus, delays in establishing the appropriate diagnosis. MRI and EEG can be of diagnostic value during acute attacks; sodium valproate and topiramate have been used to treat and prevent this condition. Without therapy, confusion usually settles within less than 24 hours. Clinicians should be made aware of this entity, and guideline makers should consider this entity as a distinct variant of migraine.

Consent

Consent was obtained from the patient.

Authors' Contributions

BT, RT, and MFHM contributed equally to the writing and preparation of this article. BT and RT wrote the initial draft of the discussion and the case presentation, respectively. BT performed the initial literature review. The draft was then reviewed, updated, and supervised by MFHM. JS was involved in the care of the patient. All the authors reviewed the initial and final draft critically and approved it for submission.

Acknowledgments

The authors acknowledge acute medical assessment and neurology teams for their involvement in the care of this patient.

References

[1] L. J. Stovner, E. Nichols, T. J. Steiner et al., "Global, regional, and national burden of migraine and tension-type headache, 1990–2016: a systematic analysis for the global burden of disease Study 2016," *Lancet Neurol*, vol. 17, no. 11, pp. 954–976, 2018.

[2] R. B. Lipton, W. F. Stewart, S. Diamond, M. L. Diamond, and M. Reed, "Prevalence and burden of migraine in the United States: data from the american migraine study II," *Headache: The Journal of Head and Face Pain*, vol. 41, no. 7, pp. 646–657, 2001.

[3] A. M. Lagman-Bartolome and C. Lay, "Pediatric migraine variants: a review of epidemiology, diagnosis, treatment, and outcome," *Current Neurology and Neuroscience Reports*, vol. 15, no. 1, 2015.

[4] I. Pacheva and I. Ivanov, "Acute confusional migraine: is it a distinct form of migraine?" *International Journal of Clinical Practice*, vol. 67, no. 3, pp. 250–256, 2013.

[5] J. Olesen, "Headache classification committee of the international headache society (ihs) the international classification of headache disorders," *Cephalalgia*, vol. 38, no. 1, p. 211, 2018.

[6] G. Gascon and C. Barlow, "Juvenile migraine, presenting as an acute confusional state," *Pediatrics*, vol. 45, no. 4, pp. 628–635, 1970.

[7] A. Ehyai and G. M. Fenichel, "The natural history of acute confusional migraine," *Archives of Neurology*, vol. 35, no. 6, pp. 368-369, 1978.

[8] W. A. Al-Twaijri and M. I. Shevell, "Pediatric migraine equivalents," *Pediatric Neurology*, vol. 26, no. 5, pp. 365–368, 2002.

[9] S. Schipper, F. Riederer, P. S. Sándor, and A. R. Gantenbein, "Acute confusional migraine: our knowledge to date," *Expert Review of Neurotherapeutics*, vol. 12, pp. 307–314, 2012.

[10] A. M. Farooqi, J. M. Padilla, and T. S. Monteith, "Acute confusional migraine: distinct clinical entity or spectrum of migraine biology?" *Brain Sciences*, vol. 8, no. 2, p. 29, 2018.

[11] A. Nezu, S. Kimura, N. Ohtsuki, M. Tanaka, and S. Takebayashi, "Acute confusional migraine and migrainous infarction in childhood," *Brain and Development*, vol. 19, no. 2, pp. 148–151, 1997.

[12] M. Fujita, J. Fujiwara, T. Maki et al., "The efficacy of sodium valproate and a MRA finding in confusional migraine," *Brain and Development*, vol. 29, no. 3, pp. 178–181, 2007.

[13] V. Pietrini, M. G. Terzano, G. D'Andrea, L. Parrino, A. R. Cananzi, and F. Ferro-Milone, "Acute confusional migraine: clinical and electroencephalographic aspects," *Cephalalgia*, vol. 7, no. 1, pp. 29–37, 1987.

34

Long-Term Sequelae in Young Convalescent COVID-19 Patients

Ayumi Nakamura[1] **Thomas J. Farrer**[1,2] **and Andy Liu**[2]

[1]Department of Psychiatry and Behavioral Sciences, Duke University Medical Center, Durham, NC, USA
[2]Department of Neurology, Duke University Medical Center, Durham, NC, USA

Correspondence should be addressed to Andy Liu; andy.liu@duke.edu

Academic Editor: Isabella Laura Simone

As of March 2022, over 78 million cases of COVID-19 and 900,000 deaths have been reported in the United States. The consequences in the acute phase due to the SARS-COV-2 infection are well defined. Beyond the direct effects of severe acute respiratory syndrome coronavirus-2 (SARS-CoV-2) involving the lung parenchyma, the post-viral complications within the central nervous system are still largely unknown, and a comprehensive evaluation regarding the long-term neuropsychological sequelae from this disease is not well characterized. An increasing number of patients previously diagnosed with COVID-19 have now presented with ongoing symptoms of inattention, executive function, and memory difficulties. These symptoms are collectively and commonly known by the public as 'brain fog', with many expressing concerns over their inability to engage in the workplace due to these symptoms. Here, we describe three patients who were seen in the Memory Disorders Clinic at Duke University to characterize the long-term neuropsychological symptoms, neuropsychological test results and brain MRI findings after infection with SARS-CoV-2 in a cohort of patients under the age of 60.

1. Introduction

In December 2019, a novel coronavirus known as Severe Acute Respiratory Syndrome coronavirus 2 (SARS-CoV-2) was identified in Wuhan, located in the Hubei Province of China. On January 31, 2020, the World Health Organization (WHO) issued a global health emergency, and the disease resulting from SARS-CoV-2, coronavirus disease 2019 (COVID-19), was declared a pandemic on March 11, 2020.

SARS-CoV-2, a positive-sense single-stranded RNA virus that primarily manifests with respiratory complications, was isolated from airway epithelial cells in patients [1]. The symptoms of COVID-19 that develop 2–14 days after exposure to SARS-CoV-2 include fever, chills, shortness of breath, fatigue, anosmia, or ageusia, and the course of illness can range from mild to severe illness requiring hospitalization. Characterization of the SARS-CoV-2 viral genome *via* next-generation sequencing led to the identification of the angiotensin-converting enzyme 2 (ACE2) receptor as the receptor that is recognized by SARS-CoV-2 [2]. The SARS-CoV-2 spike protein binds to the ACE2 receptor in airway epithelia and lung parenchyma and uses the receptor as an access point to enter host cells, thereby mediating infection and acute lung injury [3]. In addition to invasion of the respiratory tract, SARS-CoV-2 also has the potential to invade the nervous system [4]. The ACE2 receptor is expressed widely throughout the brain in both neurons and glia in the subfornical organ, paraventricular nucleus, nucleus of the tractus solitarius, and rostral ventrolateral medulla [5]. Consistent with the ability of other coronaviruses to infect brainstem neurons *via* the ACE2 receptor to contribute to dyspnea and respiratory failure in patients, SARS-CoV-2 may act through similar mechanisms [5, 6].

Those who recover from COVID-19 can manifest several extrapulmonary symptoms. Data from previous epidemics and outbreaks with coronaviruses, including SARS-CoV-1 (in 2003) and Middle East Respiratory Syndrome (MERS), have shown a diverse array of neuropsychiatric sequelae [7, 8], though the exact mechanism by which this occurs remains unclear. Recent reports of patients who were diagnosed with COVID-19 have revealed the neuroinvasive potential of SARS-CoV-2. Infection with this coronavirus can result in a myriad of neurological and psychiatric complications post-infection [7]. These complications include an increased incidence of anosmia, ageusia, headaches, cerebrovascular accidents, meningoencephalitis, as well as cognitive dysfunction [7, 9–12] and were recently coined under the collective term of post-acute sequelae of SARS-CoV-2 infection, or PASC. Though the acute manifestations of COVID-19 are well characterized [13–15], the long-term cognitive consequences in long-haulers, who experience a post-viral syndrome weeks or even months after the initial onset of symptoms, are only beginning to be recognized [7, 16, 17]. Here, we report the development of cognitive dysfunction in a series of individuals younger than age 60 who were diagnosed with and subsequently recovered from COVID-19 infection.

2. Case Presentation

2.1. Case #1. A 19-year-old Caucasian female with a history of multiple concussions, migraine headaches, autonomic dysregulation and unexplained fevers presented to the Memory Disorders Clinic five months after recovering from SARS-CoV-2 infection for evaluation of cognitive difficulties. In addition to endorsing dysgeusia and dysnomia, she reported a variety of psychiatric symptoms and behavioral changes, including persistent anxiety and depression, apathy, and irritability features that she did not experience pre-COVID-19. She also self-reported 'brain fogginess' described as difficulty concentrating (including on her schoolwork) and delayed thought process during the entire course of her illness with COVID-19. During a follow-up visit nine months after initial infection, the patient continued to struggle with word-finding difficulties and engaging in planning tasks or multitasking. She reported fatigue and apathy but noted that some of her symptoms, including her depression, had improved. She denied any history of seizures, stroke, anoxia injuries, or surgical intervention to the brain for any reason. The patient also denied having motor symptoms, gait disturbance, lateralized sensory/motor weakness, vision difficulty, auditory or visual hallucinations, obstructive sleep apnea, or REM sleep disinhibition. In terms of sleep health, she indicated that she averages 10 hours of sleep per night. She denied any pain but reported that her migraine frequency is approximately two migraines per week. She also endorsed a history of four reported concussions, one of which included a loss of consciousness at the age of 12.

2.2. Case #2. A 56-year-old South Asian-American female with a history of hypertension, type 2 diabetes, hypothyroidism, mixed connective tissue disorder, and lupus on Plaquenil presented to the Memory Disorders Clinic with language and memory difficulties after developing COVID-19 syndrome with a positive SARS-CoV-2 RT-PCR result one month earlier. She reported progressively worsening memory loss since five years prior that was noted to worsen after recovering from her recent SARS-CoV-2 infection. The patient replaced common words with sound-alike words and endorsed difficulty searching for the correct terminology. Additionally, she reported difficulty in recalling conversations and losing her train of thought when discussing topics with other individuals. She often double checked that she closed the garage door or turned off the stove in the kitchen. Though she had not gotten lost while driving, she had incidents in which she was driving and did not know where she was or where she was headed. The patient works as a physician assistant in neurology; however, her language difficulties have not impaired her ability to function at work and interact with patients.

2.3. Case #3. A 50-year-old African-American female with a history of depression, hypertension, and migraines presented to the clinic with a chief complaint of inattention and difficulties in executive function after she tested positive for SARS-CoV-2 five months prior to her initial clinic visit. She described her memory difficulties as 'drawing blanks', including entering a room and not recalling why she entered the room in the first place or recalling passwords at her workplace. Her family noted concerns that she was forgetting conversations and she self-reported misplacing various items and having to think about where those items might be located.

3. Diagnostic Results

3.1. Case #1. A Montreal Cognitive Assessment (MoCA) performed during the patient's initial visit to the Memory Disorders Clinic revealed a score of 28/30, with a score of 30/30 on a repeat testing four months later. Given mild executive dysfunction that did not impair her daily function, along with normal results on the MoCA, the patient was diagnosed with subjective cognitive impairment. Neuropsychological testing showed mild executive function difficulty with a low-average score on digit-symbol substitution, but other executive functions and overall neurocognitive function was considered normal. She endorsed mild depression and anxiety on self-report measures. Furthermore, examination of the brain MRI revealed normal findings without evidence of restriction diffusion, white matter or brain matter atrophy, and hyperintensity or hemorrhage. The patient's NeuroQuant Age-Related Atrophy Report showed a hippocampal occupancy in the 68th percentile. Given limited data for age-matched controls, the NeuroQuant Triage Brain Atrophy Report was not available for this patient.

3.2. Case #2. The patient scored a 29/30 on the MoCA during her visit, and given reported inattention and executive dysfunction that did not impair her daily function with a normal range on neuropsychological screening, she was diagnosed with subjective cognitive impairment. Results from formal neuropsychological testing performed one month after the initial clinic visit showed overall normal cognitive function except for mildly reduced processing speed of unclear clinical significance. There was no report of emotional distress on questionnaires. MRI of the brain performed three months after the clinic visit was normal without any evidence of restricted diffusion, hemorrhage, infarcts, or intracranial masses. Evaluation for hippocampal atrophy with NeuroQuant revealed a hippocampal volume in the 99th percentile and a hippocampal occupancy score in the 51st percentile. Further, atrophy was noted in the left lateral oribitofrontal as well as both left and right lateral occipital regions on the NeuroQuant Triage Brain Atrophy Report (Figure 1).

3.3. Case #3. The patient underwent a MoCA during her visit to the Memory Disorders Clinic and scored a 26/30. She was diagnosed with subjective cognitive impairment as daily function was not impaired by her executive function, memory, and inattention symptoms. Neuropsychological testing completed a month later revealed reassuring results with the exception of difficulties in verbal memory. She endorsed mild depression and anxiety on self-report measures. An MRI of the brain a month after the initial visit was normal. NeuroQuant analysis revealed a hippocampal volume in the 63rd percentile and a hippocampal occupancy score in the 70th percentile, along with evidence of atrophy in the left posterior superior temporal sulcus, left entorhinal cortex, and the left and right lateral occipital regions of the brain.

4. Discussion

In this case report, we describe three patients under the age of 60 who presented to the Memory Disorders Clinic at Duke University with complaints of cognitive dysfunction after recovery from SARS-CoV-2 infection. We sought to address several key questions, including the collection of neurologic and cognitive PASC symptoms, how long symptoms potentially last in this patient population, and whether any objective findings could be identified on imaging or neuropsychological testing. The patients, all of whom were diagnosed with subjective cognitive impairment, noted improvements in their cognition at the time of the clinic visit or on follow-up visits, and two were able to return to work after a period of leave. Assessment of their cognitive function, either with a MoCA screening tool or follow-up neuropsychological testing, revealed reassuring results (Table 1). Overall, these findings from neuropsychological testing suggest that in a young cohort of patients who develop cognitive sequelae from SARS-CoV-2 infection, their symptoms continue to improve with time. Analysis of the brain MRI of each of the three patients in this case report revealed normal hippocampal volume adjusted to age-related controls. Case #2 showed evidence of atrophy in the orbitofrontal cortex, which may be suggestive of executive dysfunction, though executive function was largely normal on neuropsychological testing. Further, cases #2 and #3 revealed atrophy in the occipital regions of the cortex, although this is of unclear significance. Longitudinal assessment with ongoing follow-up neuropsychological testing and brain imaging will better reveal the long-term clinical trajectory of these cognitive symptoms. This will also help determine if these patients are at risk for the development of a neurodegenerative disorder later in life.

Several reports have previously outlined the various symptoms that persist months after acute SARS-CoV-2 infection. The most common PASC symptoms that were noted two to six months post-infection included fatigue, dyspnea, anosmia/ageusia, anxiety, and depression [12, 18, 19], with studies suggesting more frequent incidence of PASC symptoms in those with severe disease hospitalized for COVID-19 [19]. Common neurological manifestations that have been reported in long-haulers include sleep disturbances, headaches, fatigue, cognitive impairment, and difficulties in sustaining attention [20–22]. While these studies examined the collection of PASC symptoms after initial infection in large cohorts of patients, no studies have yet stratified the symptomatology between younger and older cohorts.

The National Institute for Health and Care Excellence (NICE) in the U.K. has published guidelines to assess the clinical features of the long-term consequences of SARS-CoV-2 infection. NICE defines three stages reflecting symptomatic recovery, including the following: (1) acute COVID-19, which refers to symptoms up to 4 weeks or 28 days after the onset of infection with SARS-CoV-2; (2) ongoing symptomatic COVID-19, generally defined as symptoms ranging from four to 12 weeks after onset of infection; and (3) post-COVID-19, referring to symptoms associated with SARS-CoV-2 infection that continue for 12 weeks or greater [23]. Symptoms persisting beyond the acute phase of SARS-CoV-2 infection are commonly referred to as "long-COVID", while a "long hauler" refers to a patient who has recovered from acute SARS-CoV-2 infection experiencing persistent symptoms [23, 24]. In February 2021, the National Institutes of Health in the U.S. defined the collection of symptoms associated with long-COVID as PASC to identify the potential causes, treatment and prevention of those suffering from these long-term effects of COVID-19. However, the broad clinical phenotype and unknown duration of PASC requires further investigation to comprehensively characterize this syndrome.

With an increase in the number of cases and hospitalization rates due to the surge in variants, there continues to be an increasing number of patients who develop persistent symptoms beyond the acute phase of infection. Several crucial questions such as follows remain: (1) Does the severity of cognitive dysfunction secondary to SARS-CoV-2 correlate with severity of disease in young cohorts? Younger patients generally tend to have fewer medical comorbidities and are at reduced risk for more severe infection compared to the older population. Certainly, PASC symptoms have been identified in both patients with mild disease requiring outpatient treatment as well as in those hospitalized with more severe illness, but risk has been noted to be greater in those with severe COVID-19 [20]. (2) Are females at increased risk of developing cognitive dysfunction after recovery from SARS-CoV-2

MORPHOMETRY RESULTS

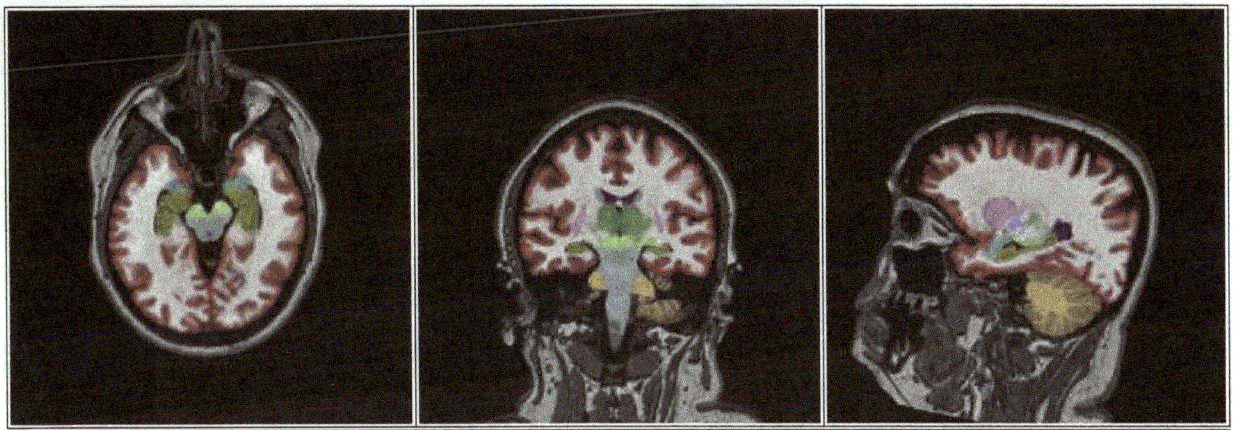

Brain Structure	Volume (cm³)	% of ICV (5%-95% Normative Percentile)	Normative Percentile
Hippocampal Occupancy Score (HOC)	0.86	N/A	51
Hippocampi	8.07	0.63 (0.45 - 0.59)	99
Superior Lateral Ventricles	11.29	0.88 (0.66 - 2.99)	13
Inferior Lateral Ventricles	1.30	0.10 (0.05 - 0.14)	73

AGE AND SEX MATCHED REFERENCE CHARTS

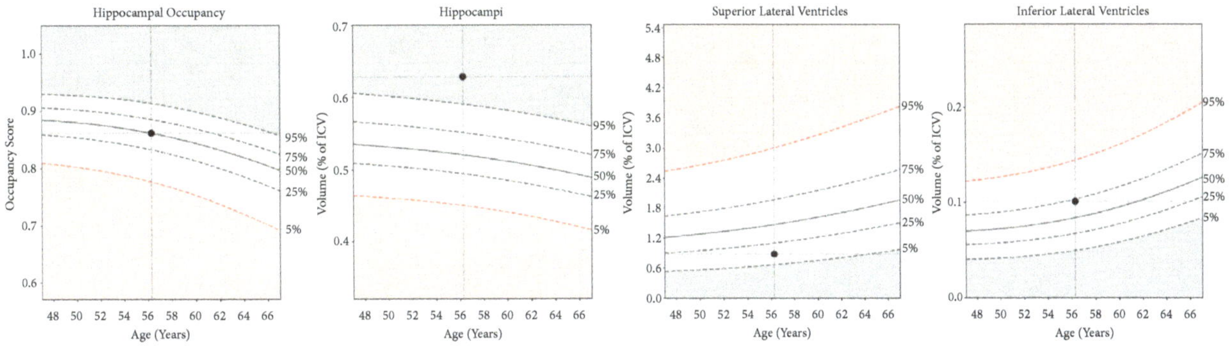

(a)

Figure 1: Continued.

MORPHOMETRY RESULTS

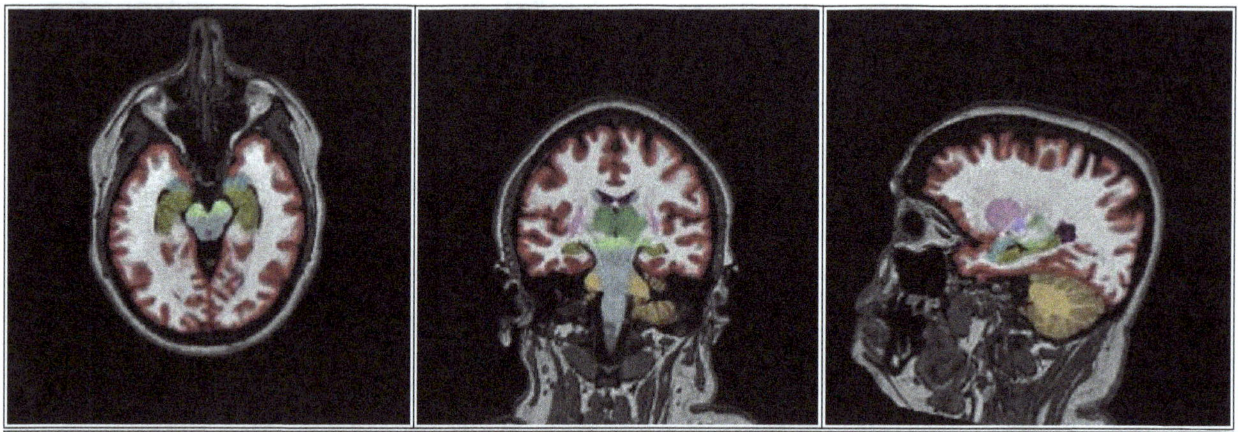

Intracranial Volume (ICV) (cm^3)	1283.14

Brain Structure	LH Volume (cm^3)	LH Volume (% of ICV)	RH Volume (cm^3)	RH Volume (% of ICV)	Asymmetry Index (%)*
Forebrain Parenchyma	438.48	34.17	449.01	34.99	-2.37
Cortical Gray Matter	215.46	16.79	221.20	17.24	-2.63
Superior Lateral Ventricle	5.49	0.43	5.80	0.45	-5.40
Inferior Lateral Ventricle	0.55	0.04	0.75	0.06	-30.73
Hippocampus	4.00	0.31	4.07	0.32	-1.59
Amygdala	1.59	0.12	1.45	0.11	8.96
Caudate	2.50	0.19	2.62	0.20	-4.62
Putamen	5.73	0.45	5.72	0.45	0.26
Pallidum	0.79	0.06	0.71	0.06	11.17
Thalamus	5.85	0.46	6.39	0.50	-8.79
Cerebellum	59.00	4.60	57.54	4.48	2.52

(b)

FIGURE 1: Continued.

MORPHOMETRY RESULTS

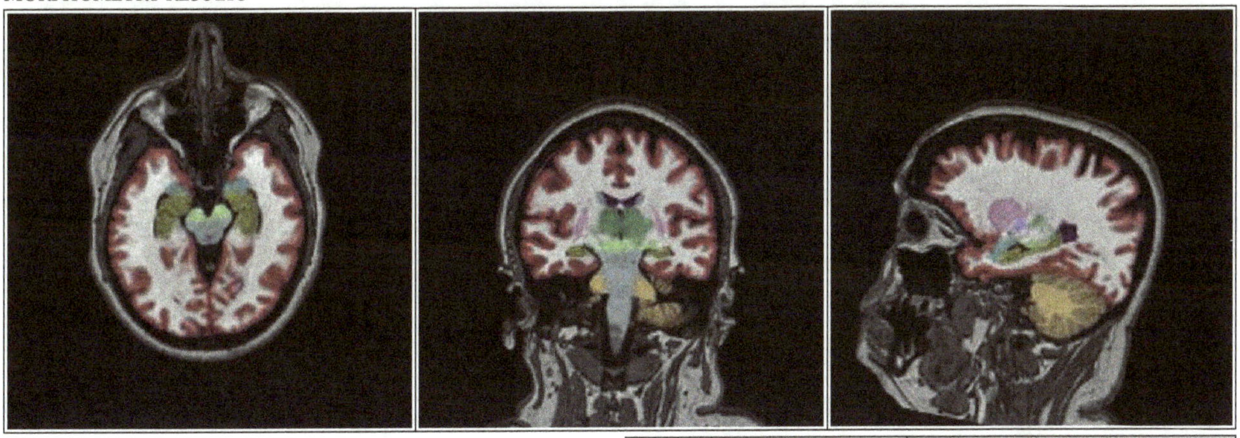

Structure	Total Volume (cm^3)	Percentile
Intracranial Volume	1283	-
Whole Brain	1022	66
Forebrain Parenchyma	887	63

Total Volumes	Percentiles		
	Left	Right	Total
Cerebral White Matter	71	78	75
Cortical Gray Matter	29	40	35
Ventricles	13	16	14
Cerebral WM Hypointensities*	2	1	2
Subcortical Structures			
Cerebellar White Matter	84	92	89
Cerebellar Gray Matter	59	45	53
Brainstem	-	-	11
Thalamus	36	81	61
Ventral Diencephalon	95	93	95
Basal Ganglia			
Putamen	99	99	99
Caudate	71	67	70
Nucleus Accumbens	59	44	52
Pallidum	79	60	72
Cingulate	32	30	29
Anterior Cingulate	8	29	18
Posterior Cingulate	97	81	93
Isthmus Cingulate	19	17	17

Cortical Brain Regions	Percentiles		
	Left	Right	Total
Frontal Lobes	38	58	49
Superior Frontal	59	62	61
Middle Frontal	47	44	44
Inferior Frontal	73	66	70
Lateral Orbitofrontal	4	33	9
Medial Orbitofrontal	33	15	20
Paracentral	41	87	67
Primary Motor	44	88	71
Parietal Lobes	61	72	66
Primary Sensory	24	57	37
Medial Parietal	87	59	79
Superior Parietal	58	76	70
Inferior Parietal	39	55	47
Supramarginal	81	82	86
Occipital Lobes	2	8	3
Medial Occipital	44	53	48
Lateral Occipital	1	2	1
Temporal Lobes	60	39	51
Transverse Temporal + Superior Temporal	50	72	63
Posterior Superior Temporal Sulcus	98	95	98
Middle Temporal	37	8	17
Inferior Temporal	65	21	42
Fusiform	35	45	39
Parahippocampal	98	96	98
Entorhinal Cortex	25	11	14
Temporal Pole	72	51	64
Amygdala	87	81	86
Hippocampus	99	99	99

(c)

Figure 1: a-c. NeuroQuant report for case #2.

infection compared to males? As findings from recent studies suggest a predominance of PASC in females [21], it will be crucial to determine whether cognitive dysfunction also has a female: male predominance, and what the contributing risk factors are. (3) Does the landscape of cognitive symptoms differ in younger *versus* older patients, and is the timeline of these symptoms different between these two populations? Further, are there any significant changes on brain MRI that occur longitudinally after recovery from SARS-CoV-2 infection? (4) Given concerns over emerging COVID-19 variants, do the characteristics of cognitive symptoms depend on the specific variant? (5) Finally, what role does vaccination play in mitigating the effects in both who previously developed and recovered from COVID-19 illness and those who have not been infected with SARS-CoV-2 but are still at risk? While these questions are beyond the scope of our study, there is a dire need to elucidate the pathophysiology and identify the risk factors and treatment modalities for those suffering from persistent symptoms secondary to SARS-CoV-2.

Table 1: Neuropsychological findings in the three cases after recovery from SARS-CoV-2 infection.

Demographics	Case 1	Case 2	Case 3
Age	56	19	49
Sex	Female	Female	Female
Education	18	13	18
Race	Asian	W/non-Hisp	Black
Tests			
TOPF (Actual)	107	111	90
Intellectual Functioning WAIS-IV			
FSIQ (SS)	103	123	NA
GAI (SS)	102	132	101
VCI (SS)	100	143	98
PRI (SS)	105	115	104
WMI (SS)	114	111	NA
PSI (SS)	92	100	NA
Executive Functioning			
TMT A (Raw) T	21 (58)	17 (59)	26 (49)
TMT B (Raw) T	50 (53)	36 (59)	74 (47)
WCST Categories (Raw)	6	6	6
Digit Span	34 (63)	30 (53)	31 (57)
Coding	53 (47)	57 (40)	70 (53)
Language			
BNT (Raw) T	44 (21)	57 (53)	52 (41)
FAS (Raw) T	39 (43)	33 (39)	60 (64)
Animal (Raw) T	19 (43)	23 (52)	25 (60)
Vocabulary (Raw) T	37 (50)	49 (70)	43 (53)
Similarities (Raw) T	29 (57)	35 (80)	30 (57)
Verbal Memory CVLT-II			
Total Learning (Raw) T	60 (63)	63 (60)	37 (36)
Delayed Recall (Raw) T	13 (55)	14 (55)	6 (30)
Visual Memory BVMT-R			
Total Learning (Raw) T	NA	29 (61)	25 (52)
Delayed Recall (Raw) T	NA	12 (66)	12 (65)
Mood			
BDI-II	7	17	18
BAI	8	8	13
NA = Not administered			

5. Methods

Clinical neuropsychological evaluations of these individuals included a fixed flexible battery. Neuropsychological tests were administered in standard fashion according to test manuals. Publisher information and additional details about these tests can be found elsewhere [25]. A master's-level psychometrist administered the neuropsychological tests under the supervision of a clinical neuropsychologist. The neuropsychological test results in Table 1 include raw scores, standard scores (SS), and T-scores, as well as raw scores and T-scores where applicable. A standard score has a mean of 100 and a standard deviation of 15. A *T* score has a mean of 50 and a standard deviation of 10. It is to be noted that because this was a fixed flexible battery there are times in which certain subtests were not administered due to a patient's tolerance for testing or due to difficulties with psychometric properties of the test. If a test was not administered, it was indicated on the table with NA.

Test measures included the following:

The Test of Premorbid Functioning (TOPF) is an assessment tool to estimate premorbid cognitive ability that requires an examinee to read a list of phonetically irregular words. The TOPF provides multiple possible scores, including a predicted score and achieved score. Table 1 includes an actual achieved score.

Wechsler Adult Intelligence Scale - Fourth Edition (WAIS-IV) is a measure of intellectual function used to derive a full-scale IQ score and four indices based on verbal comprehension, perceptual reasoning, working memory, and processing speed.

Trail Making Test (A&B) : Part A of this test assesses simple visual sequencing, psychomotor speed, and general processing speed by requiring the examinee to quickly draw lines sequentially in a numerical order from 1–25. Part B of the test is similar but requires alphanumeric sequencing (e.g., 1, A, 2, B, 3, C, etc.). Part B is considered more complex and measures cognitive flexibility. These tests are sensitive to neurological impairment and are often categorized as measures of executive function. The raw score on Table 1 is the total time to completion.

Wisconsin Card Sorting Test (WCST): This test assesses an individual's strategic planning and ability to utilize environmental feedback and problem solve. It is a common measure of executive function. It is sensitive to frontal lobe damage, particularly related to dorsolateral prefrontal regions. There are multiple subscores that can be derived from this test but the table presents the number of categories generated out of 6 possible categories.

California Verbal Learning Test - Second Edition (CVLT-II): As a test of verbal episodic memory, this test assesses for verbal learning and recall by requiring an examinee to repeat back a list of words over multiple trials and to recall as many words as possible after a delay.

Brief Visuospatial Memory Test - Revised (BVMT-R): As a visual memory test assessing episodic memory, this test requires an examinee to recall shapes and to draw them in the same location presented on a page. This test includes learning trials, a delayed recall trial, and a recognition memory trial.

Boston Naming Test (BNT): This is a common test of confrontational object naming in which an examinee is presented with simple line drawings and asked to name the item. Phonemic and semantic cues are often provided for individuals who cannot identify the object. Table 1 includes a raw score out of 60 items.

Controlled Oral Word Associations Test (FAS) and Category Naming (Animal Fluency): Verbal fluency measures required individuals to rapidly name as many objects as they can that either begin with a certain letter or fall under a certain semantic category. These are one minute trials. Phonemic fluency is mediated by frontal regions, whereas semantic fluency is mediated by left temporal and inferior parietal regions.

Beck Depression Inventory - Second Edition (BDI-II) and Beck Anxiety Inventory (BAI): These self-report questionnaires assess for symptoms of depression occurring over the most recent 2 weeks and symptoms of anxiety occurring over the most recent week.

Acknowledgments

The authors would like to thank Dr. Allen Song for his clinical guidance on the radiology findings for each of the three patients in this case report. This work was performed as part of a project of Duke University.

References

[1] N. Zhu, D. Zhang, W. Wang et al., "A novel coronavirus from patients with pneumonia in China, 2019," *New England Journal of Medicine*, vol. 382, no. 8, pp. 727–733, 2020.

[2] R. Lu, X. Zhao, J. Li et al., "Genomic characterisation and epidemiology of 2019 novel coronavirus: implications for virus origins and receptor binding," *The Lancet*, vol. 395, no. 10224, pp. 565–574, 2020.

[3] P. Zhou, X.-L. Yang, X.-G. Wang et al., "A pneumonia outbreak associated with a new coronavirus of probable bat origin," *Nature*, vol. 579, no. 7798, pp. 270–273, 2020.

[4] A. M. Baig, A. Khaleeq, U. Ali, and H. Syeda, "Evidence of the COVID-19 virus targeting the CNS: tissue distribution, host-virus interaction, and proposed neurotropic mechanisms," *ACS Chemical Neuroscience*, vol. 11, no. 7, pp. 995–998, 2020.

[5] L. Steardo, L. Steardo Jr., R. Zorec, and A. Verkhratsky, "Neuroinfection may contribute to pathophysiology and clinical manifestations of COVID-19," *Acta physiologica (Oxford, England)*, vol. 229, Article ID e13473, 2020.

[6] Y. C. Li, W. Z. Bai, and T. Hashikawa, "The neuroinvasive potential of SARS-CoV2 may play a role in the respiratory failure of COVID-19 patients," *Journal of Medical Virology*, vol. 92, no. 6, pp. 552–555, 2020.

[7] E. A. Troyer, J. N. Kohn, and S. Hong, "Are we facing a crashing wave of neuropsychiatric sequelae of COVID-19? Neuropsychiatric symptoms and potential immunologic mechanisms," *Brain, Behavior, and Immunity*, vol. 87, pp. 34–39, 2020.

[8] J. P. Rogers, E. Chesney, D. Oliver et al., "Psychiatric and neuropsychiatric presentations associated with severe coronavirus infections: a systematic review and meta-analysis with comparison to the COVID-19 pandemic," *The Lancet Psychiatry*, vol. 7, no. 7, pp. 611–627, 2020.

[9] J. Helms, S. Kremer, H. Merdji et al., "Neurologic features in severe SARS-CoV-2 infection," *New England Journal of Medicine*, vol. 382, no. 23, pp. 2268–2270, 2020.

[10] L. Mao, H. Jin, M. Wang et al., "Neurologic manifestations of hospitalized patients with coronavirus disease 2019 in wuhan, China," *JAMA Neurology*, vol. 77, no. 6, pp. 683–690, 2020.

[11] A. S. Nordvig, K. T. Rimmer, J. Z. Willey et al., "Potential neurological manifestations of COVID-19," *Neurology: Clinical Practice*, vol. 2020, 2020.

[12] J. K. Logue, N. M. Franko, D. J. McCulloch et al., "Sequelae in adults at 6 Months after COVID-19 infection," *JAMA Network Open*, vol. 4, no. 2, Article ID e210830, 2021.

[13] D. Wang, B. Hu, C. Hu et al., "Clinical characteristics of 138 hospitalized patients with 2019 novel coronavirus-infected pneumonia in wuhan, China," *JAMA*, vol. 323, no. 11, pp. 1061–1069, 2020.

[14] W.-j. Guan, Z.-y. Ni, Y. Hu et al., "egClinical Characteristics of Coronavirus Disease 2019 in China," *New England Journal of Medicine*, vol. 382, no. 18, pp. 1708–1720, 2020.

[15] N. Chen, M. Zhou, X. Dong et al., "Epidemiological and clinical characteristics of 99 cases of 2019 novel coronavirus pneumonia in Wuhan, China: a descriptive study," *The Lancet*, vol. 395, no. 10223, pp. 507–513, 2020.

[16] M. Taquet, S. Luciano, J. R. Geddes, and P. J. Harrison, "Bidirectional associations between COVID-19 and psychiatric disorder: retrospective cohort studies of 62 354 COVID-19 cases in the USA," *The Lancet Psychiatry*, vol. 2020, 2020.

[17] A. Varatharaj, N. Thomas, M. A. Ellul et al., "Neurological and neuropsychiatric complications of COVID-19 in 153 patients: a UK-wide surveillance study," *The lancet. Psychiatry*, vol. 7, pp. 875–882, 2020.

[18] A. Carfì, R. Bernabei, F. Landi, and C.-P.-A. C. S. G. Gemelli Against, "Persistent symptoms in patients after acute COVID-19," *JAMA*, vol. 324, no. 6, pp. 603–605, 2020.

[19] C. Huang, L. Huang, Y. Wang et al., "6-month consequences of COVID-19 in patients discharged from hospital: a cohort study," *The Lancet*, vol. 397, no. 10270, pp. 220–232, 2021.

[20] M. Taquet, J. R. Geddes, M. Husain, S. Luciano, and P. J. Harrison, "6-month neurological and psychiatric outcomes in 236 379 survivors of COVID-19: a retrospective cohort study using electronic health records," *The Lancet Psychiatry*, vol. 8, no. 5, pp. 416–427, 2021.
[21] E. L. Graham, J. R. Clark, Z. S. Orban et al., "Persistent neurologic symptoms and cognitive dysfunction in non-hospitalized Covid-19 long haulers," *Ann Clin Transl Neurol*, vol. 2021, 2021.
[22] A. Nalbandian, K. Sehgal, A. Gupta et al., "Post-acute COVID-19 syndrome," *Nature MedicineNature Medicine*, vol. 27, no. 4, pp. 601–615, 2021.
[23] P. Venkatesan, "NICE guideline on long COVID," *Lancet Respiratory Medicine*, vol. 9, Article ID 129, 2021.
[24] C. Del Rio, L. F. Collins, and P. Malani, "Long-term health consequences of COVID-19," *JAMA*, vol. 2020, 2020.
[25] D. B. Howieson, E. D. Bigler, D. Tranel, and M. D. Lezak, *Neuropsychological Assessment*, OUP USA, UK, 2012.

35

The Big Yawning: Pathological Yawning as a Symptom of Neuromyelitis Optica Spectrum Disorders

Veronika Spahlinger,[1] Annette Niessen,[1] Sebastian Rauer,[2] Stefan Krämer,[3] and Matthias Reinhard[1]

[1]*Department of Neurology and Clinical Neurophysiology, Medical Center Esslingen, Academic Teaching Hospital of the University of Tübingen, Tübingen, Germany*
[2]*Department of Neurology and Neurophysiology, University Medical Center Freiburg, University of Freiburg, Freiburg, Germany*
[3]*Department of Radiology and Nuclear Medicine, Medical Center Esslingen, Academic Teaching Hospital of the University of Tübingen, Tübingen, Germany*

Correspondence should be addressed to Matthias Reinhard; m.reinhard@klinikum-esslingen.de

Academic Editor: Majaz Moonis

Pathological yawning is rarely observed in cerebral or spinal diseases. A 67-year-old woman was admitted with a seven-day progressive hemisyndrome with left-sided limb ataxia and hypesthesia. The patient yawned with a high frequency, partially in salve-like episodes. MRI showed a cervical myelitis over more than three vertebral segments up to the lower medulla and Aquaporin-4-antibodies were positive (diagnostic criteria for a Neuromyelitis optica spectrum disorder were fulfilled). Under treatment with methylprednisolone, followed by plasmapheresis and immunoadsorption, clinical symptoms were regressive and the frequency of yawning completely normalized. When observing pathological yawning, even in the absence of other cerebral or brainstem symptoms, one should be aware of NMOSD as a possible cause.

1. Introduction

Yawning is an everyday phenomenon. Pathological yawning is defined by a yawning rate higher than commonly accepted without triggers like fatigue or boredom. Various anatomical structures such as the insula, thalamus, hypothalamus, and brainstem reticular formation as well as the locus coeruleus are involved in the initiation and procedure of yawning [1]. As a symptom, pathological yawning can occur as part of epileptic seizures, premigraine, and strokes or as side effects of medications [2].

2. Case Presentation

A 67-year-old woman was admitted to our hospital with a seven-day progressive hemisyndrome with left-sided limb ataxia and hypesthesia. On admission, the patient yawned with a high frequency (>3/minute) and partially in salve-like episodes (>8 yawns). There was no increased level of fatigue or boredom. Yawning was accompanied by nausea and vomiting. There were no cranial nerve deficits. The cranial MRI showed moderate leukoaraiosis not suggestive of inflammation and a signal enhancement of the coregistered myelon up to the lower medulla. The cervical MRI then revealed the full extent of the cervical myelitis over more than three vertebral segments (see Figures 1(a) and 1(b)). The cerebrospinal fluid (CSF) showed a slight pleocytosis with lymphocytes (7 cells) without elevation of CSF protein. CSF-restricted oligoclonal IgG bands were present. The visual evoked potentials were normal on both sides. The diagnostic criteria for a NMOSD were fulfilled: positive test for AQP4-IgG and acute myelitis [3]. There was no evidence for alternative diagnoses such as other systemic autoimmune, infective, vascular, neoplastic, or paraneoplastic disease. The patient had a history of autoimmune hepatitis with increased ANA titer, which was inactive under long-term treatment with low-dose azathioprine. Under initial

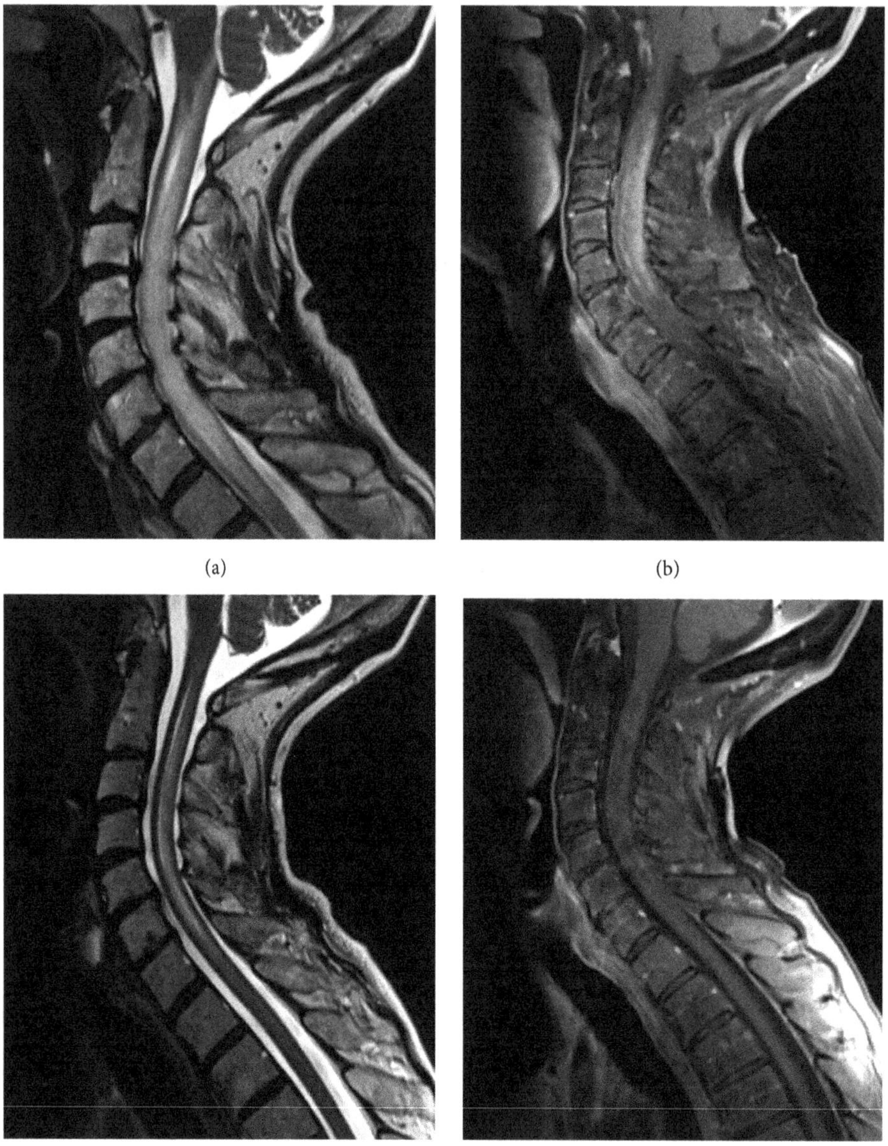

(a) (b) (c) (d)

FIGURE 1: (a) Distinct oedema of the cervical spinal cord on T2-weighted sequences with spinal cord swelling and expansion into the brainstem. (b) Distinct gadolinium enhancement of the cervical spinal cord on T1-weighted sequences with cord swelling. (c) Regressive edema in the cervical spinal cord after 5 days of methylprednisolone followed by plasmapheresis and immunoadsorption. (d) Regressive gadolinium enhancement in the cervical spinal cord after therapy.

high-dose treatment with methylprednisolone, followed by plasmapheresis and immunoadsorption, clinical symptoms of ataxia and hypesthesia and the spinal cord enhancement on MRI were regressive within 10 days (see Figures 1(c) and 1(d)). Consequently, the frequency of yawning normalized and no more salves of yawning were observed. Treatment with rituximab was initiated.

3. Discussion

This case shows pathological yawning as a symptom of NMOSD. So far, one series of 9 NMOSD patients with pathological yawning lasting over a period of at least two weeks was described [4]. Our case supports this previous notion of excessive yawning with NMOSD. The phenomenon of pathological yawning in NMOSD may be underrecognized by both patients and physicians because yawning is a regular physiological phenomenon. Only 2 of the previously reported 9 cases did not show other brainstem symptoms; one of them, however, exhibited hypothalamic symptoms. All these patients had abnormal brain MRI with inflammatory lesions in the hypothalamus and/or brainstem. In the present case, yawning existed only for a few days and dissolved rapidly after immune therapy. Interestingly, in our patient, no other brainstem or hypothalamic symptoms were observed apart from nausea and vomiting. MRI only showed involvement of the lower medulla including the area postrema but no other inflammatory brainstem or hypothalamic lesion. This might be due to treatment initiation prior to radiologically visible extension of the disease to more rostral structures.

Differential diagnoses for pathological yawning include ischemic stroke (in the upper brainstem, insula, or caudate nucleus [1, 5, 6], autonomic epileptic seizures [7], parkinsonism, intracranial hypertension due to infections or brain tumors, and side effects of medications (e.g., serotonin reuptake inhibitors and apomorphine) [2]. We could not find such factors in the present case as an alternative explanation.

Pathological yawning is not frequently observed in other chronic inflammatory central nervous system diseases apart from a single case report in multiple sclerosis [8]. It thus seems to be a rather characteristic clinical sign of NMOSD, which could be explained by the fact that brain regions with high aquaporin-4 expression are also those being involved in the mechanism or control of yawning. Assuming an increased local temperature with extensive NMOSD inflammation in the myelon and lower brainstem, an additional factor to the increased yawning frequency could be the thermoregulatory function of yawning via suggested brain cooling effects [9]. The fact that yawning subsided following administration of methylprednisolone, which decreases temperature of inflammatory tissue, supports this hypothesis.

In conclusion, when observing pathological yawning, even in the absence of other cerebral or brainstem symptoms, one should be aware of NMOSD as a possible cause.

Consent

Written informed consent was obtained from the patient.

References

[1] H. Krestel, C. Weisstanner, C. W. Hess et al., "Insular and caudate lesions release abnormal yawning in stroke patients," *Brain Structure & Function*, vol. 220, no. 2, pp. 803–812, 2015.

[2] H. A. G. Teive, R. P. Munhoz, C. H. F. Camargo, and O. Walusinski, "Yawning in neurology: a review," *Arquivos de Neuro-Psiquiatria*, vol. 76, no. 7, pp. 473–480, 2018.

[3] D. M. Wingerchuk, B. Banwell, J. L. Bennett et al., "International consensus diagnostic criteria for neuromyelitis optica spectrum disorders," *Neurology*, vol. 85, no. 2, pp. 177–189, 2015.

[4] M. A. Lana-Peixoto, D. Callegaro, N. Talim et al., "Pathologic yawning in neuromyelitis optica spectrum disorders," *Multiple Sclerosis and Related Disorders*, vol. 3, no. 4, pp. 527–532, 2017.

[5] L. Cattaneo, L. Cucurachi, E. Chierici, and G. Pavesi, "Pathological yawning as a presenting symptom of brain stem ischaemia in two patients," *Journal of Neurology, Neurosurgery, and Psychiatry*, vol. 77, no. 1, pp. 98–100, 2006.

[6] O. C. Singer, M. C. Humpich, H. Lanfermann, and T. Neumann-Haefelin, "Yawning in acute anterior circulation stroke," *Journal of Neurology, Neurosurgery, and Psychiatry*, vol. 78, no. 11, pp. 1253-1254, 2007.

[7] A. Nicotra, N. M. Khalil, P. Owbridge et al., "Pathological yawning as an ictal seizure manifestation in the elderly," *BMJ Case Reports*, 2012, bcr0120125618.

[8] T. Postert, D. Pöhlau, S. Meves, I. Nastos, and H. Przuntek, "Pathological yawning as a symptom of multiple sclerosis," *Journal of Neurology*, vol. 243, no. 3, pp. 300-301, 1996.

[9] A. C. Gallup and O. T. Eldakar, "The thermoregulatory theory of yawning: what we know from over 5 years of research," *Frontiers in Neuroscience*, vol. 6, article no 188, 2013.

36

Diffuse Gonococcal Infection (DGI) in a Patient with Treatment-Refractory Acetylcholine Receptor Antibody-Positive (AChR+) Generalized Myasthenia Gravis (gMG) Treated with Eculizumab

Nakul Katyal,[1] **Latika Nirola**,[2] **Naureen Narula**,[3] **and Raghav Govindarajan**[1]

[1]*Department of Neurology, University of Missouri, Columbia, MO, USA*
[2]*Guru Gobind Singh Medical College and Hospital, Faridkot, Punjab, India*
[3]*Department of Pulmonology and Critical Care Medicine, Staten Island University Hospital, New York, NY, USA*

Correspondence should be addressed to Nakul Katyal; katyal.nakul@gmail.com

Academic Editor: Dominic B. Fee

Patients receiving complement inhibitor, eculizumab, are at high risk for infections with encapsulated organisms such as *Neisseria* due to impaired opsonophagocytic activity. Impaired complement immunity may increase the risk for dissemination of asymptomatic *Neisseria gonorrhoeae.* Disseminated Gonococcal Infection (DGI) is a rare but potentially life-threatening complication associated with eculizumab. Physicians should obtain adequate sexual histories from the patients and educate them on safe sexual practices. Here, we describe a case of DGI in a 32-year-old African American female patient with acetylcholine receptor antibody-positive (AChR+) generalized myasthenia gravis (gMG), receiving eculizumab.

1. Introduction

Eculizumab is a recombinant humanized monoclonal antibody that binds to complement component C5 and prevents conversion to the proinflammatory C5a and eventually membrane attack complex (MAC) formation [1]. Eculizumab has been approved for management of patients with paroxysmal nocturnal hemoglobinuria (PNH) and atypical haemolytic uremic syndrome (HUS) [2]. In a phase 3, randomized, double-blind, placebo-controlled study (REGAIN) and its open-label extension, eculizumab was shown to be effective in patients with treatment-refractory acetylcholine receptor antibody-positive (AChR+) generalized myasthenia gravis (gMG) [3]. In 2017, eculizumab was approved by the Food and Drug Administration (FDA) for the treatment of AChR+ gMG [4]. Patients receiving eculizumab are at high risk for infections with encapsulated organisms such as *Neisseria* due to impaired opsonophagocytic activity [5]. Administration of meningococcal vaccines, therefore, is recommended before beginning treatment [6]. Despite vaccination, meningococcal disease has been reported in recipients of eculizumab [7, 8]. In vitro data have shown that eculizumab impairs meningococcal killing in whole blood even in subjects vaccinated against the relevant meningococcal serogroup [5, 7, 8]. Similarly, impaired complement immunity with eculizumab may increase the risk for dissemination of *Neisseria gonorrhoeae.* Here, we describe a case of Disseminated Gonococcal Infection (DGI) in a 32-year-old African American female patient with AChR+ gMG receiving eculizumab.

2. Case Report

A 32-year-old African American female with a past medical history of deep vein thrombosis (DVT) and AChR+ gMG status after thymectomy, on pyridostigmine (60 mg three times a day) and eculizumab, presented to the Emergency Room (ER), a week after sustaining a mechanical fall while walking carrying her child on an ice-covered pavement. During the fall, her child landed on her left knee. The patient was first started on eculizumab 2 years ago (June 2018) after receiving both the monovalent and quadrivalent meningococcal vaccines as per Advisory Committee on Immunization Practices (ACIP) guidelines. She was on eculizumab for a year but then stopped it (June 2019) due to significant improvement in her MG symptoms. She was off all MG treatments for a year and half but was restarted on eculizumab (Nov 2020) due to worsening fatigue, axial weakness, and dysphagia. Her last dose was 8 days before presentation to the ER.

At the time of presentation to the ER, she complained of 8/10, sharp pain, localized to the left knee, worse with movement, and better with rest. Her vital signs were unremarkable. Examination was remarkable for left knee tenderness to palpation and limited active and passive range of motion. Laboratory workup showed elevated White Blood Cell (WBC) count to 12,000/L with 72% neutrophils, elevated Erythrocyte Sedimentation Rate (ESR) to 111 mm/hour, elevated alkaline phosphatase to 162 Units/L, and C reactive protein (CRP) to 17.19 mg/dl. Urinary *N. gonorrhoeae* testing with a Nucleic Acid Amplification Technique (NAAT) showed a positive result. She denied any change in her sexual contacts or history of Sexually Transmitted Diseases (STDs). We suspect she acquired the infection from her husband who was later tested positive. X-ray of the left knee showed moderate effusion without evidence of fracture. Arthrocentesis of the left knee showed a cloudy, yellow-colored fluid with a WBC of 50,000/mcL, with 95% neutrophils, Red Blood Cell (RBC) count of 3000/mcL, and no crystals. She was diagnosed with septic arthritis of the left knee and underwent irrigation and debridement of the left knee that drained 5 cc of purulent fluid. Postoperatively, the patient was started on vancomycin (1250 mg Intravenous (IV) every 8 hours) and cefepime (2 gram IV every 8 hours). The left knee aspirate and left knee operative cultures remained negative.

On day 2 of hospitalization, blood culture from day 0 grew Gram-Positive Cocci (GPC) in the cluster, later confirmed as *N. gonorrhoeae*. She was then diagnosed with Disseminated Gonococcal Infection (DGI) likely related to recent eculizumab use (8 days before presentation). After obtaining antibiotic sensitivity testing results, on day 3 of hospitalization, vancomycin and cefepime were deescalated to ceftriaxone. She developed facial swelling after receiving the first dose of ceftriaxone that was treated with IV diphenhydramine. The patient was then switched to ertapenem 1 gram IV every 24 hours which she tolerated without any side effects. Further testing for STDs including Human Immunodeficiency Virus (HIV), syphilis, trichomonas, and chlamydia was negative. A repeat blood culture from day 2 was negative, and the patient was discharged home to complete four weeks of ertapenem therapy which she has since completed. The repeat ESR after 4 weeks trended down to 62.

3. Discussion

Our study described the complication of DGI in a patient with gMG on eculizumab. Previous studies have described similar complications of DGI in patients with PNH and HUS on eculizumab [9]. To our best knowledge, our case is the first one to describe this complication in a patient with AChR+ gMG, treated with eculizumab.

Gonorrhea is the second most commonly reported notifiable disease in the United States [9, 10]. In 2018, a total of 583,405 cases of gonorrhea were reported in the United States [10]. Persons aged 15–44 years accounted for 91.6% of the reported gonorrhea cases [10]. Although urethral gonorrhea can cause profuse discharge and pain, gonococcal infections of the cervix, pharynx, and rectum are often asymptomatic [9–11]. In approximately 0.5–3% of gonorrhea cases, the bacterium can enter the bloodstream and cause DGI [9, 12]. Patients receiving eculizumab are at high risk for infections with encapsulated organisms such as *N. gonorrhoeae* due to impaired opsonophagocytic activity [5].

A case study by Crew et al. reviewed the FDA pre- and postmarketing safety reports of gonococcal infections among patients receiving eculizumab [9]. The study described 9 cases of gonococcal infections in patients receiving eculizumab for either PNH or HUS [9]. Eight out of nine patients were females, and seven out of nine were <30 years of age [9]. Eight of the nine patients were classified as having DGI and were hospitalized [9]. A diagnostic workup of cerebrospinal fluid sampling was conducted on three patients for meningitis, but none was diagnosed, one patient had a trans-thoracic echocardiogram which was negative for valvular vegetation, and two patients required vasopressor support for the concern of septic shock [9]. Seven patients continued the therapy after the infection while one discontinued [9]. All gonococcal infections resolved except in one case where the patient had developed endocarditis and thrombotic complications and died [9].

Vaccines containing group B *N. meningitidis* outer-membrane vesicles (OMV) may provide protection against a significant proportion of *N. gonorrhoeae*, but the mechanisms for the same have not yet been elucidated and the vaccination has not been approved for use in gonococcal infection [13]. Therefore, despite vaccination against *N. meningitidis*, these patients are still at a potential risk for developing gonococcal disease. CDC recommends annual screening for gonorrhea in all young sexually active women <25 years of age and older women who are at an increased risk [9, 11]. As of now, the screening recommendations for gonorrhea in patients receiving eculizumab do not differ from those for the general population [9]. In our case, the patient acquired the infection from her significant other who was later educated and treated of *N. gonorrhoeae*. Physicians are encouraged to obtain adequate sexual histories of patients and educate them on safe sexual practices, regular use of condoms, and avoiding unprotected sexual contact [9]. In addition, patients should be educated about the increased risk of gonococcal infection and DGI with eculizumab. Healthcare professionals should keep DGI in their differential diagnosis, especially in a patient with skin or joint involvement [9].

4. Conclusions

DGI is a rare but potentially life-threatening complication associated with use of complement inhibitor, eculizumab. Physicians should obtain adequate sexual histories from the patients and educate the patients and, if possible, their partners on safe sexual practices.

Abbreviations

AChR+: Acetylcholine receptor antibody-positive
gMG: Generalized myasthenia gravis
DGI: Disseminated gonococcal infection
PNH: Paroxysmal nocturnal hemoglobinuria
HUS: Atypical haemolytic uremic syndrome
MAC: Membrane attack complex
FDA: Food and Drug Administration
DVT: Deep vein thrombosis
ER: Emergency room
STD: Sexually transmitted disease
CRP: C-reactive protein
ESR: Erythrocyte sedimentation rate
NAAT: Nucleic acid amplification technique
WBC: White blood cell
RBC: Red blood cell.

References

[1] T. C. Thomas, S. A. Rollins, R. P. Rother et al., "Inhibition of complement activity by humanized anti-C5 antibody and single-chain Fv," *Molecular Immunology*, vol. 33, no. 17-18, pp. 1389–1401, 1996.

[2] US Food and Drug Administration, "Drugs@FDA: soliris (BLA 125166)," 2018, https://www.accessdata.fda.gov/scripts/cder/daf/index.cfm?event=BasicSearch.process.

[3] J. F. Howard Jr., K. Utsugisawa, M. Benatar et al., "Safety and efficacy of eculizumab in anti-acetylcholine receptor antibody-positive refractory generalised myasthenia gravis (REGAIN): a phase 3, randomised, double-blind, placebo-controlled, multicentre study," *The Lancet Neurology*, vol. 16, no. 12, pp. 976–986, 2017.

[4] "Alexion Pharmaceuticals," *Soliris (Eculizumab)*, Alexion Pharmaceuticals, Cheshire, CT, USA, 2018, https://www.accessdata.fda.gov/drugsatfda_docs/label/2018/125166s426lbl.pdf.

[5] M. Konar and D. M. Granoff, "Eculizumab treatment and impaired opsonophagocytic killing of meningococci by whole blood from immunized adults," *Blood*, vol. 130, no. 7, pp. 891–899, 2017.

[6] CDC, *Meningococcal ACIP Recommendations*, US Department of Health and Human Services, CDC, Atlanta, GA, USA, 2017, https://www.cdc.gov/vaccines/hcp/acip-recs/vacc-specific/mening.html.

[7] N. Cullinan, K. M. Gorman, M. Riordan, M. Waldron, T. H. J. Goodship, and A. Awan, "Case report: benefits and challenges of long-term eculizumab in atypical hemolytic uremic syndrome," *Pediatrics*, vol. 135, no. 6, pp. e1506–e1509, 2015.

[8] L. A. McNamara, N. Topaz, X. Wang, S. Hariri, L. Fox, and J. R. MacNeil, "High risk for invasive meningococcal disease among patients receiving eculizumab (soliris) despite receipt of meningococcal vaccine," *Morbidity and Mortality Weekly Report*, vol. 66, no. 27, pp. 734–737, 2017.

[9] P. E. Crew, W. E. Abara, L. McCulley et al., "Disseminated gonococcal infections in patients receiving eculizumab: a case series," *Clinical Infectious Diseases*, vol. 69, no. 4, pp. 596–600, 2019.

[10] Centers for Disease Control and Prevention, "Sexually transmitted diseases surveillance," 2018, https://www.cdc.gov/std/stats18/gonorrhea.htm.

[11] K. A. Workowski, G. A. Bolan, and Centers for Disease Control and Prevention, "Sexually transmitted diseases treatment guidelines, 2015," *Morbidity and Mortality Weekly Report. Recommendations and Reports*, vol. 64, pp. 1–137, 2015.

[12] E. W. Hook and H. H. Handsfield, "Gonococcal infections in the adult," in *Sexually Transmitted Diseases*, K. K. Holmes, P. F. Starling, W. E. Stamm et al., Eds., pp. 627–645, McGraw-Hill Medical, New York, NY, USA, 4th edition, 2008.

[13] H. Petousis-Harris and F. J. Radcliff, "Exploitation of *Neisseria meningitidis* group B OMV vaccines against *N. gonorrhoeae* to inform the development and deployment of effective gonorrhea vaccines," *Frontiers in Immunology*, vol. 10, p. 683, 2019.

37

Transient, Recurrent Central Nervous System Clinical Manifestations of X-Linked Charcot-Marie-Tooth Disease Presenting with Very Long Latency Periods between Episodes: Is Prolonged Sun Exposure a Provoking Factor?

Andria Tziakouri,[1] Konstantinos Natsiopoulos,[2] Kleopas A. Kleopa,[3] and Costas Michaelides[1]

[1]*Department of Neurology, American Medical Center, Nicosia 2047, Cyprus*
[2]*Department of Radiology, American Medical Center, Nicosia 2047, Cyprus*
[3]*Neurology Clinics and Neuroscience Laboratory, The Cyprus Institute of Neurology and Genetics and Cyprus School of Molecular Medicine, Nicosia 1683, Cyprus*

Correspondence should be addressed to Andria Tziakouri; atziakouri@gmail.com

Academic Editor: Isabella Laura Simone

Charcot-Marie-Tooth disease is one of the most common inherited neurological disorders affecting the peripheral nervous system. The common clinical manifestations of the disease are distal muscle weakness and atrophy, often associated with a characteristic steppage gait and foot deformities. Transient acute and recurrent or chronic central nervous system manifestations, predominantly, dysarthria, dysphagia, motor weakness, and ataxia, have been recognized as a feature of the X-linked type 1 of CMT (CMTX1). The CNS symptoms occur typically in young age and often precede the clinical manifestation of the polyneuropathy. Several predisposing factors such as exercise, fever, and returning from areas of high altitude have been described as triggers of the CNS symptoms; however, in many cases, a substantial cause remains undetermined. In this report, we describe a patient with three attacks of transient CNS deficits at the ages of 11, 21, and 38 years, respectively, which were also accompanied by transient white matter abnormalities on MRI. Two of the attacks occurred after prolonged exposure to sunlight. In our knowledge, this is the first documented case with such long latency periods between CNS attacks as well as the only report describing intense sun exposure as a possible provoking factor.

1. Introduction

Charcot-Marie-Tooth disease (CMT) is a genetically and clinically heterogeneous group of inherited neuropathies affecting the peripheral nervous system. It is one of the most common neurological disorders with a prevalence of 1 in 2500 people, and it is characterized by progressive distal muscle weakness and atrophy with characteristic steppage gait, foot deformities (pes cavus), hyporeflexia, and sensory impairment [1, 2].

CMT is predominantly inherited in an autosomal dominant manner; however, there are 6 types of X-linked inheritance (CMTX1-6), out of which CMTX1 is the most common [3]. More than 400 mutations have been documented to cause CMTX1, all affecting the *GJB1* gene which encodes for the connexin32 protein (Cx32), a gap junction protein expressed mainly in the myelinating Schwann cells of the peripheral nerves, accounting for the main manifestations of peripheral neuropathy in CMTX1, as well as in the oligodendrocytes of the central nervous system (CNS) [2, 4, 5].

The phenotype of the disease is similar to that of other CMT1 types; however, transient CNS deficits causing stroke-like symptoms have been reported for the last 20 years in patients with CMTX1 which are also accompanied by transient white matter abnormalities on magnetic resonance imaging (MRI). The most common symptoms include dysarthria, motor weakness, ataxia, and dysphagia [1–3]. These episodes are sometimes associated with predisposing factors such as exercise, fever, and returning from areas of high altitude though in many cases a substantial cause remains undetermined [6, 7]. In many patients, these CNS manifestations even precede the diagnosis of CMTX1 [2, 8].

In this report, we describe a patient with CMTX1 presenting with three recurrent attacks of transient CNS deficits over a period of 20 years. The first episode occurred before an established CMTX diagnosis. The second and third episodes occurred after long periods of direct, strong sunshine exposure during the prolonged hours of work at a beach in Cyprus and his summer holidays on a Greek island, respectively. To the best of our knowledge, similar cases with such a long latency period between CNS attacks as well as the possibility of intense sun exposure representing a provoking factor have not been documented before in the English literature.

2. Case Report

A 38-year old man presented with dysarthria lasting for about one hour, two days after returning from holidays from the island of Corfu, where he had spent several days exposed to strong sunshine. The day after the presentation, the symptoms of dysarthria recurred and lasted about two hours before completely resolving. There were no other neurological symptoms such as headache, dizziness, confusion, or weakness (except from the baseline weakness due to the polyneuropathy). During his holidays, he was exposed to the sun for more hours than usual, but he did not report excessive use of alcohol or other substances.

The patient was examined on the second day of symptom appearance when he was found to be afebrile with no other signs of infection. His dysarthria had resolved, and the rest of his neurological examination was normal with the exception of the baseline weakness of the lower extremities due to his polyneuropathy.

Blood tests including inflammatory parameters as well as an immunological screen were normal and so was urine analysis and cerebrospinal fluid (CSF) analysis. CSF oligoclonal bands were absent.

Magnetic resonance imaging (MRI) of his brain was obtained (Figure 1) which showed a diffuse symmetric deep white matter involvement of the centrum semiovale posterior frontal and parietal, with T2/FLAIR hyperintensity and restricted diffusion an ADC map images (first row of images).

The findings extended continuously to the splenium of the corpus callosum (second row of images). No major mass effect was recognized. No hemorrhagic changes on T2/GRE images and no postcontrast enhancement on enhanced T1 images were seen (not shown here).

Due to the transient recurrence of the symptoms on the second day of presentation, the patient was treated empirically with corticosteroids (1 gram of intravenous methylprednisone per day for 3 consecutive days). His neurological examination returned to baseline.

Repeat MRI examination performed one month later showed significant symmetric improvement of the findings on T2, FLAIR, and DWI images (Figure 1). The FLAIR abnormalities were hardly recognized on the second MRI and had improved both in volume of involvement and intensity. Subtle increased signal could still be traced on DWI images, with no actual restricted diffusion on ADC map images (ADC map normalization).

Further questioning revealed two similar episodes in the past, one at the age of eleven years and one at the age of 21 years. The first episode preceded the diagnosis of CMTX, which was established at the age of sixteen, following the diagnosis of his older brother. The c.381C>G base change in the *GJB1* gene resulting in the Ile127Met amino acid substitution in Cx32 was identified in this family. He had experienced recurrent episodes of weakness of the right lower extremity lasting 2-3 hours over the course of 3 days. The medical history had revealed no evidence of infection, travel, intense exercise, or presence of any other provoking factor. MRI was not available at that time, and no medical record of laboratory examinations could be obtained.

Ten years later, at the age of twenty-one, the patient experienced a more severe episode of dysarthria lasting 4-5 hours. Over the course of the next 4 days, he continued to experience transient dysarthria attacks which subsequently progressed to paresis of the right lower limb. At that time, he had once again been exposed to strong sunshine for prolonged periods of time in the days prior to the presentation due to his work at the beach. Once again, laboratory investigation was entirely normal and he was treated with corticosteroids.

The MRI which, at that time, reported it as a possible acute disseminated encephalomyelitis (ADEM) in retrospect showed very similar findings to the one performed at our institution. The follow-up MRI was done one month later and revealed significant improvement.

3. Discussion

The first clinical manifestations of CMT in our patient were 2 consecutive episodes of dysarthria which occurred years before the diagnosis was established. As described in other reports, this provides evidence that CMT should be included in the differential diagnosis of transient CNS symptoms and should be investigated with an electrophysiology examination which can reveal decreased conduction velocities even before the manifestation of peripheral nervous system (PNS) symptoms [4, 6]. After a 10-year gap, our patient experienced similar episodes which progressed to severe lower right limb weakness and were associated with transient white matter abnormalities on MRI. Remarkably, the third episode occurred only 20 years later. This is to our knowledge the first patient to be documented with such a long latency period between CNS episodes. It is worth noting that neither the mother nor the brother of the patient ever experienced any CNS symptoms related to their disease. The same disease-causing mutation found in this family was previously

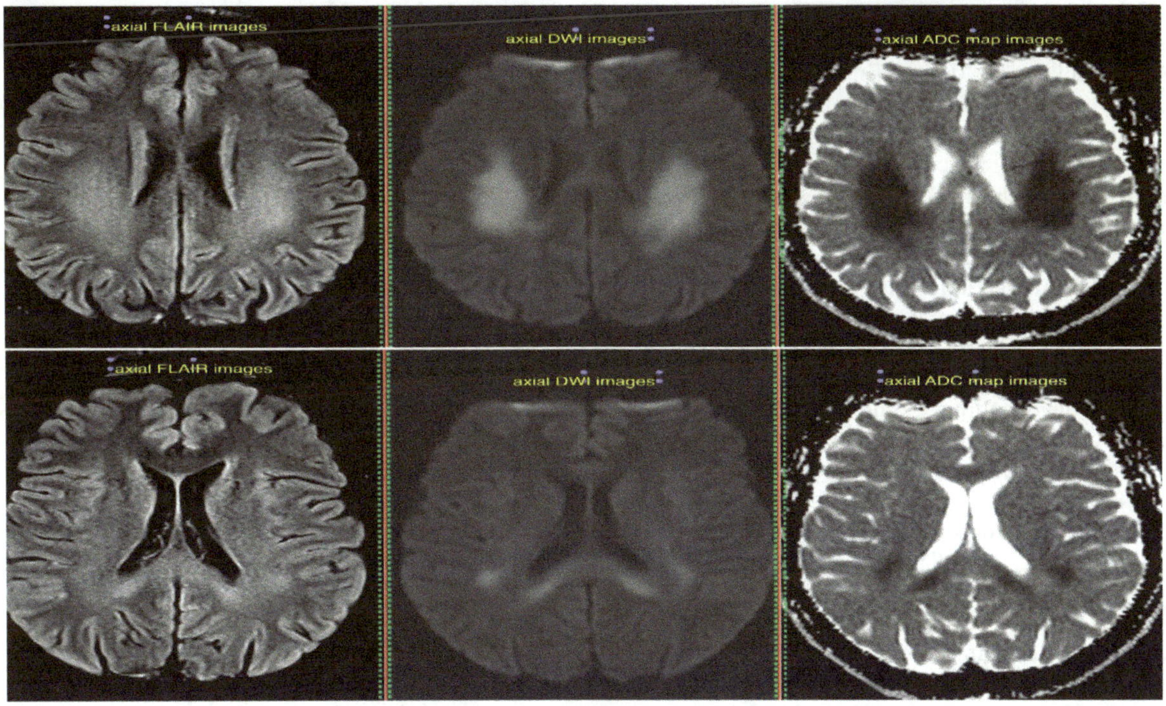

(a)

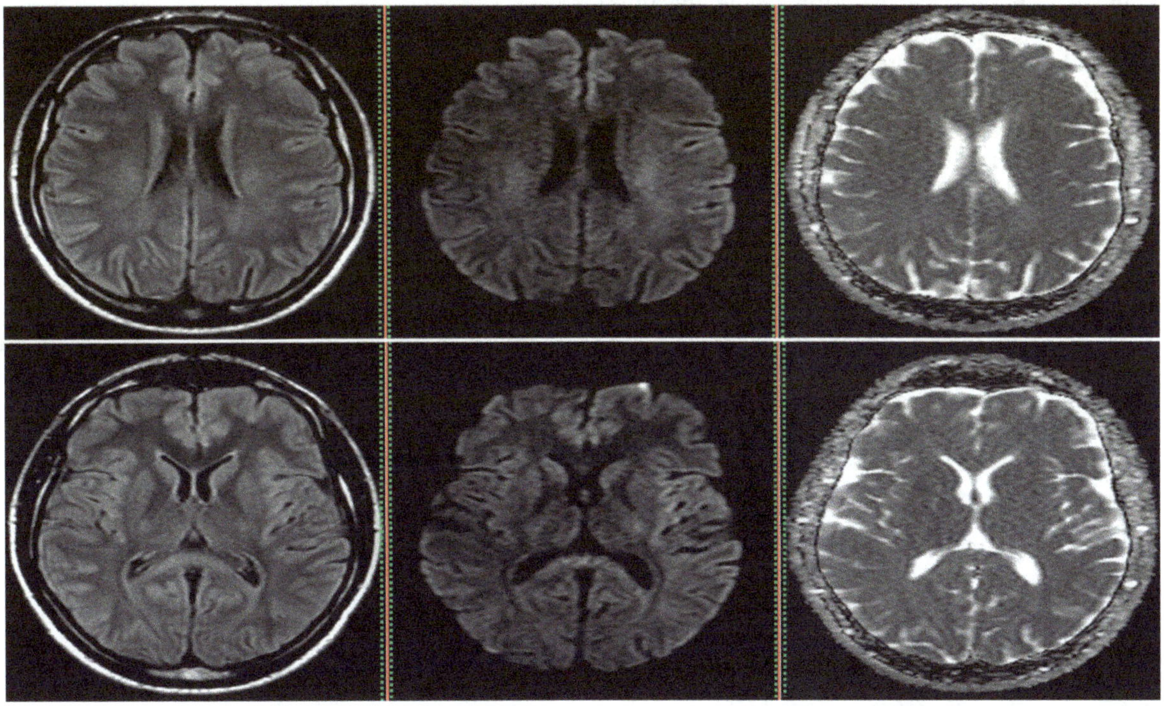

(b)

Figure 1: (a) Axial fluid-attenuated inversion recovery (FLAIR) and diffusion-weighted magnetic resonance imaging (DWI) upon symptom presentation showed diffuse symmetric deep white matter involvement of the centrum semiovale posterior frontal and parietal, with T2/FLAIR hyperintensity and restricted diffusion (first row of images), which extend continuously to the splenium of the corpus callosum (second row of images). (b) Follow-up MRI 1 month after presentation showed significant symmetric improvement of the findings on FLAIR and DWI images. The FLAIR abnormalities had improved both in volume and intensity; subtle increased signal could still be traced on DWI images, with no actual restricted diffusion on ADC map images.

reported by Nicholson et al.; however, no clinical CNS manifestations were described in affected patients [9].

The availability of MRI during the last 2 episodes revealed the typical association between the CNS symptoms and transient white matter abnormalities predominantly seen in the splenium of the corpus callosum extending to the centrum semiovale bilaterally [10, 11]. Restricted diffusion is also sometimes observed on MRI, and it is thought to be the result of dysfunctional gap junctions caused by Cx32 mutations. Cx32 forms gap junctions between the noncompact layers of myelin of peripheral myelinated fibers; however, growing evidence suggests that the same Cx32 mutations might disrupt the gap junction-mediated coupling between astrocytes and oligodendrocytes and along the myelin sheath formed by oligodendrocytes in the CNS, thus impairing the homeostasis of oligodendrocytes and white matter as a whole [1, 8, 12].

This is thought to occur during situations of metabolic stress. For example, proinflammatory cytokines that rise during fever or systemic illness, decreases in the pH of the CSF as seen after reacclimation from high altitudes, or hyperventilation and intense exercise are all examples of stressors thought to provoke the clinical manifestation of the CNS episodes [2, 13, 14]. The time interval seen between the stressor and the episodes can be attributed to the time needed for the gap junctions to shift their functions in order to re-establish homeostasis, thereby increasing the susceptibility to injury of Cx32-deficient oligodendrocytes in the white matter. It is suggested that, during normal circumstances, the intact gap junctions compensate for the impaired connexins [10]. However, in the absence of functional Cx32 gap junction channels, the stress-induced impairment of other gap junctions formed by astrocytic Cx43 and oligodendrocytic Cx47 result in clinical manifestations [15, 16]. Interestingly, none of the provoking factors recognized so far could be identified in our patient's case, but there was a relation between intense sun exposure for several days prior to the development of the last two episodes, something which could share the same triggering mechanism as fever in previously reported cases.

4. Conclusion

This case report adds to the growing literature of transient CNS manifestations seen sometimes in CMTX1 that clinicians should be aware of. It demonstrates that CNS manifestations can occur prior to the clinical manifestations of peripheral neuropathy of CMTX1 and that they can be recurrent with very long latency periods between episodes. Lastly, it highlights that prolonged exposure to strong sunshine may be a risk factor for the development of these CNS manifestations, something that had not been reported before.

Disclosure

This manuscript has been presented as a poster at the 6th Congress of the European Academy of Neurology.

Acknowledgments

The authors would like to thank Dr. Zamba-Papanicolaou Eleni of the Cyprus Institute of Neurology and Genetics, for useful comments on the manuscript.

References

[1] Y. Zhao, Y. Xie, X. Zhu, H. Wang, Y. Li, and J. Li, "Transient, recurrent, white matter lesions in X-linked Charcot-Marie-tooth disease with novel mutation of gap junction protein beta 1 gene in China: a case report," *BMC Neurology*, vol. 14, p. 156, 2014.

[2] M. Al-mateen, A. K. Craig, and P. F. Chance, "The central nervous system phenotype of X-linked charcot-marie-tooth disease," *Journal of Child Neurology*, vol. 29, no. 3, pp. 342–348, 2014.

[3] Y. Wang and F. Yin, "A review of X-linked Charcot-Marie-tooth disease," *Journal of Child Neurology*, vol. 31, no. 6, pp. 761–772, 2016.

[4] A. Sagnelli, G. Piscosquito, L. Chiapparini et al., "X-linked Charcot-Marie-tooth type 1: stroke-like presentation of a novel *GJB1* mutation," *Journal of the Peripheral Nervous System*, vol. 19, no. 2, pp. 183–186, 2014.

[5] M. Lee, I. Nelson, H. Houlden et al., "Six novel Connexin32 (*GJB1*) mutations in X linked Charcot-Marie-tooth disease," *Journal of Neurology, Neurosurgery & Psychiatry*, vol. 73, no. 3, pp. 304–306, 2002.

[6] Q. Wen, L. Cao, C. Yang, and Y. Xie, "The electrophysiological features in X-linked charcot-marie-tooth disease with transient central nervous system deficits," *Frontiers in Neurology*, vol. 9, p. 461, 2018.

[7] M. Panas, N. Kalfakis, C. Karadimas, and D. Vassilopoulos, "Episodes of generalized weakness in two sibs with the C164T mutation of the connexin 32 gene," *Neurology*, vol. 57, no. 10, pp. 1906–1908, 2001.

[8] G. Kim, K. M. Kim, S. Suh, C. Ki, and B. Eun, "Charcot-Marie-tooth disease masquerading as acute demyelinating encephalomyelitis-like illness abstract," *Pediatrics*, vol. 134, no. 1, pp. e270–e273, 2014.

[9] G. A. Nicholson, L. Yeung, and A. Corbett, "Efficient neurophysiologic selection of X-linked Charcot-Marie-Tooth families: ten novel mutations," *Neurology*, vol. 51, no. 5, pp. 1412–1416, 1998.

[10] A. Basu and P. F. Chinnery, "Recurrent stroke-like episodes in X-linked Charot-Marie-tooth disease," *Neurology*, vol. 77, no. 12, pp. 1205-1206, 2011.

[11] J. M. U-King-Im, E. Yiu, E. J. Donner, and M. Shroff, "MRI findings in X-linked Charcot-Marie-Tooth disease associated with a novel connexin 32 mutation," *Clinical Radiology*, vol. 66, no. 5, pp. 471–474, 2011.

[12] R. A. Taylor, E. M. Simon, H. G. Marks, and S. S. Scherer, "The CNS phenotype of X-linked Charcot-Marie-Tooth disease: more than a peripheral problem," *Neurology*, vol. 61, no. 11, pp. 1475–1478, 2003.

[13] C. K. Abrams and S. S. Scherer, "Gap junctions in inherited human disorders of the central nervous system," *Biochimica et Biophysica Acta (BBA)-Biomembranes*, vol. 1818, no. 8, pp. 2030–2047, 2012.

[14] H. L. Paulson, J. Y. Garbern, J. Y. Garbern, T. F. Hoban et al., "Transient central nervous system white matter abnormality in X-linked Charcot-Marie-Tooth disease," *Annals of Neurology*, vol. 52, no. 4, pp. 429–434, 2002.
[15] I. Sargiannidou, G.-H. Kim, S. Kyriakoudi, B.-L. Eun, and K. A. Kleopa, "A start codon CMT1X mutation associated with transient encephalomyelitis causes complete loss of Cx32," *Neurogenetics*, vol. 16, no. 3, pp. 193–200, 2015.
[16] M. Olympiou, I. Sargiannidou, K. Markoullis et al., "Systemic inflammation disrupts oligodendrocyte gap junctions and induces ER stress in a model of CNS manifestations of X-linked Charcot-Marie-Tooth disease," *Acta Neuropathologica Communications*, vol. 4, no. 1, p. 95, 2016.

38

Sellar Metastasis of Cervical Adenocarcinoma

Krishnan Ravindran,[1] Brandon M. Zsigray,[1] Michael P. Wemhoff,[1] John D. Spencer,[1] Ewa Borys,[2] Chirag R. Patel,[3] and Anand V. Germanwala[1,3]

[1]*Department of Neurological Surgery, Loyola University Medical Center, Maywood, Illinois, USA*
[2]*Department of Pathology, Loyola University Medical Center, Maywood, Illinois, USA*
[3]*Department of Otolaryngology Stritch School of Medicine, Loyola University Medical Center, Maywood, Illinois, USA*

Correspondence should be addressed to Anand V. Germanwala; agermanwala@gmail.com

Academic Editor: Shahid Nimjee

Background. Pituitary metastasis of cervical adenocarcinoma is an exceedingly rare phenomenon. *Case Description.* The authors present a case of a 66-year-old female with cervical adenocarcinoma who was discovered to have a rapidly growing intrasellar mass in the work-up of adrenal insufficiency and hypothyroidism. The patient underwent subsequent endoscopic endonasal subtotal resection of the mass. Histopathological analysis of the resected lesion demonstrated features consistent with metastatic mucinous adenocarcinoma of the cervix. While initially neurologically asymptomatic following surgery, the patient developed an oculomotor nerve palsy several weeks following surgical debulking, at which time neuroimaging revealed marked regrowth and suprasellar extension of the metastatic lesion. *Conclusions.* While metastatic cervical adenocarcinoma to the sella is rare, it should be considered in the differential based on the history of the patient.

1. Introduction

Metastatic lesions to the sella are believed to comprise only 1% of all pituitary lesions, of which the most common sites of primary tumor origin are the breast and lung [1–3]. Compression of parasellar anatomical structures may produce symptoms such as visual field loss, headache and ophthalmoplegia [4]. Cerebral metastasis of cervical malignancy is uncommon [5]. To our knowledge, only one other case of cervical carcinoma with pituitary metastasis has been reported in a nonautopsy setting [6]. Here, we report a case of sellar metastasis in a patient with cervical adenocarcinoma that was debulked endoscopically, highlight the clinical findings and natural history of this rare presentation, and review the literature.

2. Case Presentation

A 66-year-old female with a history of mucinous adenocarcinoma of the cervix presented to the neurosurgery outpatient clinic for evaluation of a sellar mass found during workup of adrenal insufficiency and hypothyroidism. The patient did not have unusual headaches or vision problems. Three months prior to discovery of the sellar mass, she was diagnosed with stage IIb mucinous adenocarcinoma of the cervix and was treated with chemotherapy. At the time of neurosurgery clinic presentation, she was neurologically intact, including full visual fields. Laboratory work-up demonstrated pituitary insufficiency with central hypothyroidism.

The initial magnetic resonance imaging (MRI) revealed a 1.8 × 1.1 cm contrast-enhancing mass within the sella, with extension to the suprasellar cistern and optic chiasm abutment. Preoperative imaging obtained the following month in preparation for surgery demonstrated that the mass had grown to 2.2 × 1.5 cm (Figure 1).

The patient underwent an endoscopic endonasal approach for resection of the intradural sellar mass. Intraoperative findings demonstrated a very firm, infiltrative, vascular mass with dense adherence to surrounding structures, including the dura, medical cavernous walls, and diaphragma. Intraoperative frozen section pathology was consistent with metastatic carcinoma. The tumor was debulked until normal appearing pituitary tissue was identified and the margin of tumor adherence to

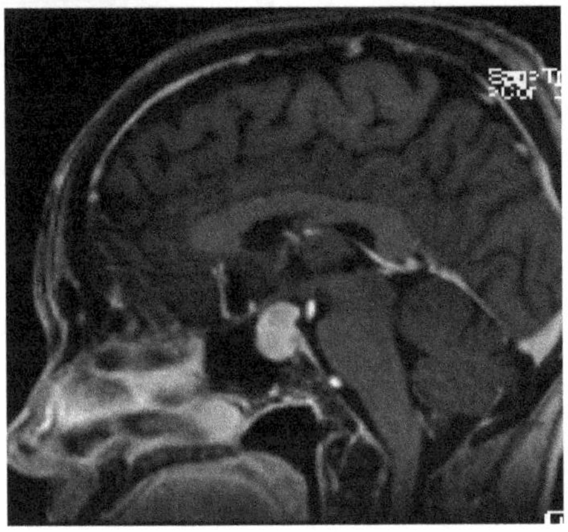

Figure 1: Preoperative sagittal MRI with contrast demonstrating the homogenously contrast enhancing sellar/suprasellar mass with mass effect on the optic chiasm.

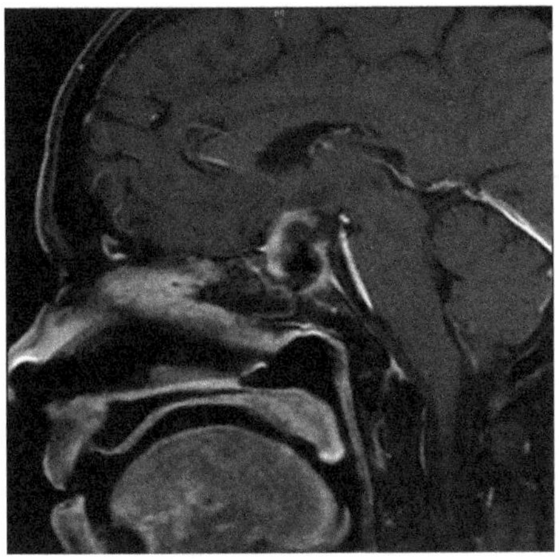

Figure 2: Immediately postoperative sagittal MRI with contrast showing subtotal resection through an endoscopic endonasal approach.

the diaphragma was reached. Postoperatively, the patient did well without new hormonal deficiencies or vision problems. A subtotal resection (>80%) was achieved (Figure 2). Gross histology and immunohistochemical staining ultimately confirmed the diagnosis of metastatic mucinous adenocarcinoma of the cervix (Figures 3 and 4).

The patient's immediate postoperative course was unremarkable. Given the diagnosis and intraoperative/postoperative findings of subtotal resection, adjuvant chemoradiation therapy was encouraged but the patient refused additional treatment. She was discharged home two days after surgery. She developed decreased left eye visual acuity and ptosis one week after surgery. A CT of the head at this time did not show any intracranial hemorrhage and a repeat MRI showed new enhancement suggestive of tumor recurrence within the sellar and suprasellar regions. The patient was started on steroids but declined any further treatment, including repeat surgery. Her ophthalmic symptoms ultimately progressed to a complete left cranial nerve III palsy four weeks after surgery. Follow-up MR imaging at five weeks after surgery revealed significant progression of the tumor to 2.9 × 2.4 cm with significant suprasellar extension (Figure 5). Though a computed tomography scan of the chest, abdomen, and pelvis at this time demonstrated no new neoplastic burden, a radiotracer bone scan demonstrated likely new metastatic lesions in the skull, bilateral humeri, bilateral acetabula, bilateral femurs, and the lumbosacral vertebrae. After further discussion with her gynecologic oncologist and radiation oncology, the patient again refused pursuing any further treatment, including palliative radiation or systemic therapies and elected to pursue home hospice. The patient died approximately two months after surgery.

3. Discussion

Metastases to the sellar region have been hypothesized to occur either hematogenously, such as from the pituitary stalk or cavernous sinus, or via leptomeningeal spread [7]. Pituitary metastasis typically occurs late in disease course, carrying a poor prognosis [8]. Metastases appear to display a predilection for the posterior lobe, likely owing to greater vascularity of the posterior lobe from the hypophyseal arteries, as compared to the anterior lobe, which is supplied by the portal system [6, 8]. Indeed, it has been suggested that metastatic involvement of the anterior lobe is in fact due to contiguous extension from the posterior lobe [9].

Pituitary adenomas and metastatic lesions to the parasellar region are nearly indistinguishable on neuroimaging. On plain film X-ray images, sellar enlargement or deformity and erosion of the sellar floor may be seen in both metastatic and benign lesions [10]. On MRI, contrast enhancement has been reported to be a prominent feature more commonly observed in metastatic lesions [10]. Metastatic lesions may also exhibit a "dumbbell" appearance due to indentation at the level of the diaphragm [11]. In this case, extension to the suprasellar cistern was seen with "minimal" bony invasion, also previously described as a predominant feature of metastatic lesions [10, 11]. Interestingly, despite radiological evidence of optic chiasm displacement on preoperative MRI, the patient's visual fields remained intact, though the patient progressed to suffer poor visual acuity and a left oculomotor nerve palsy following tumor debulking over a few weeks. It has been suggested that oculomotor nerve dysfunction may be a distinguishing clinical feature between metastatic and primary lesions given that compression of the intracavernous segment of this nerve by pituitary adenomas is rare [11].

Cervical carcinoma typically disseminates locally via the lymphatics to the retroperitoneal lymph nodes; distant hematogenous metastasis most commonly occurs to the liver, lung, and bone [12]. Cerebral metastasis is rare with an estimated prevalence of 0.5-1.0% and portends a particularly poor prognosis [5]. One study found that in postmortem examination of 60 patients with sellar lesions, 3 cases of primary cervical carcinoma were observed, none of which demonstrated sellar metastasis [2]. To our knowledge, only one other case of cervical carcinoma metastasis to the

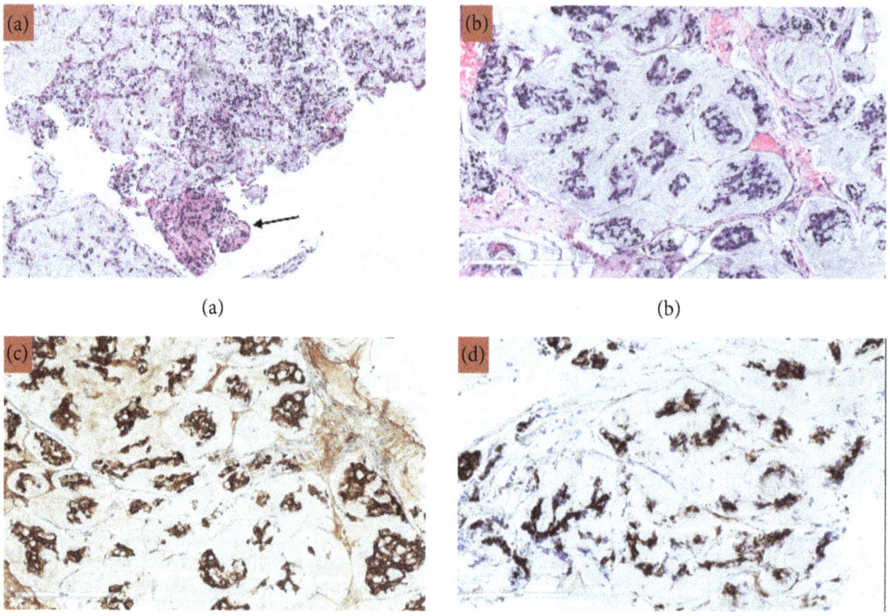

(a) (b) (c) (d)

Figure 3: (a) Frozen section tissue showing interface between mucinous adenocarcinoma metastasis and adjacent adenohypophysis (arrow), H&E, 40x. (b) Metastatic mucinous adenocarcinoma showing clusters of moderately pleomorphic epithelial cells floating in pools of mucin separated by fibrovascular septae of variable thickness, H&E, 200x. (c) Cytokeratin CK8/18 is positive in tumor cells; immunohistochemical stain, 200x. (d) p16 shows nuclear positivity; immunohistochemical stain, 200x.

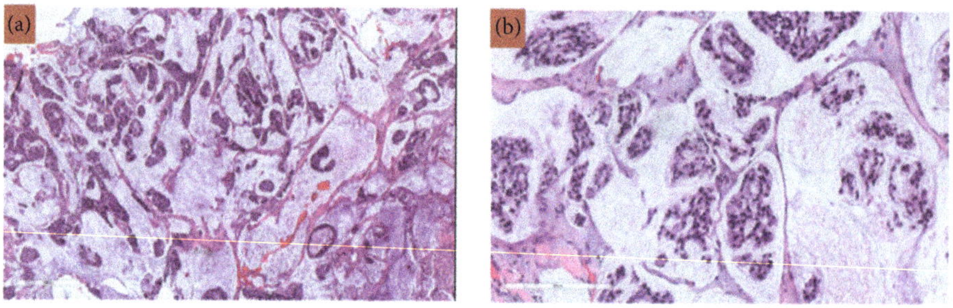

(a) (b)

Figure 4: (a, b) Cervical biopsy showing a moderately differentiated mucinous/colloid adenocarcinoma. H&E, 40x (a) and 200x (b).

pituitary has been reported [6]. In a 2000 study, Salpietro and colleagues described a sellar/suprasellar metastasis of an epidermoid cervical carcinoma in a 44-year-old female who presented with diabetes insipidus and diplopia. Radiation therapy of the primary cervical lesion had been done two years prior to presentation. Despite transsphenoidal debulking, the patient's condition deteriorated in the context of widespread metastatic disease to the lung and bone, and the patient died within several months.

For brain metastasis from cervical cancer, combination therapy of either chemotherapy or stereotactic radiosurgery followed by whole-brain irradiation has been shown to extend median survival to up to 4.6 months [13, 14]. The majority of these studied cases have been squamous cell carcinomas with an intraparenchymal location. Additionally, the majority of these lesions have been histologically poorly differentiated with high tumor grade [15]. Multimodality therapies are generally recommended with adjuvant chemoradiation therapy following maximal safe surgical resection. This case highlights the importance of initiating multimodality therapy expeditiously.

4. Conclusion

While cerebral metastases of cervical malignancies have been described, metastasis of well-differentiated cervical malignancy to the pituitary region is rare. However, this should be considered in the differential diagnosis of patients with this history and based on the clinical presentation. The development of rapid endocrinopathies, oculomotor dysfunction, and quick radiographic progression suggest a more aggressive neoplasm. Maximally safe resection should be performed,

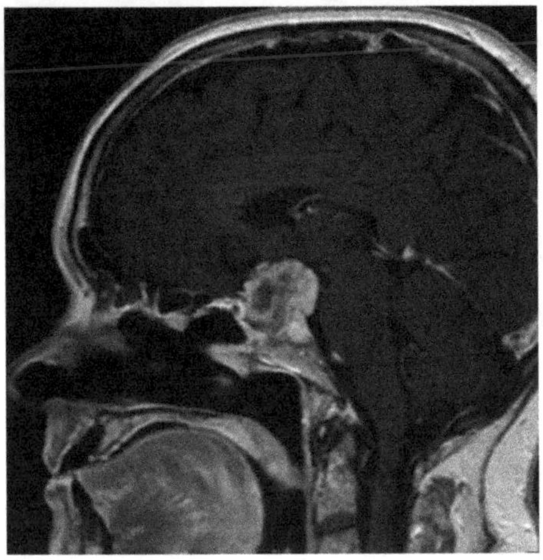

Figure 5: Postoperative sagittal MRI with contrast five weeks after surgery showing significant tumor recurrence.

including decompression of the optic apparatus, followed by efficient consideration for adjuvant therapy.

References

[1] R. J. Teears and E. M. Silverman, "Clinicopathologic review of 88 cases of carcinoma metastatic to the pituitary gland," *Cancer*, vol. 36, no. 1, pp. 216–220, 1975.

[2] U. Roessmann, B. Kaufman, and R. L. Friede, "Metastatic lesions in the sella turcica and pituitary gland," *Cancer*, vol. 25, no. 2, pp. 478–480, 1970.

[3] J. Gsponer, N. De Tribolet, J.-P. Déruaz et al., "Diagnosis, treatment, and outcome of pituitary tumors and other abnormal intrasellar masses. Retrospective analysis of 353 patients," *Medicine*, vol. 78, no. 4, pp. 236–269, 1999.

[4] M. Castle-Kirszbaum, T. Goldschlager, B. Ho, Y. Y. Wang, and J. King, "Twelve cases of pituitary metastasis: a case series and review of the literature," *The Pituitary Society*, vol. 21, no. 5, pp. 463–473, 2018.

[5] L. Kumar, R. K. Tanwar, and S. P. Singh, "Intracranial metastases from carcinoma cervix and review of literature," *Gynecologic Oncology*, vol. 46, no. 3, pp. 391-392, 1992.

[6] F. M. Salpietro, A. Romano, C. Alafaci, and F. Tomasello, "Pituitary metastasis from uterine cervical carcinoma: A case presenting as diabetes insipidus," *British Journal of Neurosurgery*, vol. 14, no. 2, pp. 156–159, 2000.

[7] T. Altay, K. M. Krisht, and W. T. Couldwell, "Sellar and parasellar metastatic tumors," *International Journal of Surgical Oncology*, vol. 2012, Article ID 647256, 9 pages, 2012.

[8] D. R. Fassett and W. T. Couldwell, "Metastases to the pituitary gland," *Neurosurgical Focus*, vol. 16, no. 4, p. E8, 2004.

[9] O. B. Leramo, J. D. Booth, B. Zinman, C. Bergeron, A. A. Sima, and T. P. Morley, "Hyperprolactinemia, hypopituitarism, and chiasmal compression due to carcinoma metastatic to the pituitary," *Neurosurgery*, vol. 8, no. 4, pp. 477–480, 1981.

[10] J. Komninos, V. Vlassopoulou, D. Protopapa et al., "Tumors metastatic to the pituitary gland: case report and literature review," *The Journal of Clinical Endocrinology & Metabolism*, vol. 89, no. 2, pp. 574–580, 2004.

[11] O. Schubiger and D. Haller, "Metastases to the pituitary-hypothalamic axis - An MR study of 7 symptomatic patients," *Neuroradiology*, vol. 34, no. 2, pp. 131–134, 1992.

[12] V. Carlson, L. Delclos, and G. H. Fletcher, "Distant metastases in squamous-cell carcinoma of the uterine cervix," *Radiology*, vol. 88, no. 5, pp. 961–966, 1967.

[13] J. C. Chura, K. Shukla, and P. A. Argenta, "Brain metastasis from cervical carcinoma," *International Journal of Gynecological Cancer*, vol. 17, no. 1, pp. 141–146, 2007.

[14] S.-B. Chung, K.-I. Jo, H.-J. Seol, D.-H. Nam, and J.-I. Lee, "Radiosurgery to palliate symptoms in brain metastases from uterine cervix cancer," *Acta Neurochirurgica*, vol. 155, no. 3, pp. 399–405, 2013.

[15] H. Li, X. Wu, and X. Cheng, "Advances in diagnosis and treatment of metastatic cervical cancer," *Journal of Gynecologic Oncology*, vol. 27, no. 4, p. e43, 2016.

39

Meningoencephalitis with *Streptococcus equi* Subspecies *equi* Leading to a Dural Arteriovenous Fistula

Jeroen Kerstens,[1,2] **Busra Durmus**,[1] **Stijn Lambrecht**,[3] **Ingrid Baar**,[4] **Margareta M. Ieven**,[3] **Thijs Van Der Zijden**,[5] **Paul M. Parizel**,[5,6] **Tomas Menovsky**,[7] **Martin M. Y. Lammens**,[8] **and Philippe G. Jorens**[4]

[1]*Antwerp University Hospital, University of Antwerp, Department of Neurology, Edegem 2650, Belgium*
[2]*AZ Middelheim, ZNA, Lindendreef 1, 2020, Antwerp, Belgium*
[3]*Antwerp University Hospital, University of Antwerp, UZGent, UGent, Dept of Chemistry, 9000 Gent, Belgium*
[4]*Antwerp University Hospital, University of Antwerp, Department of Critical Care Medicine, Edegem 2650, Belgium*
[5]*Antwerp University Hospital, University of Antwerp, Department of Radiology, Edegem 2650, Belgium*
[6]*Royal Perth Hospital, University of Western Australia, Medical School, Perth, WA, Australia*
[7]*Antwerp University Hospital, University of Antwerp, Department of Neurosurgery, Edegem 2650, Belgium*
[8]*Antwerp University Hospital, University of Antwerp, Department of Pathology, Edegem 2650, Belgium*

Correspondence should be addressed to Philippe G. Jorens; philippe.jorens@uza.be

Academic Editor: Dominic B. Fee

Invasive infection with Lancefield group C streptococci in humans is extremely rare, with the vast majority of clinical isolates belonging to *Streptococcus dysgalactiae* subsp. *equisimilis*. We report a case of meningoencephalitis in a 69-year-old man caused by *Streptococcus equi* subsp. *equi*, a microbe that causes strangles in *Equus caballus* (i.e., the horse). This is only the fourth infection with this subtype of the central nervous system (CNS) reported in humans. The invasiveness of these bacteria, known to be capable of releasing strongly immunogenic exotoxins, is illustrated by white matter lesions that are present in the acute phase. This patient initially recovered well after treatment with antibiotics and glucocorticoids. However, the patient was readmitted 5 months later with multiple intraparenchymatous cerebral haemorrhages. Cerebral angiography confirmed the presence of a suspected superficial dural arteriovenous fistula (DAVF), which is seldom reported after CNS infection. The invasiveness of these bacteria was illustrated by white matter lesions present in the acute phase and the occurrence of a de novo dural arteriovenous fistula in the follow-up period.

1. Introduction

Lancefield group C streptococci (GCS) are a serological subgroup of beta-hemolytic streptococci [1]. Two of the 5 subspecies belong to the normal commensal flora of the human upper airway and are frequently asymptomatic colonizers of the skin, gastrointestinal tract, and female genital tract. The latter three (*S. equi* subsp. *zooepidemicus*, *S. equi* subsp. *ruminatorum*, and *S. equi* subsp. *equi)* are part of the commensal flora of the upper respiratory tract of horses, where they also cause various respiratory tract infections, and, in the case of *S. equi* subsp. *equi*, a highly contagious suppurative lymphadenitis (strangles) occurs [2]. Invasive GCS infection in humans is rare. Sporadically implicated in soft tissue infections and pharyngitis, the vast majority of clinical isolates belong to *S. dysgalactiae* subsp. *equisimilis* [3].

We report a unique case of human meningoencephalitis by *S. equi* subsp. *equi*, which was further complicated by occurrence of a de novo dural arteriovenous fistula (DAVF).

2. Case Presentation

A 69-year-old Caucasian male was admitted to the emergency department of our hospital after returning from a one-month vacation to Myanmar that included horseback riding. The patient had not taken malaria prophylaxis and did not receive any vaccinations prior to his departure. The patient's medical history was remarkable for gout, ciguatera, and neurosurgical reconstruction of the skull after a basilar skull fracture. The latter occurred 5 years before this event (after a fall from a horse), and it was complicated by cerebrospinal fluid (CSF) leakage and right-sided glossopharyngeal and vagal nerve damage, which resulted in right-sided vocal cord paralysis with hoarseness and sporadic aspiration. The patient did not take any medications and did not smoke, but he drank wine regularly.

For the last few days, the patient had been increasingly tired and somnolent, with complaints of headache, left-sided ear pain, and night sweats. One day prior to admission, the patient had become increasingly confused. On the day of his admission, he was found by his wife lying on the floor of his home, confused, agitated, shivering, and incontinent of urine. At the emergency department, the patient's temperature was 39.2 °C, and his heart rate was 111 beats per minute, with a respiratory rate of 20 breaths per minute and a blood pressure of 161/88 mmHg. The patient's peripheral oxygen saturation was 87%, and his Glasgow Coma Scale was scored as 9 (E2 M5 V2). Clinical examination revealed fasciculations of the face and lower legs and crepitation over the right lower lung on pulmonary auscultation. There was no purpura or nuchal rigidity.

At that time, blood results revealed a leukocyte count of 34 900 × 10^9/l (normal: 4 300–10 000) (>95% being neutrophils) and a C-reactive protein (CRP) level of 204 mg/l (normal value <3). A chest X-ray revealed no abnormalities. A CT scan of the brain showed only nonspecific white matter lesions but no haemorrhage or oedema. Lumbar puncture examination revealed a leukocyte count of 1160/mm^3 (almost all neutrophils), a normal glucose level, and a total protein level of 128 mg/dl (normal value 15–40) accompanied by an elevated lactate level of 6.1 meq/l. Gram stain showed irregularly shaped cocci. Bacterial meningitis was suspected, and after obtaining two sets of blood cultures, empirical therapy with 2 g of intravenous ceftriaxone every 12 h, 2 g of ampicillin every 4 h and 10 mg/kg of acyclovir every 8 h was initiated. Shortly after starting the antibiotic therapy, the patient became more somnolent and developed a left-sided hemiplegia, left-sided central facial palsy, and right-sided head and eye deviation, and the patient was admitted to the intensive care unit (ICU). Because of increasingly obstructive respirations and an increasing oxygen need by the next day, the patient was intubated and ventilated.

Cerebrospinal fluid (CSF) cultures showed β-hemolytic colonies; blood and CSF cultures were positive for *Streptococcus equi*. Intravenous treatment with 2 g of ceftriaxone every 12 h was continued for 21 days, while ampicillin and acyclovir were discontinued. In vitro testing confirmed a sensitivity to ceftriaxone. Fluid-attenuated inversion recovery images (FLAIR) showed a "dirty CSF" appearance in the right parietal region (Figure 1(a), white arrow). Axial (Figure 1(b)) and sagittal (Figure 1(c)) T1-weighted images after the intravenous administration of gadolinium-chelate revealed a focal area of superficial contrast enhancement overlying the cerebral cortex, presumably representing a thickened pia mater and opacification of the left mastoid. In view of the MRI lesions and the left hemiplegia, one gram of intravenous methylprednisolone once daily was added to the treatment for 3 days with gradual tapering afterwards because meningoencephalitis with accompanying cerebral vasculitis was suspected [4]. After 4 days, the patient was weaned from the ventilator and extubated. Initially, the patient remained very agitated and disoriented and was temporarily treated with 25 mg of twice daily quetiapine and 100 mg of daily trazodone. Nine days after admission to the ICU, the patient was transferred to the neurology department. Later, this *Streptococcus equi* was identified as *S. equi* subspecies *equi* (at the National Reference Center for Invasive Non-Group B Beta-Hemolytic Streptococci, Belgium).

The patient initially recovered completely and had no complaints apart from mild gait disturbances and lightheadedness at a follow-up appointment 3 months after discharge. Because of the patient's prior medical history of basilar skull fracture and opacification of the left mastoid on brain MRI, despite a lack of clinical evidence of acute otitis or mastoiditis, an additional CT scan of the base of the skull was performed to rule out possible portals of entry for central nervous system (CNS) infection. The CT scan revealed only an asymmetrical widening of the left squamosal suture; therefore, we opted for a conservative approach.

One month later (5 months after the initial referral), the patient was readmitted with intracranial bleeding, and consecutive CT scans showed multiple right-sided cerebral haemorrhages, with the largest located precentrally in the frontal lobe with small perilesional parietal and temporal haemorrhages accompanied by a left hemiparesis and aphasia (Figure 2(a)). CT angiography examination (Figure 2(b), para-axial MPR) showed multiple tortuous, engorged pial veins of the right hemisphere. Cerebral angiography confirmed the presence of a suspected superficial dural arteriovenous fistula (Figure 2(c), lateral projection of right internal carotid artery injection, large black arrow) in the right parietal region. The arterial feeders were mainly meningeal branches originating from the right ophthalmic artery and transosseous feeders from the right superficial temporal and occipital arteries (Figure 2(d), lateral projection right external carotid artery injection); in addition, there was limited arterial supply to the fistula from the left middle meningeal artery across the midline (not shown). Venous drainage was through a large, right temporal draining vein (large white arrow) with reflux into multiple tortuous, superficial frontotemporal veins, as shown in Figure 2(b), indicating a fistula with high risk of haemorrhage.

Comparison of the axial T2-weighted images of MRI examinations at initial admittance (Figure 2(e)) and at the second admission (Figure 2(f)) showed the new finding of dilated pial veins (encircled), demonstrating de novo development of the dural AV fistula.

The dural AV fistula was excised by the neurosurgeon. Microscopy of the resected dura showed a previously

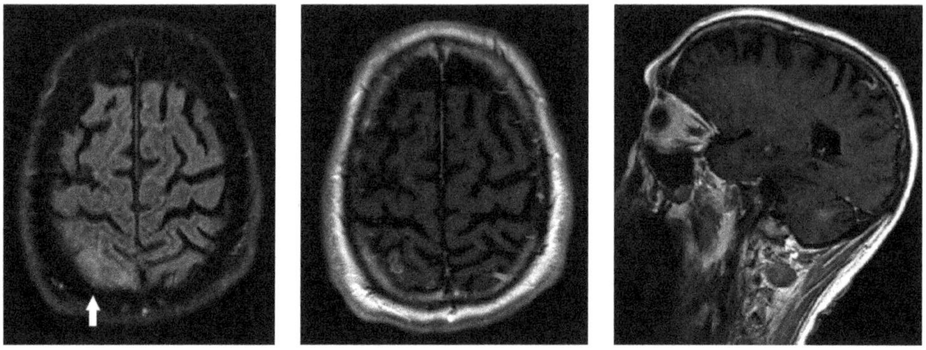

(a) (b) (c)

FIGURE 1: Fluid-attenuated inversion recovery images (FLAIR) showed a "dirty CSF" appearance in the right parietal region ((a), white arrow). Axial (b) and sagittal (c) T1-weighted images after the intravenous administration of gadolinium-chelate revealed a focal area of superficial contrast enhancement overlying the cerebral cortex, presumably representing a thickened pia mater.

damaged vein with inflammatory remnants and granulation tissue in its wall (Figures 3(a) and 3(b)). The patient was discharged to home with a hemiparesis that was still present. Seven months later, after this second event, the patient's GCS was 15/15, and the hemiparesis had almost completely disappeared.

3. Discussion

S. equi subsp. *equi* infects the horse in which it causes a contagious disease called strangles [5]. Transmission occurs from horse to horse and indirectly by contact with water troughs, feed buckets, stalls, trailers, and grooming equipment. Flies can also act as vectors [5].

This microbe produces immunogenic capsular proteins, i.e., the SeM protein, which inhibits the ability of neutrophils to phagocytose bacteria [6]. This protein indeed binds fibrinogen and immunoglobulin G to inhibit the deposition of C3b, which further causes phagocytes to be destroyed [7]. *S. equi* is also able to release streptolysin S and streptokinase, further damaging cell membranes [8]. Several important genes involved with *S. equi* pathogenesis are also found in *S. pyogenes*, known to cause severe central nervous destruction by releasing exotoxins [9]. These immunogenic factors certainly contributed to the "cerebritis" as seen in this patient.

Occlusive arterial vasculitis or septic cortical thrombophlebitis may accompany bacterial meningitis and meningoencephalitis [10], with focal neurological signs because of necrosis of the cerebral tissue. Inflammation and thrombosis of both arteries and small cortical veins may be caused either by the accumulation of inflammatory cells between the endothelium and the internal elastic lamina of small arteries (to the point of obliteration of the lumen) or by the direct invasion of blood vessel walls by organisms. Autopsy data obtained from patients with pneumococcal meningoencephalitis indicate that perivascular or nodular inflammatory muffs appear in the white matter, accompanied by obliterating vasculitis, glial satellitosis, neuronophagy, and foci of demyelination of varied and irregular sizes [11]. We postulated that the intraparenchymal lesion documented on the diffusion-weighted MRI of our patient reflected ischaemia with cytotoxic oedema secondary to necrotising vasculitis [12, 13]. Although some of the improvement may have been caused by the evolution under antibiotic treatment, the administration of glucocorticoids, as proposed in isolated cases of cerebral parenchymal injury, such as cerebral vasculitis meningoencephalitis, certainly contributed to the recovery [4]. Remarkably, 5 months after the initial infection, a de novo dural arteriovenous fistula (DAVF) was observed at the site of the initial lesions and presented as a parenchymal haemorrhage. Dural arteriovenous fistulas (DAVFs) are a rare type of acquired intracranial vascular malformations consisting of the creation of a pathological shunt but are most commonly found in the region of the transverse, sigmoid, and cavernous sinuses, as was the case in our patient [14, 15]. DAVFs are typically supplied by meningeal arteries and exhibit venous drainage either directly into the dural venous sinuses or via cortical and meningeal veins. The aetiology of these lesions remains controversial. Although the causal role of venous thrombosis is supported by the association of DAVFs with hypercoagulable states and hormonal causes, a history of intracranial surgery, radiation exposure, pregnancy, trauma, or infection have all been proposed as sources of DAVFs [14, 15]. DAVFs have rarely been reported months after prior viral meningitis and bacterial meningitis [16, 17]. In our case, we assumed that destruction by these aggressive exotoxins and local thrombosis caused a profound inflammatory response in the brain that further evolved into symptomatic DAVF. Remnants of inflammation and reparation signs were still present in a dural vein when excision was performed.

A human CNS infection caused by GCS is very rare, with fewer than 50 cases reported in the literature [1,18–26]. Almost all cases of bacterial meningitis are caused by subspecies of *zooepidermicus*; complications have occurred in these cases, which are most commonly distant infection foci, such as endophthalmitis and endocarditis. Considering the *S. equi* subspecies *equi*, only a few cases were reported as an invasive infection in humans, and only three (apart from ours) involved the CNS [19, 23, 26]. In these cases, direct contact with horses could be pinpointed. To the best of our

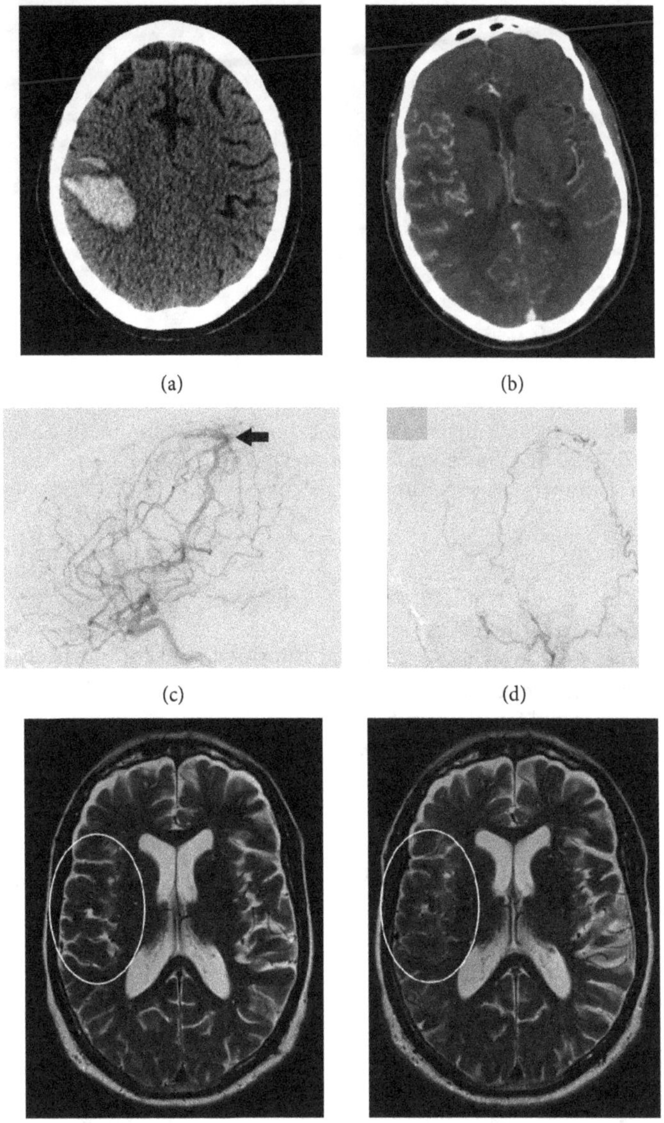

(a) (b) (c) (d) (e) (f)

FIGURE 2: During readmission five months after the initial referral, consecutive CT scans showed multiple right-sided cerebral haemorrhages, the largest being located precentrally in the frontal lobe ((a), para-axial nonenhanced). CT angiography examination ((b), para-axial MPR) showed multiple tortuous, engorged pial veins of the right hemisphere. Cerebral angiography confirmed the presence of a suspected superficial dural arteriovenous fistula ((c), lateral projection of right internal carotid artery injection, large black arrow) in the right parietal region. The arterial feeders were mainly meningeal branches originating from the right ophthalmic artery and transosseous feeders from the right superficial temporal and occipital arteries ((d), lateral projection right external carotid artery injection); in addition, there was limited arterial supply to the fistula from the left middle meningeal artery, across the midline (not shown). Venous drainage was through a large, right temporal draining vein (large white arrow), with reflux into multiple tortuous, superficial frontotemporal veins, as shown in Figure 2(b), indicating a fistula with a high risk of haemorrhage. Comparison of axial T2-weighted images of MRI examinations at initial admittance (e) and at the second admission (f) showed the new finding of dilated pial veins (encircled), demonstrating the de novo development of the dural AV fistula.

knowledge, our patient presented here is only the fourth reported case of human CNS infection with *S. equi* subsp. *equi*, and this patient is only the second case in an adult patient and the first reported case of meningoencephalitis with a DAVF.

The first case was published in 2003 by Elsayed et al. [19]. They reported a 13-year-old Canadian boy who lived on a horse farm with a medical history of resection of a petrous intracranial inflammatory mass at age 9; he presented with a 2-day history of fever, increasing neck stiffness, headache, anorexia, nausea, vomiting, lethargy, photophobia, bilateral deafness, and ataxia. The patient was diagnosed with bacterial meningitis that was empirically treated with cefotaxime and vancomycin, and the patient was switched to penicillin G after CSF cultures were positive for a multisensitive *S. equi* subsp. *equi*. The patient developed

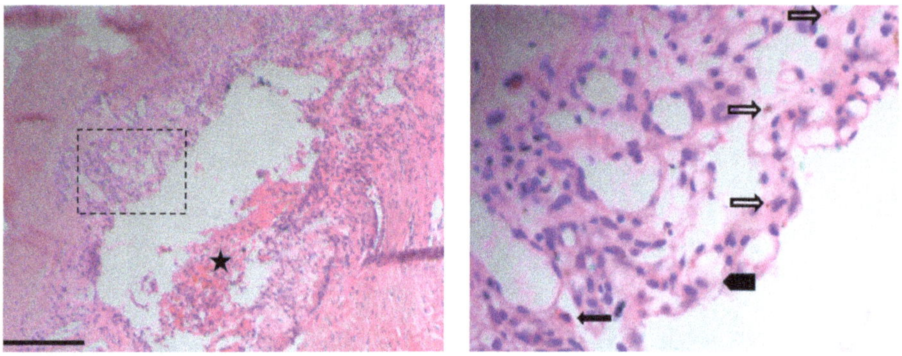

FIGURE 3: Histopathology of the excised dura with lymphocytic inflammatory remnants around a damaged venous sinus (a). In the upper part of the vessel wall (see also insert (b)) there is granulation tissue with many newly formed capillaries, lymphocytes, macrophages (thick arrow), a few eosinophils (thin black arrow) and some iron debris (thin open arrow). (Haematoxylin-Eosin Staining, bar = 1 mm; asterisk = peripheral blood).

noncommunicating hydrocephalus that required ventriculoperitoneal shunting but recovered with only a mild residual ataxia and severe bilateral sensorineural hearing loss for which he received a cochlear implant. Popescu et al. [23] later reported a second case of a 75-year-old female admitted with fever and stupor who was successfully treated with 10 days of intravenous ceftriaxone and dexamethasone. She later stated that her neighbours were horse owners and she had visited their farm within two weeks prior to her admission. Very recently, a 13-year-old-boy with systemic lupus erythematosus who presented with sepsis and meningitis after contact with a sick pony has been described [26]. Although he recovered fully following eight weeks of intravenous ceftriaxone and oral rifampicin, the clinical course was complicated by a subdural empyema requiring neurosurgical evacuation [26].

In our patient, recent contact with infected horses in Myanmar was presumably the cause of the disease, and prior surgery was a possible route of entry.

In summary, we report a rare case of *S. equi* subsp. *equi* meningoencephalitis that initially recovered well after treatment with antibiotics and glucocorticoids. The cerebral lesions seen on MRI not only caused meningitis but also meningoencephalitis, and the postinfectious dural AV fistula accompanied by intraparenchymal bleeding illustrated the aggressive nature of the toxins released by this bacterium with a further inflammatory reaction.

Abbreviations

CT: Computed tomography
CSF: Cerebrospinal fluid
CNS: Central nervous system
DAVF: Dural arteriovenous fistula
GCS: Group C Streptococci.

Consent

Informed consent has been obtained from the patient that this information may be published.

Disclosure

This case report was written and prepared according to the most recent CARE guidelines.

Authors' Contributions

Jeroen Kerstens, Busra Durmus, Ingrid Baar, Thijs Van Der Zijden, Tomas Menovsky, and Philippe G Jorens took care of the patient. Jeroen Kerstens, Busra Durmus, Stijn Lambrecht, and Philippe G Jorens initially wrote the manuscript. Stijn Lambrecht and Margareta Ieven were responsible for the identification and typing of the *Streptococcus*. Paul Parizel and Thijs Van Der Zijden performed and interpreted the radiological investigations. Tomas Menovsky excised the dural arteriovenous fistula. Martin Lammens performed the histological examination. All co-authors read, approved and reviewed the manuscript.

Acknowledgments

The authors are indebted to the nurses and staff who took care of the patient. The authors thank the National Reference Center for Invasive Non-Group B Bèta-Hemolytic Streptococci (Nationaal Referentiecentrum voor Invasieve β-hemolytische Streptokokken niet behorend tot groep B) for their help with species subtyping. The secretarial assistance of Hilde Fleurackers is greatly acknowledged.

References

[1] A. Rajasekhar and C. J. Clancy, "Meningitis due to group C Streptococcus: a case report and review of the literature," *Scandinavian Journal of Infectious Diseases*, vol. 42, no. 8, pp. 571–578, 2010, PMID: 20632899.

[2] J. F. Timoney, "The pathogenic equine streptococci," *Veterinary Research*, vol. 35, no. 4, pp. 397–409, 2004, PMID: 15236673.

[3] A. Jensen and M. Kilian, "Delineation of *Streptococcus dysgalactiae*, its subspecies, and its clinical and phylogenetic relationship to *Streptococcus pyogenes*," *Journal of Clinical Microbiology*, vol. 50, no. 1, pp. 113–126, 2012, PMID: 22075580.

[4] P. G. Jorens, P. M. Parizel, H. E. Demey et al., "Meningoencephalitis caused by *Streptococcus pneumoniae*: a diagnostic and therapeutic challenge," *Neuroradiology*, vol. 47, no. 10, pp. 758–764, 2005, PMID: 16151706.

[5] C. R. Sweeney, J. F. Timoney, J. R. Newton, and M. T. Hines, "Streptococcus equi infections in horses: guidelines for treatment, control, and prevention of strangles," *Journal of Veterinary Internal Medicine*, vol. 19, no. 1, pp. 123–134, 2005, PMID: 15715061.

[6] J. F. Timoney, P. Suther, S. Velineni, and S. C. Artiushin, "The antiphagocytic activity of SeM of Streptococcus equi requires capsule," *Journal of Equine Science*, vol. 25, no. 2, pp. 53–56, 2014, PMID: 25013359.

[7] C. Kelly, M. Bugg, C. Robinson et al., "Sequence variation of the SeM gene of Streptococcus equi allows discrimination of the source of strangles outbreaks," *Journal of Clinical Microbiology*, vol. 44, no. 2, pp. 480–486, 2006, PMID: 16455902.

[8] J. Flanagan, N. Collin, J. Timoney, T. Mitchell, J. A. Mumford, and N. Chanter, "Characterization of the haemolytic activity of *Streptococcus equi*," *Microbial Pathogenesis*, vol. 24, no. 4, pp. 211–221, 1998, PMID: 9533893.

[9] P. G. Jorens, A. Vander Borght, B. Ceulemans et al., "Encephalomyelitis-associated antimyelin autoreactivity induced by streptococcal exotoxins," *Neurology*, vol. 54, no. 7, pp. 1433–1441, 2000, PMID: 10751252.

[10] M. J. DiNubile, W. Henry Boom, and F. S. Southwick, "Septic cortical thrombophlebitis," *Journal of Infectious Diseases*, vol. 161, no. 6, pp. 1216–1220, 1990, PMID: 2189005.

[11] J. Magnus, P. M. Parizel, B. Ceulemans, P. Cras, M. Luijks, and P. G. Jorens, "*Streptococcus pneumoniae* meningoencephalitis with bilateral basal ganglia necrosis," *Journal of Child Neurology*, vol. 26, no. 11, pp. 1438–1443, 2011, PMID: 21677202.

[12] R. J. Caselli, B. W. Scheithauer, J. D. O'Duffy, G. C. Peterson, B. F. Westmoreland, and P. A. Davenport, "Chronic inflammatory meningoencephalitis should not be mistaken for Alzheimer's disease," *Mayo Clinic Proceedings*, vol. 68, no. 9, pp. 846–853, 1993, PMID: 8371602.

[13] D. Laky, V. Filon, M. Radulescu, S. Socolovschi, and F. Halalau, "Up-to-date aspects of meningoencephalitis. Anatomo-clinical researches," *Romanian journal of morphology and embryology = Revue roumaine de morphologie et embryologie*, vol. 38, no. 3-4, pp. 107–114, 1992, PMID: 1342197.

[14] T. R. Miller and D. Gandhi, "Intracranial dural arteriovenous fistulae," *Stroke*, vol. 46, no. 7, pp. 2017–2025, 2015, PMID: 25999384.

[15] Y. Serulle, T. R. Miller, and D. Gandhi, "Dural arteriovenous fistulae," *Neuroimaging Clinics of North America*, vol. 26, no. 2, pp. 247–258, 2016, PMID: 27154607.

[16] J. Hai, L. Zhang, J. F. Wan, S. H. Su, F. Wang, and G. Y. Zhang, "A dural arteriovenous fistula in cavernous sinus developed from viral meningitis," *Acta Neurologica Belgica*, vol. 111, no. 2, pp. 146–148, 2011, PMID: 21748936 DIO:.

[17] S. Tsutsumi, Y. Yasumoto, M. Ito, H. Oishi, H. Arai, and A. Yoritaka, "Atypical dural Arteriovenous fistula associated with meningitis," *Neurologia Medico-Chirurgica*, vol. 48, no. 2, pp. 68–71, 2008, PMID: 18296875.

[18] M. Clarke, H. Enuh, J. Saverimuttu, and J. Nfonoyim, "Streptococcus group C meningitis with cavernous sinus thrombosis," *Infection and Drug Resistance*, vol. 6, pp. 79–81, 2013, PMID: 23966796.

[19] S. Elsayed, O. Hammerberg, V. Massey, and Z. Hussain, "*Streptococcus equi* subspecies equi (Lancefield group C) *meningitis in a child*," *Clinical Microbiology and Infection*, vol. 9, no. 8, pp. 869–872, 2003, PMID: 14616711.

[20] D. W. Eyre, J. Kenkre, I. C. J. W. Bowler, and S. J. McBride, "*Streptococcus equi* subspecies zooepidemicus meningitis-a case report and review of the literature," *European Journal of Clinical Microbiology & Infectious Diseases*, vol. 29, no. 12, pp. 1459–1463, 2010, PMID: 20820836.

[21] D. Madzar, M. Hagge, S Moller et al., "Endogenous endophthalmitis complicating *Streptococcus equi* subspecies zooepidemicus meningitis: a case report," *BMC Res Notes*, vol. 8, p. 184, 2015 PMID: 25940309.

[22] L. R. Minces, P. J. Brown, and P. J. Veldkamp, "Human meningitis from *Streptococcus equi* subsp. zooepidemicus acquired as zoonoses," *Epidemiology and Infection*, vol. 139, no. 3, pp. 406–410, 2011, PMID: 20492747.

[23] G.-A. Popescu, R. Fuerea, and E. Benea, "Meningitis due to an unusual human pathogen: *Streptococcus equi* subspecies *equi*," *Southern Medical Journal*, vol. 99, no. 2, pp. 190-191, 2006, PMID: 16509563.

[24] G. Torano Peraza, I. Arias Portales, A. Castillo Marshall, and G. Brossard Elejo, "First case of meningitis from *Streptococcus equi* subsp. zooepidemicus in Cuba," *Revista Cubana de Salud Publica*, vol. 41, no. 1, pp. 165–168, 2015.

[25] A. Van Samkar, M. C. Brouwer, A. Van der Ende, and D. Van de Beek, "Streptococcus equi meningitis," *Clinical Microbiology and Infection*, vol. 22, no. 1, pp. e3–e4, 2016, PMID: 26369601.

[26] P. Torpiano, N. Nestorova, and C. Vella, "*Streptococcus equi* subsp. Equi meninigitis, septicemia and subdural empyema in a child," *ID Cases*, vol. 21, p. e00808, 2020.

An Intracranial Extradural Dermoid Cyst Presenting with Two Dermal Sinuses and an Abscess in a Child

Aysha Albastaki,[1] Reem AlThawadi,[1] Janan Alajaimi,[1] Khawla F. Ali,[1] and Talal Almayman[2]

[1]*Royal College of Surgeons in Ireland-Medical University of Bahrain, Busaiteen, Bahrain*
[2]*King Hamad University Hospital, Al Sayh, Bahrain*

Correspondence should be addressed to Aysha Albastaki; aysha.a97@hotmail.com

Academic Editor: Dominic B. Fee

Dermoid cysts account for only a small fraction of intracranial masses, with extradural dermoid cysts being considered a much rarer entity than those located intradurally. Intracranial dermoid cysts vary in clinical presentations: some maybe asymptomatic whilst others harbor features of raised intracranial pressure, neurological deficits, or even aseptic meningitis. Dermoid cysts may also present with cutaneous lesions. Herein, we report a rare case of a 1-year-old female presenting with a midline, scalp abscess. Brain MRI revealed an intracranial, extradural tumor, with features suggestive of a dermoid cyst, unusually located in the crista galli, and complicated by the formation of two cutaneous sinus tracts. After identification and characterization by MRI, bitemporal craniotomy was performed with complete excision of the mass and sinus tracts. Histological analysis confirmed dermoid cyst as the final diagnosis. Postoperatively, the patient recovered fully and had no evidence of recurrence in subsequent visits. The case mentioned above highlights the rarity of such a presentation for an intracranial extradural dermoid cyst and the vitality of early imaging for midline cutaneous lesions for identification of intracranial extensions and avoidance of detrimental consequences.

1. Introduction

Dermoid cysts are benign lesions lined by the squamous epithelium that congenitally arise as a result of failure of the ectoderm to separate from the neural tube. These cysts might also form subsequent to trauma that led to the sequestration and inclusion of ectodermal tissue [1].

Embryologically, dermoid cysts are derived from two germ cell layers: the ectoderm and the mesoderm. Dermoid cysts typically appear along the midline plane of the human body, corresponding to sites of embryonic fusion [2].

Intracranial dermoid cysts are relatively rare, benign tumors, which make up 0.025% to 0.04% of all intracranial tumors, and are seen in 1 in 2500 live births [3]. Two-thirds of all intracranial cysts arise in the posterior fossa, with the remaining third usually located intradurally in the parasellar and midline frontobasal region [2, 4]. Extradural dermoid cysts, on the other hand, are considered a much rarer entity [5, 6].

Herein, we report a rare case of an extradural, intracranial dermoid cyst, located on the crista galli, presenting with a scalp abscess and complicated by the formation of two dermal sinuses. We review and discuss in details the current literature in view of this rarity.

2. Case Presentation

A 1-year-old female presented to the Department of Pediatric Surgery with a progressively enlarging forehead swelling for the past 3 weeks. On examination, the swelling was erythematous, tender, fluctuant, 3×4 cm in diameter, and located to the right of the midline, consistent with the diagnosis of an abscess. Concurrently, a smaller lesion on the nasal bridge containing a few hair strands was present. The nasal lesion, per the mother's report, had been present since birth.

A brain MRI was also performed to rule out any possible intracranial extension of the lesion, given its midline location. The MRI revealed an intracranial, extradural tumor, with radiological features suggestive of a dermoid cyst. Additionally, the lesion was complicated by the formation of two dermal sinus tracts, with one opening into the forehead and the other into the nasal region (Figure 1).

Subsequently, the patient underwent surgical drainage, with a small incision made at the medial aspect of the right eyebrow, revealing copious amounts of pus.

The decision to surgically excise the intracranial mass and debride both the frontal and nasal dermal sinuses was agreed upon by both neurosurgery and ENT departments. Intraoperatively, a sutar bitemporal incision of the scalp was performed, followed by bitemporal craniotomy, exposing the dura mater. The frontal mass, overlying the crista galli, was identified with one tract that led to the forehead and another extending to the nasal lesion (Figure 2). Because the mass was fused with the parietal dura, extra care was taken to precisely excise it using a sharp surface cut in order to avoid cerebrospinal fluid (CSF) leakage. Although the mass was fused with the outermost layer of the dura, dural invasion was highly unlikely as ruled out by both radiological evidence and the absence of any symptoms in the patient suggestive of chemical meningitis. The mass was successfully excised, intact with no rupture or CSF leakage, and the dermal sinus that led to the forehead was removed. The lower nasal sinus tract was excised by ENT, and the overlying skin was sutured. Lastly, a Hemovac drain was applied and the bone flap was reconstructed. The subcutaneous layer of the scalp skin was approximated with absorbable sutures, and the overlying skin was closed with proline interrupted sutures.

Histopathology reports on the specimen obtained intraoperatively confirmed the diagnosis of a dermoid cyst with a chronically inflamed dermal sinus tract. Postoperatively, the patient had full recovery with no complications. During subsequent follow-up visits to the neurosurgery clinic, there were no clinical features suggestive of possible recurrence.

3. Discussion

3.1. Background. Intracranial dermoid and epidermoid cysts have not been acknowledged until E. Bostroem first recognized in 1897 the epithelial origin of the "tumeur perlees" that was described by Cruveilhier in 1829 [7, 8]. Ever since these discoveries, several reports of dermoid and epidermoid cysts have been published [9].

Intracranial dermoids and epidermoids are rare benign congenital tumors compromising 0.4% to 1.9% in several large series of intracranial tumors [10, 11]. Dermoids, however, appear less frequently than epidermoids with a ratio of 1 : 1.2–1.9 and account for only 0.025% to 0.04% to of all intracranial tumors [3, 12].

Location of head and neck dermoid cysts, both extradural and intradural, has been mainly reported in the fontanels, petrous apex, Eustachian tube, periorbital or perinasal soft tissue, cavernous sinus, anterior cranial fossa, or in the skull suture located near the skin where they connect directly to a dermal sinus [5, 6, 13, 14]. Head and neck dermoid cysts rarely originate from the skull base, the infratemporal region, supratentorial, or the fourth ventricle [15–18].

Extradural intracranial dermoid cysts, when compared to those located intradurally, are a much rarer entity [5, 6]. Only one case was reported of a dermoid cyst located in the vicinity of the foramen ovale [13]. To our knowledge, this is the first report of a dermoid cyst lying on the crista galli with two dermal sinuses.

3.2. The Origins of Dermoid Cysts. The embryologic origins of dermoid cysts have been controversial due to the unknown mechanism of formation of such dysraphisms. Dermoid cysts are made up of both ectodermal and mesodermal elements and form either as a result of incomplete closure of the neural tube during the third to fifth week of fetal development or due to traumatic implantation of skin elements [13, 15, 19].

As the fetus develops, anomalous closure of the neural folds in the midline results in an aberrant adhesion between the ectoderm and the underlying neural tube. This incomplete separation forms a cyst dwelling of a well-differentiated stratified squamous epithelium, hair follicles, apocrine, sebaceous and sweat gland, smooth and stratified muscle, cartilage, bone, minor salivary glands, nerves, and lymph nodes [4, 19, 20].

The provenance of intracranial dermoid cyst cells may be explained by two main theories. Firstly, it has been proposed that dermoid cysts might originate from multipotent embryonic stem cells. The other theory, however, states that the cysts might arise from the translocation of epithelial cells that have migrated from the otic vesicles or developing neurovasculature. Although these stem cells were not found in the dura, they can still form an extradural cyst by proliferation in combination with epithelial cell migration during the extradural neurovasculature process [4].

3.3. Clinical Presentation of Dermoid Cysts. The average time between the onset of symptoms and diagnosis of dermoid cysts has been reported at 8.5 years within the previous century, allowing copious time for a variety of clinical symptoms to appear [21, 22]. However, with the recent advances in diagnostic imaging, the diagnosis of dermoid cysts has become possible in its preclinical stages and as early as infancy [13, 23, 24].

Given that intracranial dermoid cysts are space-occupying lesions, their clinical presentation depends on the size and location of the tumor. Symptoms, if present, are often nonspecific and may include headaches, dizziness, or seizures. Papilledema is unlikely to occur, and the patients' spinal tap is clear in more than half of the cases [10, 25]. Patients with dermoid cysts might also be asymptomatic

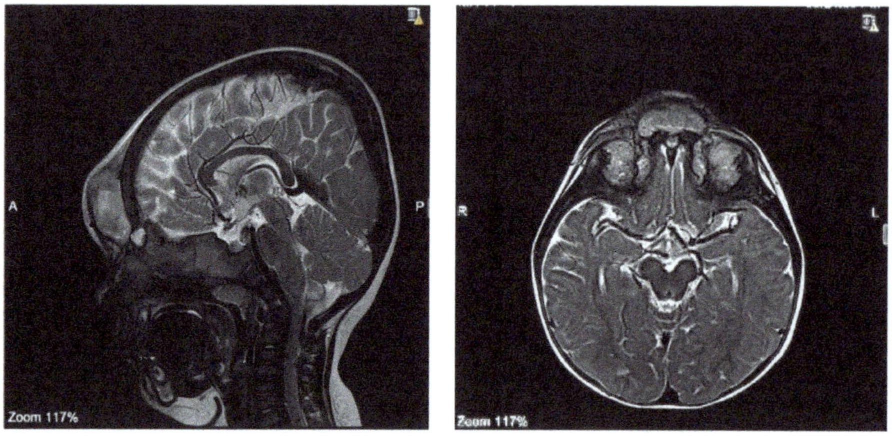

(a) (b)

Figure 1: The patient's brain MRI in the T2-weighted sequence. The intracranial mass connected to the sinus tract and opening into the forehead abscess are shown in a (a) sagittal plane and (b) transverse plane.

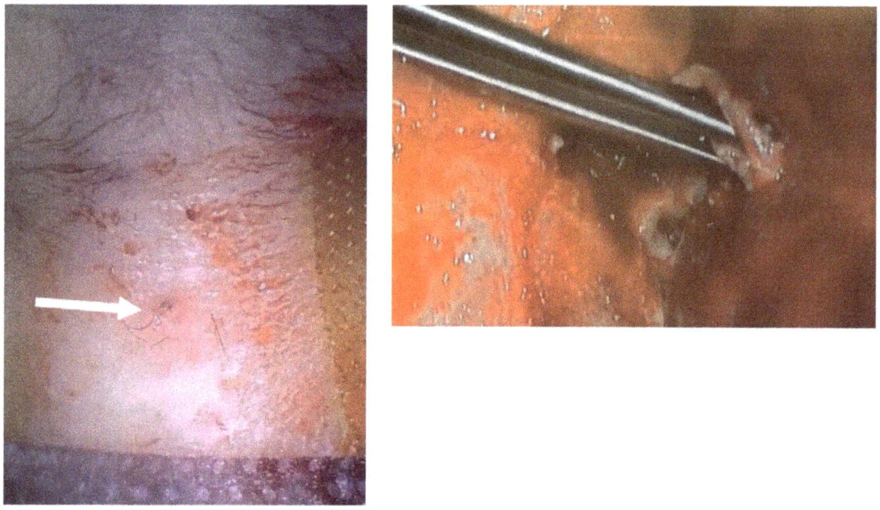

(a) (b)

Figure 2: Gross appearance of the lesion. (a) The cutaneous lesion with a few hair strands on the nasal bridge (white arrow). (b) Intraoperative image showing the sinus tract that was leading to the forehead, being held by the surgical forceps.

with the only clinical sign being a cutaneous lesion, as was the case presented in this report. This, hence, highlights the importance radiological imaging at determining the presence of any intracranial extension to midline lesions.

Despite their benign nature, dermoid cysts have a high rate of morbidity and mortality if rupture was to occur [26]. Rupture, whether spontaneous or traumatic, results in the lipid content of the cyst, a chemical irritant, to be released into the subarachnoid space and ventricles [27–29]. Following rupture, patients would present with severe aseptic or chemical meningitis leading to transient cerebral ischemia secondary to vasospasm and eventually leading to infarction, coma, and death [30–33]. The rupture of the cyst might also lead to chronic granulated arachnoiditis, aqueductal stenosis, or ventriculitis [23, 34]. However, with the early radiological detection of dermoid cysts, devastating events such as the latter are rarely reported.

Other complications of dermoid cysts include the development of dermal sinuses, which are channels connecting the dermoid cyst with the skin. Lesions as such most commonly present in the lumbar and occipital regions [35]. Intracranial extension of the nasal dermal sinuses is a rare entity, with the first case being reported in 1951 by Matson and Ingraham [36].

The differential diagnosis of dermoid cysts includes a wide range of pathologies, such as epidermoid cysts, lipomas, teratomas, cystic craniopharyngiomas, and arachnoid cysts [26, 32, 37]. The differentiation between these multiple lesions can be achieved by the aid of radiological imaging. However, for definitive diagnosis, histological examination of the lesion is necessary.

3.4. Diagnosis of Dermoid Cysts. Both CT and MRI scans are considered to be the diagnostic methods of choice for dermoid cysts. The radiological features associated with dermoid cysts include the characteristic signal intensities, absence of perilesional oedema, and the presence of well-defined margins to the cyst.

CT scans can easily depict dermoid cysts as discrete lesions of low density, a characteristic which is consistent with their fatty content. Mass effects are usually minimal relative to the size of the lesions. In addition, peripheral calcifications may be spotted in the lucent area [12]. The wall of the cyst can partially enhance after administering CT-iodinated contrast material [32]. However, enhancement is generally uncommon and if present, usually only exists as a thin peripheral rim [38]. However, on rare occasions, dermoid cysts may appear as hyperdense lesions on a CT scan [39, 40]. This unusual feature of hyperdensity is thought to be due to a combination of microcalcification, blood products, and saponification, and this is more likely to occur in the posterior fossa, for reasons which are unknown [38].

On MRI scans, dermoid cysts have variable signal characteristics [38]. They tend to appear as hyperintense lesions on T1-weighted imaging due to their lipid content and as a heterogeneous lesion on T2-weighted imaging owing to their various contents that include bones, cartilage, and calcifications [26, 32, 33]. Hence, as aforementioned, the signal intensity on MRI images can be influenced by the variety of contents present within the dermoid cysts [13, 41, 42].

Other imaging modalities, such as plain skull film, may show a well-defined, lucent lesion with ring-like or egg shell calcification, as well as bony defects, if present.

3.5. Management of Dermoid Cysts. Complete surgical resection of dermoid cysts is the only effective treatment for prevention of future recurrence and/or complications [30]. Resection has to be carefully performed to avoid spilling of contents intracranially. In some instances, complete resection might be difficult due to the cyst's extensive fibrous adhesions into the adjacent neurovascular structures [13]. Despite this, total resection of the cyst along with the adhesions and sinuses is crucial as to avoid recurrences.

4. Conclusions

In summary, we reported a rare case of an extradural, intracranial dermoid cyst, located on the crista galli, presenting with a scalp abscess and complicated by the formation of two dermal sinuses. The case highlights the rarity of such a presentation. It also emphasizes the necessity of early radiological imaging in the evaluation of midline, scalp lesions for determination of the presence or absence of intracranial extension. The latter constitutes a critical prevention method against future catastrophic intracranial events.

References

[1] E. Mathes and N. W. Kittler, "Skin nodules in newborns and infants," 2020, https://www-uptodate-com.ezproxy.rcsi-mub.com/contents/skin-nodules-in-newborns-and-infants?sectionName=Dermoid%20cysts%20and%20sinuses&topicRef=1734&anchor=H3&source=see_link#H3.

[2] B. Goldstein and A. Goldstein, "Approach to the patient with a scalp disorder," 2019, https://www-uptodate-com.ezproxy.rcsi-mub.com/contents/approach-to-the-patient-with-a-scalp-disordersearch=intracranial%20dermoid%20cyst%26source=search_result%26selectedTitle=2%7E150%26usage_type=default%26display_rank=2.

[3] R. Stendel, T. A. Pietilä, K. Lehmann, R. Kurth, O. Suess, and M. Brock, "Ruptured intracranial dermoid cysts," *Surgical Neurology*, vol. 57, no. 6, pp. 391–398, 2002.

[4] S.-J. Ko, K.-J. Park, D.-H. Park, and S.-H. Kang, "Extradural dermoid cyst located in the lateral sphenoid ridge," *Brain Tumor Research and Treatment*, vol. 2, no. 1, p. 39, 2014.

[5] M. Ammirati, M. Delgado, H. W. Slone, and A. Ray-Chaudhury, "Extradural dermoid tumor of the petrous apex," *Journal of Neurosurgery*, vol. 107, no. 2, pp. 426–429, 2007.

[6] J. N. S. J. Blythe, P. J. Revington, and R. Nelson, "Anterior cranial fossa dermoid cyst: case report," *British Journal of Oral and Maxillofacial Surgery*, vol. 45, no. 8, pp. 661–663, 2007.

[7] E. Bostroem, "Ueber die pialen epidermoide. dermoide und lipome und duralen dermoidez entbl.allgpath.pathanat," 2020, https://ci.nii.ac.jp/naid/10004932672/.

[8] J. Cruveilhier, "Anatomie pathologique du corps humain, ou descriptions, avec figures lithographiées et coloriées, des diverses altérations morbides dont le corps humain est susceptible," 2020, https://books.google.com.bh/books?hl=en&lr=&id=O2n-nQEvkk4C&oi=fnd&pg=PT12&dq=Cruveilhier.

[9] E. Hamel, R. A. Frowein, and A. Karimi-Nejad, "Intracranial intradural epidermoids and dermoids," *Neurosurgical Review*, vol. 3, no. 4, pp. 215–219, 1980.

[10] J. S. Tytus and J. Pennybacker, "Pearly tumours IN relation to the central nervous system," *Journal of Neurology, Neurosurgery & Psychiatry*, vol. 19, no. 4, pp. 241–259, 1956.

[11] K. J. Zülch, "Brain tumors," 2010, https://books.google.com.bh/books?hl=en&lr=&id=KKrzBgAAQBAJ&oi=fnd&pg=PA1&ots=ynwcDB7RHq&sig=AUSZ81ydvlfBGLq89tEAvecnswM&redir_esc=y#v=onepage&q&f=false.

[12] J. Handa, H. Handa, Y. Nakano, and T. Mukai, "Radiolucent intracranial dermoid cyst. Report of an unusual case," *Neuroradiology*, vol. 17, no. 4, pp. 211–214, 1979.

[13] K. S. Jin, B. H. Jin, R. K. Hwa et al., "Skull base dermoid cyst in the right infratemporal fossa diagnosed using the dixon technique: a case report and review of literature," *ScienceOn*, vol. 21, no. 2, 2017.

[14] K. N. North, J. H. Antony, and I. H. Johnston, "Dermoid of cavernous sinus resulting in isolated oculomotor nerve palsy," *Pediatric Neurology*, vol. 9, no. 3, pp. 221–223, 1993.

[15] C. Filomena, Y. Nonaka, M. Matsuda et al., "Extradural dermoid cyst of the anterior infratemporal fossa. Case report," *Journal of Neurological Surgery Reports*, vol. 76, no. 2, pp. e195–e199, 2015.

[16] P. Perrini, P. Di Russo, and A. Iannelli, "Dermoid cyst of the lateral wall of the cavernous sinus presenting with isolated abducens nerve palsy," *Acta Neurochirurgica*, vol. 155, no. 4, pp. 741-742, 2013.

[17] W. M. Bogdanowicz and D. H. Wilson, "Dermoid cyst of the fourth ventricle demonstrated on brain scan," *Journal of Neurosurgery*, vol. 36, no. 2, pp. 228–230, 1972.
[18] C. S. Maccarty, M. E. Leavens, J. G. Love, and J. W. Kernohan, "Dermoid and epidermoid tumors in the central nervous system of adults," *Surgery, Gynecology & Obstetrics*, vol. 108, no. 2, 2017.
[19] H. S. Al-Muhaimeed, H. Y. Abdelwahed, E. A. Elgamal, and M. M. Ashraf, "Extradural dermoid cyst of mastoid bone: a case report," *Case Reports in Otolaryngology*, vol. 2012, Article ID 548340, 5 pages, 2012.
[20] J. G. Smirniotopoulos and M. V. Chiechi, "Teratomas, dermoids, and epidermoids of the head and neck," *Radiographics*, vol. 15, no. 6, pp. 1437–1455, 1995.
[21] J. G. Love and J. W. Kennohan, "Dermoid and epidermoid tumors (cholesteatomas) of central nervous system," *Jama*, vol. 107, pp. 1876–1883, 1936.
[22] N. R. Miller and M. H. Epstein, "Giant intracranial dermoid cyst: case report and review of the literature on intracranial dermoids and epidermoids," *Canadian Journal of Neurological Sciences/Journal Canadien des Sciences Neurologiques*, vol. 2, no. 2, pp. 127–134, 1975.
[23] M. Caldarelli, L. Massimi, C. Kondageski, and C. Di Rocco, "Intracranial midline dermoid and epidermoid cysts in children," *Journal of Neurosurgery: Pediatrics*, vol. 100, no. 5, pp. 473–480, 2004.
[24] C. Arseni, L. Dănăilă, N. Carp, and P. Decu, "Cerebral dermoid tumours," *Min-Minimally Invasive Neurosurgery*, vol. 19, no. 3, pp. 104–114, 1976.
[25] J. F. Fleming and E. H. Botterell, "Cranial dermoid and epidermoid tumors," *Surgery, Gynecology & Obstetrics*, vol. 109, pp. 403–411, 1959.
[26] H. Altay, O. Kitiş, C. Calli, and N. Yünten, "A spinal dermoid tumor that ruptured into the subarachnoidal space and syrinx cavity," *Diagnostic and Interventional Radiology*, vol. 12, no. 4, 2014.
[27] I.-Y. Kim, S. Jung, T.-Y. Jung, S.-S. Kang, and T.-S. Kim, "Traumatic rupture of an intracranial dermoid cyst," *Journal of Clinical Neuroscience*, vol. 15, no. 4, pp. 469–471, 2008.
[28] S. K. Park and K. G. Cho, "Recurrent intracranial dermoid cyst after subtotal removal of traumatic rupture," *Clinical Neurology and Neurosurgery*, vol. 114, no. 4, pp. 421–424, 2012.
[29] W. E. Phillips, C. R. Martinez, and D. W. Cahill, "Ruptured intracranial dermoid tumor secondary to closed head trauma," *Journal of Neuroimaging*, vol. 4, no. 3, pp. 169-170, 1994.
[30] A. G. Osborn and M. T. Preece, "Intracranial cysts: radiologic-pathologic correlation and imaging approach," *Radiology*, vol. 239, no. 3, pp. 650–654, 2019.
[31] R. Bhatia, S. Anderson, V. Bradley, and J. A. Akinwunmi, "Neuropsychological profiling of ischemic deficit secondary to ruptured dermoid cyst: a case report," *Applied Neuropsychology*, vol. 15, no. 4, pp. 293–297, 2008.
[32] M. J. Ray, D. W. Barnett, G. J. Snipes, K. F. Layton, and M. J. Opatowsky, "Ruptured intracranial dermoid cyst," *Baylor University Medical Center Proceedings*, vol. 25, no. 1, pp. 23–25, 2012.
[33] A. R. Čatić, M. Nikšić, and Z. Kadenić, "Ruptured intracranial dermoid cyst: a case report," *Journal of Health Sciences*, vol. 2, no. 3, 2012.
[34] C. Oursin, S. G. Wetzel, P. Lyrer, H. Bächli, and K. W. Stock, "Ruptured intracranial dermoid cyst," *Journal of Neurosurgical Sciences*, vol. 43, no. 3, 2011.
[35] H. L. Brydon, "Intracranial dermoid cysts with nasal dermal sinuses," *Acta Neurochirurgica*, vol. 118, no. 3-4, pp. 185–188, 1992.
[36] D. D. Matson and F. D. Ingraham, "Intracranial complications of congenital dermal sinuses," *Pediatrics*, vol. 8, no. 4, 2010.
[37] S. K. Venkatesh, R. V. Phadke, P. Trivedi, and D. Bannerji, "Asymptomatic spontaneous rupture of suprasellar dermoid cyst: a case report," *Neurology India*, vol. 50, no. 4, 2010.
[38] S. Llopis, A. Olivas, and V. Martinez, "Intracranial dermoid cyst," *[Operative Neurosurgery]*, 2015.
[39] J. Y. Brown, A. P. Morokoff, P. J. Mitchell, and M. F Gonzales, "Unusual imaging appearance of an intracranial dermoid cyst," *AJNR. American Journal of Neuroradiology*, vol. 22, pp. 1970–1972, 2001.
[40] L. A. Tan, M. K. Kasliwal, A. Harbhajanka, R. G. Kellogg, L. D. Arvanitis, and L. F. Munoz, "Hyperdense suprasellar mass: an unusual radiological presentation of intracranial dermoid cyst," *Journal of Clinical Neuroscience*, vol. 22, no. 7, pp. 1208–1210, 2015.
[41] G. Rubin, R. Scienza, A. Pasqualin, L. Rosta, and R. Da Pian, "Craniocerebral epidermoids and dermoids," *Acta Neurochirurgica*, vol. 97, no. 1-2, pp. 1–16, 1989.
[42] G. Wilms, J. Casselman, P. Demaerel, C. Plets, I. De Haene, and A. L. Baert, "CT and MRI of ruptured intracranial dermoids," *Neuroradiology*, vol. 33, no. 2, pp. 149–151, 1991.

41

HaNDL Syndrome Presenting with Thunderclap Headache

Melvin Parasram, Ashwin Malhotra, Andrea S. Yoo, and Saad A. Mir

NewYork-Presbyterian Hospital/Weill Cornell Medical Center, Department of Neurology, New York, New York, USA

Correspondence should be addressed to Melvin Parasram; mep9081@nyp.org

Academic Editor: Peter Berlit

Introduction. Transient headache and neurologic deficits with cerebrospinal fluid lymphocytosis (HaNDL) is defined as a secondary, nonvascular headache disorder characterized by the findings described in its name. Patients with HaNDL syndrome typically present with gradual onset migrainous headaches of moderate to severe intensity with transient neurological symptoms. *Case Report.* We discuss a patient who presented with thunderclap headache, recent transient neurologic deficits, and was ultimately diagnosed with HaNDL after an extensive neurologic evaluation. *Conclusion.* Thunderclap headache has very rarely been described in patients with HaNDL. After excluding emergent and secondary causes, HaNDL should be considered in patients with thunderclap-quality headaches, particularly when there is a history of transient neurological symptoms.

1. Background

Transient headache and neurologic deficits with cerebrospinal fluid lymphocytosis (HaNDL) is a rare, benign, and self-limiting syndrome characterized by moderate to severe headaches, stroke-like deficits, and cerebrospinal fluid (CSF) lymphocytosis [1, 2]. Patients with HaNDL develop neurologic deficits such as parasthesias, aphasia, altered mental status, and weakness. Migrainous type headaches of moderate to severe intensity often lag behind these focal symptoms [3–5]. Duration of neurological deficits can range from minutes to hours, and repeat attacks can occur for days to weeks following the initial event [2, 4]. The underlying pathophysiology is not fully elucidated, although a viral or inflammatory etiology has been suggested given the CSF lymphocytic pleocytosis [1, 2].

HaNDL often present to the emergency room with neurological emergencies since the stroke-like symptoms are alarming and severe. Computed tomography (CT) and magnetic resonance imaging (MRI) are unremarkable while perfusion studies can demonstrate focal hypoperfusion in symptomatic areas [4, 6]. Electroencephalography (EEG) is typically negative or can occasionally show focal slowing [4]. CSF analysis typically demonstrates elevated opening pressure, lymphocytic pleocytosis, elevated protein, absence of infectious causes, and negative oligoclonal bands and IgG index [7]. Management largely involves symptomatic treatment of headache and reassurance of disease course [8]. Most cases resolve within months and the frequency and severity of attacks traditionally diminish over time.

Here, we report a case of a patient with HaNDL presenting atypically with a thunderclap headache.

2. Case Report

A 32-year-old woman with a recent diagnosis of transient ischemic attack (TIA) presented to the emergency department 2.5 hours after awakening from sleep with sudden onset, thunderclap headache described as the worst headache of her life. Her headache was frontal, pressure-like, exacerbated by supine positioning, and was associated with nausea, vomiting, and photophobia. The headache reached maximal intensity within 60 seconds of onset. She denied prior history of headaches and migraines and denied recent viral illness and/or infectious symptoms. On exam, her vitals were normal and she had no focal neurologic deficits. A noncontrast CT of the head was negative for subarachnoid hemorrhage (SAH) and intracerebral hemorrhage (ICH). MRI brain revealed no evidence of stroke or blood products, but was notable for hydrocephalus and mega cisterna magna, presumed to be chronic given normal head circumference and the absence of transependymal flow. MR angiography of head and neck was negative for findings to support reversible cerebral vasoconstriction syndrome (RCVS) or dissection, and MR venogram was negative for cerebral venous sinus thrombosis (CVST). Intravenous normal saline, magnesium, and metoclopramide provided relief of headache.

She reported an admission to an outside hospital five days prior for a progressive syndrome of migratory paresthesias followed by global aphasia and right hemiparesis. During that admission, she was treated with tissue plasminogen activator given her aphasia and right hemiparesis. While in the intensive care unit, her neurological deficits resolved within 6 hours of symptom onset, but she developed a moderate intensity migrainous headache with mild photophobia and nausea. This headache resolved by the next day. Brain MRI was negative for stroke and MR angiography of head and neck was unrevealing for a dissection or other vessel pathology. Additional workup was also negative including 24 hours of video EEG monitoring, a transesophageal echocardiogram, and arterial and venous hypercoagulability studies. She was discharged on aspirin 81 mg daily for presumed transient ischemic attack.

We performed a lumbar puncture in the lateral decubitus position with extension of her lower extremities showing an opening pressure of 28 mmH_2O, 28/uL total nucleated cells with 99% lymphocytes, 1/uL red blood cell, 33.2 mg/dL total protein, 64 mg/dL glucose, negative xanthochromia, negative bacterial and fungal culture, negative cryptococcus antigen, and negative meningoencephalitis viral panel.

The patient was discharged with a diagnosis of HaNDL. Her prior diagnosis of TIA was misdiagnosed, as her initial symptoms were consistent with HaNDL syndrome. Her aspirin was discontinued. Over the next 8 weeks after discharge, she developed periodic right-sided paresthesias followed by migrainous headaches of moderate severity with photophobia and nausea that would subside within 60–120 minutes. For the headaches, she used abortive agents such as acetaminophen, nonsteroidal anti-inflammatory drugs, and metoclopramide. These episodes became less intense and less frequent over the ensuring 8 weeks until they completely abated.

3. Discussion

We report a rare case of HaNDL presenting with thunderclap headache. Thunderclap-quality headache is defined as a severe and sudden onset headache, which reaches maximal intensity in one minute or less [9]. The most common causes of thunderclap headache include aneurysmal SAH and RCVS [10, 11]. Other less common causes of thunderclap headache are cervical or intracranial arterial dissection, CVST, pituitary apoplexy, posterior reversible vasoconstriction syndrome, primary intracerebral hemorrhage, and intracerebral hemorrhage secondary to ruptured cavernous malformations or arteriovenous malformations [11].

HaNDL typically manifests with gradual onset migrainous headaches and rarely presents as thunderclap headache as in our case [7]. In a single-center study of 433 patients who presented to the hospital with acute headache complaints (including thunderclap headache), only 1 patient was diagnosed with HaNDL after workup [12]. Furthermore, in a systematic review of 219 journal articles of causes of thunderclap headache other than SAH, only 1 case report described HaNDL [13].

Our case highlights the importance of recognizing HaNDL as a potential cause of thunderclap headache in the setting of negative workup for neurologic emergencies.

Authors' Contributions

MP and SM conceptualized and designed the study. MP drafted the manuscript. MP, AM, and AY were responsible for acquisition, analysis, or interpretation of data. MP, AM, AY, and SM critically revised the manuscript for important intellectual content. SM gave administrative, technical, or material support. All authors have approved the submitted version and have agreed to be personally accountable for the authors' own contributions.

References

[1] J. D. Bartleson, J. W. Swanson, and J. P. Whisnant, "A migrainous syndrome with cerebrospinal fluid pleocytosis," *Neurology*, vol. 31, no. 10, pp. 1257–1262, 1981.

[2] M. J. Berg and L. S. Williams, "The transient syndrome of headache with neurologic deficits and CSF lymphocytosis," *Neurology*, vol. 45, no. 9, pp. 1648–1654, 1995.

[3] M.-A. Babi, A. Applebee, R. Shapiro, and W. Waheed, "Syndrome of transient headache and neurologic deficits with cerebrospinal fluid lymphocytosis presenting as acute neurological emergencies," *Cephalalgia*, vol. 37, no. 3, pp. 284–289, 2017.

[4] S. Quintas, R. López Ruiz, S. Trillo et al., "Clinical, imaging and electroencephalographic characterization of three cases of HaNDL syndrome," *Cephalalgia*, vol. 38, no. 7, pp. 1402–1406, 2018.

[5] S. Nelson, "Confusional state in HaNDL syndrome: case report and literature review," *Case Reports in Neurological Medicine*, vol. 2013, Article ID 317685, 2013.

[6] A. Yilmaz, H. Kaleagasi, O. Dogu, E. Kara, and A. Ozge, "Abnormal MRI in a patient with 'headache with neurological deficits and CSF lymphocytosis (HaNDL)'," *Cephalalgia*, vol. 30, no. 5, pp. 615–619, 2010.

[7] F. Gomez-Aranda, F. Canadillas, J. F. Marti-Masso et al., "Pseudomigraine with temporary neurological symptoms and lymphocytic pleocytosis. A report of 50 cases," *Brain*, vol. 120, no. Pt 7, pp. 1105–1113, 1997.

[8] T. Filina, K. N. Feja, and R. W. Tolan Jr, "An adolescent with pseudomigraine, transient headache, neurological deficits, and lymphocytic pleocytosis (HaNDL syndrome)," *Clinical Pediatrics*, vol. 52, no. 6, pp. 496–502, 2013.

[9] D. W. Dodick, "Thunderclap headache," *Journal of Neurology, Neurosurgery & Psychiatry*, vol. 72, no. 1, pp. 6–11, 2002.

[10] A. Ducros and M.-G. Bousser, "Thunderclap headache," *BMJ*, vol. 346, e8557 pages, 2013.

[11] Y.-C. Cheng, K.-H. Kuo, and T.-H. Lai, "A common cause of sudden and thunderclap headaches: reversible cerebral vasoconstriction syndrome," *The Journal of Headache and Pain*, vol. 15, no. 1, 13 pages, 2014.
[12] S. H. Bø, E. M. Davidsen, P. Gulbrandsen, and E. Dietrichs, "Acute headache: a prospective diagnostic work-up of patients admitted to a general hospital," *European Journal of Neurology*, vol. 15, no. 12, pp. 1293–1299, 2008.
[13] E. Devenney, H. Neale, and R. B. Forbes, "A systematic review of causes of sudden and severe headache (thunderclap headache): should lists be evidence based?" *The Journal of Headache and Pain*, vol. 15, no. 1, 49 pages, 2014.

Permissions

All chapters in this book were first published by Hindawi Publishing Corporation; hereby published with permission under the Creative Commons Attribution License or equivalent. Every chapter published in this book has been scrutinized by our experts. Their significance has been extensively debated. The topics covered herein carry significant findings which will fuel the growth of the discipline. They may even be implemented as practical applications or may be referred to as a beginning point for another development.

The contributors of this book come from diverse backgrounds, making this book a truly international effort. This book will bring forth new frontiers with its revolutionizing research information and detailed analysis of the nascent developments around the world.

We would like to thank all the contributing authors for lending their expertise to make the book truly unique. They have played a crucial role in the development of this book. Without their invaluable contributions this book wouldn't have been possible. They have made vital efforts to compile up to date information on the varied aspects of this subject to make this book a valuable addition to the collection of many professionals and students.

This book was conceptualized with the vision of imparting up-to-date information and advanced data in this field. To ensure the same, a matchless editorial board was set up. Every individual on the board went through rigorous rounds of assessment to prove their worth. After which they invested a large part of their time researching and compiling the most relevant data for our readers.

The editorial board has been involved in producing this book since its inception. They have spent rigorous hours researching and exploring the diverse topics which have resulted in the successful publishing of this book. They have passed on their knowledge of decades through this book. To expedite this challenging task, the publisher supported the team at every step. A small team of assistant editors was also appointed to further simplify the editing procedure and attain best results for the readers.

Apart from the editorial board, the designing team has also invested a significant amount of their time in understanding the subject and creating the most relevant covers. They scrutinized every image to scout for the most suitable representation of the subject and create an appropriate cover for the book.

The publishing team has been an ardent support to the editorial, designing and production team. Their endless efforts to recruit the best for this project, has resulted in the accomplishment of this book. They are a veteran in the field of academics and their pool of knowledge is as vast as their experience in printing. Their expertise and guidance has proved useful at every step. Their uncompromising quality standards have made this book an exceptional effort. Their encouragement from time to time has been an inspiration for everyone.

The publisher and the editorial board hope that this book will prove to be a valuable piece of knowledge for researchers, students, practitioners and scholars across the globe.

List of Contributors

Behnaz Ansari and Helia Hemasian
Isfahan Neuroscience Research Center, Department of Neurology, Al Zahra Research Institute, Isfahan University of Medical Sciences, Isfahan, Iran

Kavinda Dayasiri, Kaushika Thudugala and Aruni Ranaweera
Department of Paediatrics, Base Hospital Mahaoya, Maha Oya, Sri Lanka

V. Thadchanamoorthy
Faculty of Health Care Science, Eastern University, Chenkalady, Sri Lanka

N. Parthipan
Department of Radiology, Base Hospital Mahaoya, Maha Oya, Sri Lanka

Byung-chul Son
Department of Neurosurgery, Seoul St. Mary's Hospital, Seoul, The Catholic University of Korea, Republic of Korea
Catholic Neuroscience Institute, College of Medicine, The Catholic University of Korea, Seoul, Republic of Korea

Manabu Wada, Hikaru Nagasawa and Yoshitaka Yamaguchi
Department of Neurology, Yamagata Prefectural Central Hospital, 1800 Aoyagi, Yamagata, Japan

Todd D. Rozen and Hector A. Robles
Department of Neurology and Neuroradiology, Mayo Clinic Florida, Jacksonville, USA

Joseph Seemiller and Muhammad Taimur Malik
Geisinger Neuroscience Institute, Danville, PA, USA
Geisinger Commonwealth School of Medicine, Scranton, PA, USA

Komi Igneza Agbotsou
Neurology Department of Valence Hospital Center, Valence, France
Neurology Department of Campus Teaching Hospital, Lome, Togo

Damelan Kombate, Kossivi Apetse and Kpalma Duga Bakpatina-Batako
Neurology Department of Campus Teaching Hospital, Lome, Togo

Christopher Mehri, Olivier Guerrier, Albert Beschet, Karine Blanc Lasserre, Ludovic Breynaert and Victor Chan
Neurology Department of Valence Hospital Center, Valence, France

Chamara Dalugama, Udaya Ralapanawa, Shamali Abeygunawardena and Thilak Jayalath
Department of Medicine, University of Peradeniya, Peradeniya, Sri Lanka

Achila Jayasinghe
Teaching Hospital, Peradeniya, Sri Lanka

Elijah Lackey, Deepal P. Shah-Zamora, Jodi Hawes and Andy J. Liu
Duke University Department of Neurology, Duke University Medical Center 2905, 40 Medicine Circle, Durham, NC 27710, USA

Jhon Perea, María Belén Luis, Luciana Grimanesa Lázaro, Sergio Scollo, Agustina Tamargo, José Crespo, Maira Avalle, Nora Fernández Liguori and Ricardo Alonso
Department of Neurology, Sanatorio Güemes – University Hospital, Buenos Aires, Argentina

Horacio Solarz
Anatomical Pathology, Sanatorio Güemes – University Hospital, Buenos Aires, Argentina

Ravindra Singh Shekhawat, Ming Hui Yong and Shahul Hameed
Department of Neurology, National Neuroscience Institute-Singapore General Hospital, Singapore
DUKE-NUS Medical School, Singapore

Si Ying Julienne Keong and Kunihiko Chen
DUKE-NUS Medical School, Singapore

Chow Wei Too
Department of Vascular and Interventional Radiology, Singapore General Hospital, Singapore

Josef Finsterer
Klinik Landstrasse, Vienna, Austria

Jing Ming Yeo
Department of Neurology, Queen's Medical Centre, Nottingham University Hospitals NHS Trust, Derby Road, Lenton, Nottingham NG7 2UH, UK

Donald MacArthur
Department of Neurosurgery, Nottingham University Hospitals NHS Trust, Nottingham NG7 2UH, UK

Jillian Davis and Ian Scott
Department of Pathology, Nottingham University Hospitals NHS Trust, Nottingham NG7 2UH, UK

Bruno Gran
Department of Neurology, Nottingham University Hospitals NHS Trust, Nottingham NG7 2UH, UK

Antonina Obayo
Department of Medicine, Aga Khan University, Nairobi, Kenya

Sylvia Mbugua
Neurology, Department of Medicine, Aga Khan University, Nairobi, Kenya

Sayed K. Ali
Internal Medicine, Department of Medicine, Aga Khan University, Nairobi, Kenya

Ho-Man Yeung and Sarah Schmitz
Department of Medicine, Lewis Katz School of Medicine at Temple University, Philadelphia, PA, USA

Nino Kvantaliani and Christina Martin
Department of Neurology, Lewis Katz School of Medicine at Temple University, Philadelphia, PA, USA

Marcellin Bugeme
Faculty of Medicine, University of Lubumbashi, Lubumbashi, Democratic Republic of the Congo

Ousmane Cissé and Amadou Gallo Diop
Université Cheikh Anta Diop, Dakar, Senegal

Olivier Mukuku
Institut Supérieur des Techniques Médicales de Lubumbashi, Lubumbashi, Democratic Republic of the Congo

Koji Tsuzaki, Yuwa Oka and Toshiaki Hamano
Department of Neurology, Kansai Electric Power Hospital, Osaka, Japan
Division of Clinical Neurology, Kansai Electric Power Medical Research Institute, Osaka, Japan

Kenji Murakata
Department of Neurology, Kansai Electric Power Hospital, Osaka, Japan
Department of Neurology, Nakatsu Hospital, Osaka, Japan

Mayu Kamei and Akihiro Kikuya
Department of Neurology, Kansai Electric Power Hospital, Osaka, Japan

Paulo Diniz da Gama, Rafaela Ramos Smaniotto, Penélope de Lima Petuco and Wammer Alves de Almeida
Faculty of Medical Sciences of Sorocaba, PUC-SP - Campus Sorocaba, São Paulo, Brazil

Tiago Gomes de Alcantara and Rodrigo Assad Diiniz da Gama
The Conjunto Hospitalar de Sorocaba, Sorocaba, Brazil

Yara Dadalti Fragoso
Universidade Metropolitana de Santos, Santos SP, Brazil

Katharina Berger
Centre for Neurovascular Diseases Tübingen, ZNET: University of Tübingen, Tübingen, Germany
Department of Neurology & Epileptology, University of Tübingen, Tübingen, Germany
Hertie Institute for Clinical Brain Research, University Tübingen, Tübingen, Germany

Jennifer Sartor-Pfeiffer, Annerose Mengel, Ulf Ziemann and Katharina Feil
Centre for Neurovascular Diseases Tübingen, ZNET: University of Tübingen, Tübingen, Germany
Hertie Institute for Clinical Brain Research, University Tübingen, Tübingen, Germany
Department of Neurology & Stroke, University of Tübingen, Tübingen, Germany

Ulrike Ernemann and Florian Hennersdorf
Centre for Neurovascular Diseases Tübingen, ZNET: University of Tübingen, Tübingen, Germany
Department of Diagnostic & Interventional Neuroradiology, University of Tübingen, Tübingen, Germany

A. Verentzioti, A. Alexoudi, P. Patrikelis, A. Siatouni, S. Korfias, D. Sakas and S. Gatzonis
Department of Neurosurgery, National & Kapodistrian University of Athens, Evangelismos Hospital, Athens, Greece

I. Blumcke
Department of Neuropathology, University Hospital Erlangen, Germany

Laura N. Zamproni, Reinaldo T. Ribeiro and Marina Cardeal
Instituto de Neurologia Funcional, Rua Padre Machado, 42 São Paulo, SP, Brazil

Michel Sáenz-Farret, Mariana Aurora Cansino-Torres, Valeria Sandoval-Rodríguez, Rigoberto Navarro-Ibarra and Carlos Zúñiga-Ramírez
Movement Disorders and Neurodegenerative Diseases Unit, Hospital Civil de Guadalajara "Fray Antonio Alcalde", Guadalajara, Mexico

Kyle Sanchez and Steven Glener
University of Central Florida College of Medicine, 6850 Lake Nona Boulevard, Orlando, FL 32827, USA

Nathan E. Esplin
Department of Neurosurgery, Allegheny General Hospital, 320 E North Ave., Pittsburgh, PA 15212, USA

Okorie N. Okorie and Amay Parikh
Florida Hospital, 601 E Rollins Street, Orlando, FL 32803, USA

J. Finsterer
Krankenanstalt Rudolfstiftung, Messerli Institute, Vienna, Austria

Suran L. Fernando
Immunology Laboratory, New South Wales Health Pathology, Royal North Hospital, Sydney, Australia
Department of Clinical Immunology and Allergy, Royal North Hospital, Sydney, Australia
Sydney Medical School, University of Sydney, Sydney, Australia

Therese Boyle
Immunology Laboratory, New South Wales Health Pathology, Royal North Hospital, Sydney, Australia

Annika Smith
Department of Clinical Immunology and Allergy, Royal North Hospital, Sydney, Australia

John D.E. Parratt
Department of Clinical Immunology and Allergy, Royal North Hospital, Sydney, Australia
Sydney Medical School, University of Sydney, Sydney, Australia
Department of Neurology, Royal North Hospital, Sydney, Australia

L. M. Conners, A. Betcher, A. Shahinian and P. Janda
Department of Neurology, Valley Hospital Medical Center, Las Vegas, NV, USA

Vincenzo Spina, Luca Bonfiglio and Maria Chiara Carboncini
Department of Translational Research and New Technologies in Medicine and Surgery, University of Pisa, Pisa, Italy

Francesco Tomaiuolo
Auxilium Vitae, Volterra (Pisa), Italy

Lorenzo Celli
Neurology Department, ASLAL, San Giacomo Hospital, Novi Ligure (Alessandria), Italy

Luca Cecchetti
MolecularMind Lab, IMT School for Advanced Studies Lucca, Lucca, Italy

Byung-Chul Son
Department of Neurosurgery, Seoul St. Mary's Hospital, College of Medicine, The Catholic University of Korea, Seoul, Republic of Korea
Catholic Neuroscience Institute, College of Medicine, The Catholic University of Korea, Seoul, Republic of Korea

Changik Lee
Department of Neurosurgery, Seoul St. Mary's Hospital, College of Medicine, The Catholic University of Korea, Seoul, Republic of Korea

Hatem B. Afana
Orthopaedic Department, European Gaza Hospital, Gaza Strip, State of Palestine

Nidal M. M. Abuhadrous
Neurosurgery Department, European Gaza Hospital, Gaza Strip, State of Palestine

Alaa Eldin Elsharkawy
Neurosurgery Department, Bonifatius Hospital, Lingen, Germany
Neurosurgery Teaching Program, University of Traditional Medicine, Yerevan, Armenia

Alisha Khan and Amit S. Dhamoon
Department of Medicine, SUNY Upstate Medical University, Syracuse, NY, USA

Jonathan Hingre
College of Medicine, SUNY Upstate Medical University, Syracuse, NY, USA

Di Chen and Hongyun Huang
Beijing Hongtianji Neuroscience Academy, Beijing 100143, China

Haitao Xi
Department of Neurorehabilitation, Capital Medical University Affliated Beijing Rehabilitation Hospital, Beijing 100144, China

Ke Tan
Department of Neurosurgery, Capital Medical University Affliated Beijing Chaoyang Hospital, Beijing 100020, China

Amanda L. Faulkner, James David Bacon, Brian A. Fischer and Kevin W. Hatton
Department of Anesthesiology, N-202 UKMC, 800 Rose Street, Lexington, KY 40536, USA

Stephen L. Grupke
Department of Neurosurgery, 800 Rose Street, Lexington, KY 40536, USA

Bashar Tanous, Raad Tahtouh, Sundus Sardar, Sara Mohamed, Aseel Sukik and Mhd-Baraa Habib
Internal Medicine Residency Program, Internal Medicine Department, Hamad Medical Corporation, Doha, Qatar

Jamal Sajid and Mouhand F. H. Mohamed
Internal Medicine Department, Hamad Medical Corporation, Doha, Qatar

Ayumi Nakamura
Department of Psychiatry and Behavioral Sciences, Duke University Medical Center, Durham, NC, USA

Thomas J. Farrer
Department of Psychiatry and Behavioral Sciences, Duke University Medical Center, Durham, NC, USA
Department of Neurology, Duke University Medical Center, Durham, NC, USA

Andy Liu
Department of Neurology, Duke University Medical Center, Durham, NC, USA

Veronika Spahlinger, Annette Niessen and Matthias Reinhard
Department of Neurology and Clinical Neurophysiology, Medical Center Esslingen, Academic Teaching Hospital of the University of Tübingen, Tübingen, Germany

Sebastian Rauer
Department of Neurology and Neurophysiology, University Medical Center Freiburg, University of Freiburg, Freiburg, Germany

Stefan Krämer
Department of Radiology and Nuclear Medicine, Medical Center Esslingen, Academic Teaching Hospital of the University of Tübingen, Tübingen, Germany

Nakul Katyal and Raghav Govindarajan
Department of Neurology, University of Missouri, Columbia, MO, USA

Latika Nirola
Guru Gobind Singh Medical College and Hospital, Faridkot, Punjab, India

Naureen Narula
Department of Pulmonology and Critical Care Medicine, Staten Island University Hospital, New York, NY, USA

Andria Tziakouri and Costas Michaelides
Department of Neurology, American Medical Center, Nicosia 2047, Cyprus

Konstantinos Natsiopoulos
Department of Radiology, American Medical Center, Nicosia 2047, Cyprus

Kleopas A. Kleopa
Neurology Clinics and Neuroscience Laboratory, The Cyprus Institute of Neurology and Genetics and Cyprus School of Molecular Medicine, Nicosia 1683, Cyprus

Krishnan Ravindran, Brandon M. Zsigray, Michael P. Wemhoff and John D. Spencer
Department of Neurological Surgery, Loyola University Medical Center, Maywood, Illinois, USA

Ewa Borys
Department of Pathology, Loyola University Medical Center, Maywood, Illinois, USA

Chirag R. Patel
Department of Otolaryngology Stritch School of Medicine, Loyola University Medical Center, Maywood, Illinois, USA

Anand V. Germanwala
Department of Neurological Surgery, Loyola University Medical Center, Maywood, Illinois, USA
Department of Otolaryngology Stritch School of Medicine, Loyola University Medical Center, Maywood, Illinois, USA

Jeroen Kerstens
Antwerp University Hospital, University of Antwerp, Department of Neurology, Edegem 2650, Belgium
AZ Middelheim, ZNA, Lindendreef 1, 2020, Antwerp, Belgium

Busra Durmus
Antwerp University Hospital, University of Antwerp, Department of Neurology, Edegem 2650, Belgium

Stijn Lambrecht and Margareta M. Ieven
Antwerp University Hospital, University of Antwerp, UZGent, UGent, Dept of Chemistry, 9000 Gent, Belgium

Ingrid Baar and Philippe G. Jorens
Antwerp University Hospital, University of Antwerp, Department of Critical Care Medicine, Edegem 2650, Belgium

Thijs Van Der Zijden
Antwerp University Hospital, University of Antwerp, Department of Radiology, Edegem 2650, Belgium

Paul M. Parizel
Antwerp University Hospital, University of Antwerp, Department of Radiology, Edegem 2650, Belgium
Royal Perth Hospital, University of Western Australia, Medical School, Perth, WA, Australia

Tomas Menovsky
Antwerp University Hospital, University of Antwerp, Department of Neurosurgery, Edegem 2650, Belgium

Martin M. Y. Lammens
Antwerp University Hospital, University of Antwerp, Department of Pathology, Edegem 2650, Belgium

Aysha Albastaki, Reem AlThawadi, Janan Alajaimi and Khawla F. Ali
Royal College of Surgeons in Ireland-Medical University of Bahrain, Busaiteen, Bahrain

Talal Almayman
King Hamad University Hospital, Al Sayh, Bahrain

Melvin Parasram, Ashwin Malhotra, Andrea S. Yoo and Saad A. Mir
NewYork-Presbyterian Hospital/Weill Cornell Medical Center, Department of Neurology, New York, New York, USA

Index

www.ingramcontent.com/pod-product-compliance
Lightning Source LLC
LaVergne TN
LVHW082230200926
848484LV00008B/2328